Board
Stiff
Three

Preparing for the Anesthesia Orals

Christopher J. Gallagher, MD
Associate Professor
Department of Anesthesiology
State University of New York–Stony Brook
Stony Brook, New York

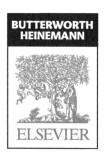

BUTTERWORTH
HEINEMANN

ELSEVIER

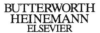

BUTTERWORTH
HEINEMANN
ELSEVIER

1600 John F. Kennedy Blvd.
Ste 1800
Philadelphia, PA 19103-2899

BOARD STIFF THREE   ISBN: 978-0-7020-3092-5
Copyright © 2009 by Butterworth-Heinemann, an imprint of Elsevier Inc.

Notice

Knowledge and best practice in this field are constantly changing. As new research and experience broaden our knowledge, changes in practice, treatment and drug therapy may become necessary or appropriate. Readers are advised to check the most current information provided (i) on procedures featured or (ii) by the manufacturer of each product to be administered, to verify the recommended dose or formula, the method and duration of administration, and contraindications. It is the responsibility of the practitioner, relying on their own experience and knowledge of the patient, to make diagnoses, to determine dosages and the best treatment for each individual patient, and to take all appropriate safety precautions. To the fullest extent of the law, neither the Publisher nor the Author assumes any liability for any injury and/or damage to persons or property arising out of or related to any use of the material contained in this book.

The Publisher

Library of Congress Cataloging-in-Publication Data
Gallagher, Christopher J.
   Board stiff three : preparing for the anesthesia orals / Christopher J. Gallagher. -- 3rd ed.
      p. ; cm.
   Includes index.
   Rev. ed. of: Board stiff too / Christopher J. Gallagher, Steven E. Hill, David A. Lubarsky. 2nd ed. c2001.
   ISBN 978-0-7020-3092-5
   1. Anesthesia--Examinations, questions, etc. I. Gallagher, Christopher J. Board stiff too. II. Title. III. Title: Preparing for the anesthesia orals.
   [DNLM: 1. Anesthesia--Examination Questions. 2. Anesthesiology--education.
WO 218.2 G162ba 2009]
   RD82.3.G35 2009
   617.9'6076--dc22

                                                                    2008032056

Acquisitions Editor: Natasha Andjelkovic
Publishing Services Manager: Tina Rebane
Project Manager: Fran Gunning
Design Direction: Lou Forgione

Transferred to Digital Printing in 2013

Acknowledgments

I am deeply grateful to all of my colleagues from Stony Brook and Miami who have shared their most interesting case scenarios and trickiest questions. From the Department of Anesthesiology at Stony Brook University, I am indebted to attending physicians Rishimani Adsumelli, MD, Carole Agin, MD, Dan Bhangoo, MD, Walter Backus, MD, Brian Durkin, DO, Igor Izrailtyan, MD, Zvi Jacob, MD, Robert Katz, MD, Ursula Landman, DO, Irina Lokshina, MD, Shaji Poovathor, MD, Eleanor Romano, DO, Joy Schabel, MD, Bharathi Scott, MD, Peggy Seidman, MD, Syed Shah, MD, Roy Soto, MD, Ellen Steinberg, MD, Francis Stellacio, MD, Andrea Voutsas, MD, and Paul Willoughby, MD. I am also indebted to our residents Anshul Airen, MD, Steve Chen, MD, Chris Collado, MD, Jian Lin, MD, Chris Martin, DO, Chris Page, MD, Igor Pikus, MD, Eric Posner, MD, Steve Probst, MD, Misako Sakamaki, MD, Matthew Tito, MD, Robert Trainer, DO, and Timothy Ueng, MD. I am also very grateful to Carlos Mijares, MD, and Wei Song, MD, from the Department of Anesthesiology, University of Miami.

CHRISTOPHER J. GALLAGHER, MD
STONY BROOK, NEW YORK

Introduction

"Hello, Elsevier?" a chastened, indebted Gallagher asked. "Look, *Board Stiff Too* is getting a little long in the tooth. What say we give it another go? This time, let's spice up the questions a little bit and have every practice board question based on a case that actually happened. I'll ask around. Everyone has done an *'Oh, my God, this is so unbelievable it could be a board question'* case. Let's make these unbelievable cases into practice test questions. Deal?"

Board Stiff rides again. This book is organized in four main parts.

Part I is a review. Ten chapters review the major points you will need to know for your oral board exam. This is not an appraisal of the whole discipline of anesthesia. It is a focused review of the things that appear on the test or things that people always ask me to review for them. For example, lots of people feel a little weak on heart cases, and they often ask me to "go over how to do a cardiac case." The chapter on hearts is the longest and addresses many topics frequently asked about, such as how big the cardiac preoperative preparation should be and who gets β-blockade. On the other hand, most people are comfortable with obstetrics, so I focus on the major topic that always appears on the exam: preeclampsia.

The final chapter in the review section is a hodgepodge of smaller topics that appear again and again:

- Managing oliguria
- What to do for increased intracranial pressure
- What to do when the patient fails to awaken
- Implications of obstructive sleep apnea
- Acute and chronic pain issues

These are subjects that do not merit entire chapters, but they are things you need to know.

Part II covers cases from real life, including stem questions and grab bags. Everyone reading this book has worked on a case "bad enough to be a board question." I hit up the residents and attendings at Stony Brook and some people at Miami (Drs. Mijares and Wei) to give me their cases that were bad enough to be board questions. These cases, arranged in the oral board format, are drawn from their experiences.

Answers are provided for all the questions. You are reminded that you should come up with your own answers before looking at our answers. We will not be there at test time. You will be, so prepare accordingly. Your answers may be different and may be better. This book is a workbook, not a textbook, and the most important thing is for you to work this book, not just read it and say, "Oh, yeah."

At the end of each exam, you will see a "How It Actually Went Down" section. This material is provided in case you are curious about how the case turned out. It is like reality television, only in book form!

Part III describes oldies but goodies. The earlier oral board format had preoperative, intraoperative, and postoperative questions for both rooms. I have been using a batch of questions in this format for years and modifying them as times change. I have included these for your perusal. The format is somewhat dated, but the questions are still valid. You will notice some overlap (how many ways are there to ask, "You cannot intubate; now what do you do?"), but repetition in learning is fine and dandy.

But wait, where are the answers to this section? They do not exist! The answers were omitted on purpose. You got plenty of answers in Part II. Now, it is time for you to practice without help. Practice often, and make sure you practice aloud. I will tell you that time and time again. You have to practice!

Part IV provides suggested topics and some final words of encouragement. Do you know the best way to prepare for the oral boards? Write an exam yourself! Brief blurbs are provided that you should work into entire exams on your own. In this way, you can look into the brains of the examiners. It is a great exercise.

Students preparing to take the exams ask me, "What should I read to fill in the gaps?" These are good sources:

- Hines R, Marschall K (eds): Stoelting's Anesthesia and Co-Existing Disease, 5th ed. Philadephia, Elsevier/Churchill Livingstone, 2008.
- The latest American Society of Anesthesiologists (ASA) refresher course (www.asahq.org/continuinged.htm). This material will bring you up to date.
- Audio Digest (www.audio-digest.org). The lectures are concise, written by the best experts, cover all the big topics, and are extremely useful for oral board preparation.

The main thing is to practice aloud. Read to fill in where you are weak, and then practice again.

Good luck to you all!

Please note that the previous printing included a DVD attached to the inside back cover with a video with simulated board scenarios to help you prepare. This video can now be accessed at http://static.us.elsevierhealth.com/gallagher_board_stiff_3_9780702030925/gallagher_board_stiff_video.mp4

Table of Contents

Part I

Review

1

Shifting Gears

The purpose of all knowledge is to impress people at cocktail parties.

KIM GALLAGHER, PhD, AUTHOR'S BROTHER

The opening quotation needs a little modification when it comes to getting board certified in anesthesiology:

For an hour or so in your not-too-distant future, the purpose of all knowledge is to impress two oral board examiners that "you know of what you speak."

It is a little clunkier than the original, but you get the idea. This chapter can help you change gears. It can get you to "quit thinking written boards" and "start thinking oral boards." Until now, your education has been geared toward the written boards:

All of the following disorders are associated with increased bleeding, except

1. Liver dysfunction
2. Idiopathic thrombocytopenic purpura
3. Transfusion reaction
4. Bronchospasm
5. Prolonged cardiopulmonary bypass

To meet that goal, you completed a bunch of practice questions in various review books, you (gasp!) actually read some textbooks, and you came up with the correct answer (4). Good for you!

As a matter of fact, if you are reading this book, you have done that phase of your life to perfection. You have *passed* the written boards. So guess what? You *know* the material that will appear on the oral boards! You have the raw material to pass the oral boards, because the oral boards are no longer in the style of "pick the one right answer from the line-up" or "pick A if 1, 2, and 3 are correct, B if 1 and 3 are correct, C if … ."

The oral boards are a test of your ability to "put it all together" and "paint a satisfactory clinical picture." This is not a trivial pursuit contest in which you pluck the soda lime equation out of your memory banks; this is a test of your case management and a discussion about what you do every day in the operating room. Instead of fielding the earlier question about increased bleeding, you will field a question on a topic such as this:

An alcoholic patient with idiopathic thrombocytopenic purpura has a transfusion reaction after a prolonged cardiopulmonary bypass run and develops refractory bronchospasm.

AAG! (Oh, that's a good one, come to think of it.) Instead of a straightforward "pick the right answer " (i.e., written boards), you are presented with a complex clinical situation (i.e., a million reasons to bleed plus bronchospasm, just to make life interesting). You must explain your plan of action, your alternative plans in case the patient does not respond appropriately, and how you will handle additional headaches.

It is tough but doable. You know the material, and now you must do three things:

- Organize your thoughts.
- Defend your reasoning.
- Adjust as conditions change.

What is the best way to prepare for this test?

- Practice aloud.
- Practice aloud.
- Practice aloud.

It is time to hear the drumbeat of this book and the recurrent theme in Board Stiff Land. Because you will be asked to deliver an *oral* plan during these *oral* boards, it stands to reason (and has been my experience for many years) that *practicing out loud* is the sine qua non of success.

Practice with your partners at work; hook up with your old attendings; go to a review course; practice with a dictation machine, and listen to yourself; or talk to yourself in the car. Do whatever it takes. Do *not* bury yourself in a book and think you can *read* your way through this test. You will have to speak up on "the big day," so make sure you speak up before the big day.

Yea, verily, I say unto you. Since the time of my own test (when the earth was still hot to the touch), through the original *Board Stiff* and its demon spawn *Board Stiff Too*, and from a bazillion practice exams, I can tell you one thing with absolute certainty:

PRACTICING ALOUD IS THE COMMON THREAD FOR SUCCESS.

This is true for the smart ones, not-so-smart ones, confident docs, shaky docs, stars, lesser lights, the first time, or the fifth time. It is as predictable as the tides and the seasons and as apparent as the sun at high noon in the Sahara: *Those who read and never practice do worse than those who practice.*

Are there exceptions? Of course! Many a *Board Stiff* nonbeliever has come to me and said, "Why should I do practice exams? I read and studied during residency, explained myself thoroughly in teaching rounds and in the operating room, and feel no need to practice. I think I can go in there cold and pass this exam by just saying what I do every day."

To that I say, "Amen!" If you did all that in residency (and you *should* have done that in residency), you are perfectly prepared. Many such people have gone into the exam cold and have passed fine and dandy, sugar candy. Bravo to them one and all.

If you want to hedge your bet, if you want to tip the balance in your favor, and if you are nervous about not hitting a home run, I go back to principles: *Those who read and never practice do worse than those who practice.* If you are looking for *the* way to improve your chances, do practice exams. Start them *now*. Do not wait for some magic date when you will have "enough time" or "enough energy." That day never comes, but *now* is always here. Do a practice exam as soon as possible. It does not matter if you do not perform perfectly on the first one or the first ten. They are for practice, and practice exams can uncover your weaknesses.

The only exam that counts is the real one, so do not sweat it if you blow a practice exam with your partner or your former attending. You often do not recognize your weak areas until you try a practice exam, and you sure as hell do not want to discover you know nothing about pediatrics during the real exam. You want to find that out a few months ahead of time, so you can brush up, fill in the gaps, and show up ready Freddy on the day of the exam.

I wish I had a dime for every person I examined who said, "Oh, hearts! Gee, I haven't done one in forever," or "Oh, pain! God, that's right; I guess I better know a little about that, huh?" or "We don't cover obstetrics at my hospital, and I've forgotten all about pre-eclampsia." If I did have a dime for every time I have heard those statements, I would be hiring and firing Donald Trump on my *own* reality show.

No kidding, you need to shift gears, and get *in* the oral board zone and get *out* of the written board zone. How so? Make every day before the exam an oral board exam practice day:

- Pick up every syringe you drew up. Can you say a few things about it?
- You did a spinal block for that transurethral prostatectomy (TURP). Can you explain why? What would you do if it went high? If it failed? If he had a low sodium level?
- Pretend someone challenges you on the Swan-Ganz catheter you put in for that pancreatectomy.
- A code blue is called over the public address system. Are you up on the latest advanced cardiac life support (ACLS) guidelines? Can you run the entire code yourself? What about biphasic versus monophasic defibrillators?

With this approach, each day becomes a board preparation day. As you change gears from the written exam to the oral exam, you may ask whether it is worth the time and money to take an oral board review course.

I run an oral board review course, Board Stiff Live, Inc. The small-group reviews have one examiner to every three or four students (Boardstifflive.com). Keep in mind this caveat: I have something to gain by saying you should take an oral board review course. I may be trying to cheat you out of your hard-earned money!

The question remains: Should you take an oral board review course? The answer is a resounding *maybe*, based on the following:

- If you trained well, studied well, and can explain yourself clearly, you do not need a review course.
- If you have ample opportunity to practice with your colleagues, you do not need a review course.
- Legions of board-certified anesthesiologists never took any review course, and they did just fine.

A REVIEW COURSE IS A LUXURY, NOT AN ABSOLUTE NECESSITY BY ANY STRETCH OF THE IMAGINATION.

That being said, some people *choose* luxuries. Do you need a Rolex to tell time? A Timex does just as well. Do you need a Lexus to get to work? A 1974 Buick Regal with 150,000 miles on it can get you to work. Do you need a 6000-ft^2 house overlooking the lake? The 3000-ft^2 house around the block will provide you shelter from the storm. However, you paid extra for those items because those were things you wanted.

The same principle applies to a review course. It may be one luxury you choose to pay for, so which one is best?

- Board Stiff Live provides the smallest student-to-teacher ratio.
- Board Stiff Live gives you the most individualized attention.
- Board Stiff Live gives you the most private exams.

You tell me! Which one do you think is best?

What is the bottom line? If I sailed through a good residency and had plenty of confidence and time to practice, I would not take a review course. If I were having trouble passing, lacked confidence, or just wanted a focused time dedicated to nothing but oral board study, I would take a review course, and I would take the best one.

2

Now You're in for It: The Exam

What's that roaring sound?

THE FIRST PERSON PADDLING A CANOE ABOVE NIAGARA FALLS

It is a good idea to know what is "down the river" before you dip your oars in the water. This chapter describes the examiners, the exam criteria, and the exam format.

THE EXAMINERS

I have worked with several different board examiners in private practice and in the hallowed halls of academe. It is a good idea to see things from their perspective as you roll into the exam (and before you pitch over the waterfall).

Examiners are not superheroes. They are not clinicians beyond the reach of mere mortals. They are practicing anesthesiologists, just like you and me. They look up stuff, ask around, have someone nearby in a jam—all the regular things that regular people do during the daily grind of operating room work.

Examiners receive the exam questions the night before and are specifically told they cannot look up anything. This means that they must draw on the knowledge they already have, just as you will have to draw on the knowledge you already have. That makes the exam fair, and it should set your mind at ease, at least a little bit. The examiners cannot dig deep in Miller's *Anesthesia* to find some obscure tidbit about infrared plasma vortex intracraniographic positron interactions with lipophilic ameboid capsules in the pseudohypoparathyroid patient with Munchausen syndrome. They know what they know. You know what you know—so have at it.

The examiners invest a lot of time and effort to do these exams, and they are paid peanuts. They are aware that they have been entrusted with an enormous responsibility.

How can our specialty be recognized unless we make sure board certification means something? That is serious stuff, and that is what guides the examiners. They do not wake up in the morning thinking, "Who can we *get* today? Let's *nitpick* the next person to death." They just want to make sure that the American Board of Anesthesiologists' imprimatur is valid.

They will pass you if you know how to do anesthesia. If you are a safe, careful, thoughtful physician who does what "most clinicians would do in a similar situation," you get to pass Go and collect $200.

One examiner summed it up quite nicely, and his words are worth keeping in mind as you prepare for your exam: "If I ask a candidate how to handle malignant hyperthermia, and he or she tells me the right way to handle it, then on what grounds am I going to flunk this person?" Apply that to everything else we do, and you have a perfect glimpse into the mind of the examiner. On what grounds are they going to flunk you

- If they ask you how to manage a preeclamptic patient, and you tell them the right way to handle a preeclamptic patient?
- If they ask you how to manage an intravascular injection of local anesthetic, and you tell them the right way to manage an intravascular injection of local anesthetic?
- If they ask you to diagnose and treat myocardial ischemia based on electrocardiographic changes in the middle of a case, and you diagnose and treat myocardial ischemia appropriately?
- If they ask you about fluid management in a burn patient, and you correctly describe the protocol?
- If they ask you about intracranial pressure issues in a head-injured patient, and you explain the issues and appropriate management?
- If they ask you about failed intubation, and you explain the correct approach?
- If they ask you about hypotension in a patient with a bleeding aneurysm, and you describe the right way to handle the patient?
- If they ask you about hypoxemia in a patient with acute respiratory distress syndrome (ARDS), and you tell them the correct way to handle the case?

If they ask you something about anesthesia, and you say the right thing (no tricks here or plot twists), you are in clover.

Do the examiners make it tough? Yes, but consider it from their point of view. If they did not make it tough, the test would be meaningless, and board certification would be meaningless.

You walk in and shake hands. You sit down.

An examiner says, "Good morning. How would you anesthetize a healthy young man with no medical problems for a hernia operation?"

You respond, "Uh, general anesthesia with a laryngeal mask airway."

The examiner says, "Okay, that's fine. Thank you for coming to your board exam. We'll be sending your certification in about 6 weeks. Have a nice day."

It is safe to say that is not going to happen. You will have some tough and thorny problems. People coming back from exams tell me all the time about their questions, and some are doozies! However, one theme has held true for the past 20 years: The exams are tough, but they are always fair.

That bears repeating. The exams are always tough, but they are always fair. They always cover topics that we should know. No returning examinee has ever accused the examiners of playing unfair.

THE CRITERIA

We next look at the things the examiners grade you on. Four criteria are used in grading your exam: judgment, adaptation, clarity, and application.

A simple example illustrates these four criteria in action.

Your patient is a 65-year-old man about to undergo transurethral prostatectomy (TURP). What kind of anesthetic will you use?

Judgment. A spinal block provides a good, dense block and gives you information about TURP syndrome and bladder rupture, because the patient can communicate with you. Your good *judgment* tells you to do a spinal.

Adaptation. The patient is on Plavix for eluting stents placed 3 months ago. This introduces a clotting issue, and a spinal block is not such a good idea. Your *adaptability* tells you to do this procedure under general anesthesia.

Clarity. Should you use an endotracheal tube or laryngeal mask airway (LMA)? The patient is at no risk for aspiration and has had nothing by mouth (NPO), so your notion of *clarity* says that you will use an LMA. You do not waffle or debate the two options endlessly; you make a clear decision and go with it.

Application. Halfway through the case, you see green liquid in the LMA. Plan A has not worked. A new complication has arisen, and you have to *apply* your knowledge of anesthesia to manage this situation. You go head down, suction, and secure the airway with an endotracheal tube.

Let's go through the four grading criteria again and address a recurrent theme in your oral board preparation. The examiners want to hear the voice of a *consultant* in anesthesia.

Judgment. A consultant has sufficient knowledge to pick the right course of action.

Adaptation. A consultant is not bound to one course of action. A consultant knows that different circumstances (here, Plavix) call for different plans.

Clarity. A consultant is not a memorizer of long lists, ready to dredge out every bit of possibly relevant information. A consultant gets to the point with a clear, concise plan or response.

Application. A consultant is sufficiently nimble after the case has started that he or she can apply accrued knowledge to changing situations. Most often in the exam, the situation is a complication or failure of the original plan. Do not worry if this happens! It does not mean you "did wrong" and are now in this jam due to your foolishness. It means the examiner has a sheet of paper with a question that asks what happens when "the local anesthetic goes intravascular," "the spinal goes high," or "the teeth get chipped." Apply your knowledge and answer!

You now know about the examiners and the criteria. We next consider the exam format.

THE EXAM FORMAT

After you apply for your oral exam, the American Board of Anesthesiology (ABA) sends you the whole format plus a sample exam. Look it over. Talk about getting stuff straight from the horse's mouth! Here it is laid out for you.

In room 1, you face two examiners, with a possible third in the room. The third person is grading the examiners, not grading you. You are given a long stem question, with all the preoperative information provided and taken care of.

Your exam consists of a long section on intraoperative questions, followed by a shorter postoperative section, after which you are finished with the stem question. The examiners then shift gears and ask you two or three shorter questions on other topics (this section of the exam has earned the sobriquet *grab bag* and is labeled as such in later chapters). Someone knocks on the door at the end of 35 minutes (it will seem as if you just got there!). Out into the hall you go, and you are given a second stem question in the next room.

In room 2, there are again two examiners, with a possible third person to grade them, not you. Your stem question is short this time, and the examiners start by asking you preoperative questions, and they then lead into the intraoperative questions; the longest section in both rooms covers intraoperative topics. There is no postoperative section in room 2. The examiners finish with the stem question and do two or three grab bags before the knock comes.

To summarize, the long stem question has intraoperative, postoperative, and grab bag sections. The short stem question has preoperative, intraoperative, and grab bag sections.

You have about 5 minutes to look over the stem questions before they let you in the room. Most people scribble furiously on the paper, hoping to put down a flurry of reminders and things they absolutely must have down. There is nothing wrong with this, and it may even do you some good. However, many people have told me that after the examiners blast the first question at you, your mind goes gazoinkel, and you never even look down at your carefully constructed notes. That is what happened to me, but by all means, write notes if that makes you feel better. What the hell are you supposed to do in those 5 minutes anyway? Pull out a Sodoku puzzle and fill that in?

So there you have the exam, with all its component parts—the examiners, the criteria, and the format.

3

Hot Tips from the School of Hard Knocks

Listen to the old guys. They've been there. Don't trust the bastards, but do listen to them.

SOMEBODY MUST HAVE SAID THIS.

Here are the four most important, time-tested, "this really helped me" tips amassed from helping people through these exams since the late 1980s. Times have changed, therapies and drugs have changed, and our thinking about anesthesia has changed, but these four tenets hold true:

1. Do not ask questions.
2. Do not complicate things.
3. Think head to toe.
4. Break down questions into their component parts.

DO NOT ASK QUESTIONS

Asking a question after getting a question is a reflex. Learn to suppress this reflex. Better yet, train yourself through practice to suppress the reflex.

Examiner: The blood pressure drops.
You: What's the heart rate?

Don't do that!

Examiner: The heart rate goes up.
You: What's the blood pressure?

What did I just say? Do not bounce questions back to the examiners. What should you do? Make your assumptions, cover the bases, and give an answer.

Examiner: The blood pressure drops.
You: Assuming this is related to blood loss from an injury, I would give fluids, send a gas, and decrease potent inhaled agents.

That's more like it!

Examiner: The heart rate goes up.
You: If the heart rate is up and the blood pressure is up, this could be light anesthesia, so I would deepen it; but if the heart rate is up and the pressure is down, it would be typical of hypovolemia, and I would replace volume.

Good for you! You gave a complete, concise answer that covered all the major things that could be going wrong, and you did not waste a lot of time asking useless questions.

DO NOT COMPLICATE THINGS

Make the patient as healthy as you can. There is no need to tack pathology on pathology.

> Examiner: This man is 1 year out from a myocardial infarction (MI).
>
> You: Well, he could have had arrhythmias and might have an automatic implantable cardioverter defibrillator (AICD). His ejection fraction could be severely impaired—heck, he might be about to arrest right now! I would intubate him in the preoperative clinic and set up extracorporeal membrane oxygenation!"

This is a bit over the top, wouldn't you say?

> Examiner: This man is 1 year out from an MI.
>
> You: Assuming he has fully recovered and is doing well clinically, with cardiology following him and adjusting his medications, I would induce him with standard induction agents.

See? You do not need to drag in problems that are not there. Make an assumption that the patient is healthy, and answer the question. The examiners may up the ante and *make* the patient sick. This is not a problem. You prove your adaptability and your skill at application (see Chapter 2), and you adjust accordingly.

> Examiner: After his MI, they placed an AICD.
>
> You: Before we went into the operating room, I would make sure the AICD was turned off, and I would put external pads on. I then would induce for his hernia repair, aware that the AICD is off, and I would be on the lookout for dangerous rhythms because I will have to jump in and shock the patient.

THINK HEAD TO TOE

As you start preparing for the orals, it seems impossible to know everything that could happen to anyone under any anesthetic. So you throw your hands up in the air and yield to despair.

But wait! Think about what makes a human being, go from head to toe, and you will understand that no matter how you slice or dice it, there are only so many things that can go wrong. There are only so many areas the examiners can focus on, because we humans have only so many pathologic conditions:

- Head: intracranial injury or tumor; cerebral perfusion
- Eye: oculocardiac reflex; open eye and full stomach debate
- Ear: nitrous oxide expands pockets; nausea and vomiting concerns
- Mouth: airway, airway, airway; lost teeth
- Neck: injured cervical spine; head injury indicating possible neck injury and vice versa; line placement and misfortunes
- Heart: ischemia; preoperative testing; left ventricular function; rhythm disturbance de jour; pacemakers and AICDs; thoracic aortic dissections and aneurysms; differential of blood pressure (high/low), heart rate (high/low)
- Lungs: aspiration; bronchospasm; "all that wheezes is not asthma"; pulmonary function tests (yes/no); arterial blood gas interpretation; lung isolation; differential diagnosis for hypoxemia

- Abdomen: baby (preeclampsia is the biggie in this department); obesity; liver dysfunction; renal failure; aortic aneurysms; severe third spacing and fluid losses with obstructions and long operations
- Extremities: blocks and attendant local anesthetic problems; trauma (causing fat emboli and blood loss); burns; peripheral vascular disease
- Age: very young (systems all immature, childhood differences from adult conditions); very old (everything goes to hell, as one look at me can confirm).

With a quick head-to-toe review and by thinking about the main "ills that flesh is heir to," you can hit on probably 90% of the questions the examiners can ask you. A great tip, based on a lot of experience with a lot of examinees, is to go over the head-to-toe review and ask yourself a simple question: Can you answer questions pertaining to these head-to-toe problems?

Unless examiners start asking us about parakeets or Martians, the previous list is pretty much everything that you could ask about anyone. There is no need to despair because the list is quite manageable!

BREAK DOWN QUESTIONS INTO THEIR COMPONENT PARTS

The questions can seem impossible at first glance, such as the one that came from a former student. Hang onto your hat.

> A pregnant woman at term is in a motor vehicle accident on her way into the hospital. Her Glasgow Coma Scale (GCS) score was 8, so she was intubated in the emergency department. You are in the elevator, taking her up to the operating room, and the endotracheal tube gets pulled out. Your laryngoscope has a burned out light bulb.

I almost fell out of my chair when I heard this. At first glance, determining what to do seems impossible. So now it is time to be systematic.

Airway, Breathing, and Circulation

Checking the airway, breathing, and circulation (ABC) is always a good place to start! You have a suboptimal situation here, so you manage the ABCs *as best* you can with *what* you have.

You cannot intubate, so mask ventilate. As soon as the elevator door opens, call for help, and get to a place where you can resecure the airway. Keep a finger on the pulse to monitor circulation.

Emergency, Urgent, or Elective Management

Emergency means life, limb, or sight are at risk. *Urgent* means delay can cause damage to life, limb, or sight. *Elective* means action can wait.

This case is an emergency. A GCS score of 8 means serious neurologic trouble and an inability to protect the airway. You move to resecure the airway and to determine a need for neurosurgical care, such as for an epidural or subdural hematoma or cervical spine injury.

Concomitant Conditions

What else does the patient have? This is where you can run into clashing objectives. In this case, the woman is pregnant, and you would like to avoid instrumenting the airway, because there is a higher fatality rate for cesarean sections under general than under regional anesthesia. However, she has a GCS score of 8, and you need to protect the airway.

You do not want to intubate, but you do want to intubate—clashing objectives. That is what makes it a board question! These "damned if you do, damned if you don't" dilemmas are a test of your understanding of complex problems.

Here are other examples of common clashing objectives:

- Asthma (want to intubate deeply) and a full stomach (no time to intubate deeply)
- Difficult airway (want to intubate while the patient is awake) and asthma (intubating while the patient is awake may trigger asthma)
- No venous access in a mentally challenged adult patient (want to breathe down) and obesity (do not want to breathe down)
- Asthma (want to give β-agonists) and cardiac ischemia (want to give β-blockers)

Stuff You Always Have To Answer

No matter what the case scenario, you will be asked about these things:

- What laboratory or other studies are needed before you proceed?
- What monitors (specifically, which invasive monitors) are needed?
- What are your plans for induction, maintenance, and emergence?
- Does the patient require placement in an intensive care unit (ICU)?

We can apply these questions to our unfortunate mommy-to-be who just got extubated in the elevator.

After she is out of the elevator and her airway is secured, you want to make sure you have blood available (type and crossmatch but can use O negative if she crashes first). Computed tomography (CT) scans of the cervical spine and head CT should be obtained if vital signs allow. Blood gas determinations should be made.

Place an arterial line (need for frequent blood gas determinations and for beat-to-beat blood pressure measurement given her precarious state) and large-bore intravenous catheters for access. Use a fetal heart rate monitor.

Because the patient is unstable, induce with etomidate. For maintenance, use intravenous agents, depending on her vital signs. Alert the pediatric department that if a cesarean section occurs, they may need to support the infant's ventilation. Until the neurologic picture is clearer, keep the patient on a ventilator at emergence.

With a GCS score of 8, boy howdy is the patient going to the ICU.

The next chapter considers our very reason for existence—managing problems with the vital signs.

4

Vital Signs Are Vital

Do you feel a pulse? I don't. I think he's dead.

THE GUY WHO DISCOVERED KING TUT'S MUMMY

I made up that quotation, but it makes a good point. When you cannot feel a pulse, and someone has been buried for 3000 years, you have good prima facie evidence that they are, in point of fact, dead. This underscores the importance of vital signs.

This chapter was originally written in the first edition of *Board Stiff*, and it is so good, we are going back in time to revisit that chapter from long, long ago, because it covers the topic as well today as it did then. Retro? Yes, but in a good way.

Prepare yourself to handle every aberration in vital signs. That is the essence of every anesthesiologist's job. In the intraoperative part of the oral exam, you will have to handle vital sign aberrations. Work on and have clear responses to the following situations:

- Tachycardia
- Bradycardia
- Hypertension
- Hypotension
- Hypoxemia
- Hypercapnia

TACHYCARDIA

Tachycardia can be primary or secondary.

Primary tachycardia (i.e., pathology inherent in the heart)
   1. Supraventricular arrhythmia
   2. Ventricular arrhythmia
Secondary tachycardia (i.e., sympathetic stimulation)
   1. Hypoxemia
   2. Hypercapnia
   3. Decreased oxygen delivery
      a. Anemia
      b. Decreased cardiac output
   4. Pain (usually associated with hypertension)
      a. Somatic (e.g., incision, fractured bone)
      b. Visceral (e.g., distended bladder)
      c. Sympathetic (e.g., tourniquet pain, which is difficult to treat)
   5. Hypovolemia (usually associated with hypotension)
      a. Absolute (e.g., dehydration, hemorrhage)
      b. Relative (e.g., tamponade, pneumothorax, positive end-expiratory pressure [PEEP])

6. Unusual possibilities
    a. Inotrope running wide open
    b. Pheochromocytoma "leaking" an inotrope
    c. Carcinoid syndrome

BRADYCARDIA

Like tachycardia, bradycardia can be primary or secondary.

Primary bradycardia (i.e., something wrong with the heart itself)
    1. Sick sinus syndrome
    2. Complete heart block
Secondary bradycardia (i.e., vagal stimulation or sympathetic suppression)
    1. Drug-induced
        a. Digoxin (i.e., too much causes heart block)
        b. Narcotics (i.e., a vagal thunderbolt)
        c. Anticholinesterases (Oops! Forgot the glycopyrrolate!)
        d. β-Blockers (i.e., sympatholysis)
        e. Dexmedetomidine (i.e., sympatholysis from α_2-stimulation)
        f. Calcium channel blockers
    2. Vagal stimulation
        a. Oculocardiac reflex
        b. Traction on viscera (e.g., pleura, peritoneum)
        c. Laryngoscopy
        d. Baroreceptor reflex (e.g., manipulation during carotid surgery)

HYPERTENSION

Hypertension goes hand in hand with tachycardia. Patients have primary hypertension (i.e., preexisting high blood pressure, such as long-standing hypertension or preeclampsia) or secondary hypertension (i.e., sympathetic stimulation, the same as with tachycardia).

Primary hypertension
    1. Long-standing hypertension (called primary hypertension)
    2. Hypertension associated with a specific disease entity
        a. Preeclampsia
        b. Kidney failure
Secondary hypertension (i.e., sympathetic stimulation)
    1. Hypoxemia
    2. Hypercapnia
    3. Pain (usually associated with tachycardia)
        a. Somatic (e.g., incision, fractured bone)
        b. Visceral (e.g., distended bladder)
        c. Sympathetic (e.g., tourniquet pain, which is difficult to treat)
    4. Unusual possibilities
        a. Inotrope running wide open
        b. Pheochromocytoma "leaking" an inotrope
        c. Carcinoid syndrome

The widespread use of β-blockers can confuse the picture. A patient under light anesthesia may not manifest a tachycardic response in conjunction with tachycardia.

HYPOTENSION

Hypotension requires a more elaborate explanation than does primary and secondary hypotension. We have to put on our physiology hats and break blood pressure down into its basic parts:

1. Preload
2. The heart itself
3. Afterload
4. The blood itself

Preload can be insufficient:

- There is not enough (e.g., bleeding, dehydration).
- There is enough, but it cannot get back to the heart because of tamponade, positive-pressure ventilation, PEEP, tension pneumothorax, aortocaval compression, a vessel pinched during surgery, or bent and twisted heart during off-pump coronary artery bypass grafting (CABG).

The *heart* itself can be insufficient:

- The muscle itself is not strong enough (e.g., cardiomyopathy, infarcted heart muscle).
- The muscle is fine, but it is not able to deliver enough blood because of bradycardia, tachycardia (i.e., too fast to fill or too fast to function, as in ventricular tachycardia or fibrillation), or valvular problems (i.e., insufficiency or stenosis).

Afterload can be insufficient:

- It is too low (e.g., anaphylaxis, vasodilators gone wild, spinal shock).

The *blood* can be insufficient:

- There is not enough of it (e.g., hematocrit of 3), and there is not enough viscosity to generate pressure in the circulatory system.

Wait a minute! Where does anesthesia fit into all of this? We cause hypotension all the time. Why is not part of the differential diagnosis of hypotension? Anesthesia is there, in that an excess of anesthetic can affect the afterload (e.g., propofol) or the heart itself (i.e., volatile anesthetics hemodynamically act as "anti-epinephrine").

HYPOXEMIA

If you are not asked about hypoxemia sometime during your oral board exam, I will personally buy you a beer at the next American Society of Anesthesiologists (ASA) meeting. If you are going to be board certified in anesthesiology, you damned well better be able to diagnose and treat hypoxemia! What follows is a "geographic" approach to nailing this question.

Go from the wall to the tubing to the endotracheal tube to the lungs. Then go from outside to inside on the patient: chest wall to pleura to parenchyma to pulmonary vasculature to the heart itself. Before you wrap it up, take a quick peek at the brain. This systematic approach covers all hypoxemic bases.

From the wall to the endotracheal tube

- Wrong gas composition: line crossover
- No gas delivery: disconnect, ventilator off, switch thrown the wrong way

Endotracheal tube to lungs

- Endobronchial or esophageal intubation
- Kink, clog, aspiration of big things such as hot dogs and other stuff you can get at a county fair
- Disconnect
- Tube went subcutaneously (i.e., tracheotomy in the wrong place)

Thorax, outermost to innermost

- Chest wall weak from residual neuromuscular blocker
- Kyphoscoliosis, flail chest, phrenic nerve damage
- Pleura: fluid (e.g., intravenous fluid, blood, chylous fluid, effusion) or air (e.g., pneumothorax)
- Parenchyma: aspiration, pneumonia, acute respiratory distress syndrome (ARDS), congestive heart failure (CHF), atelectasis, ventilation-perfusion ($\dot{V}/\dot{Q}$) mismatch from patient positioning or from one lung ventilation
- Pulmonary vasculature: emboli (e.g., clot, fat, amniotic fluid, air)
- Cardiac plumbing: right-to-left shunts (PEEP sometimes worsens this!)

Central nervous system

- Apnea from inhaled or injected anesthetic drugs
- Damage to the respiratory center
- High cervical lesion impairing the patient's ability to breathe

HYPERCAPNIA

Hypoxemia was pretty involved. Thankfully, hypercapnia is a little less taxing. The patient is making too much, getting rid of too little, or rebreathing carbon dioxide.

Making too much

- Malignant hyperthermia
- Thyrotoxicosis
- Sepsis

Getting rid of too little

- Hypoventilation from your sub-optimal anesthetic
- You are setting the ventilator wrong, or if the patient is breathing on his own, you are overdosing him on the muscle relaxant, narcotics, or inhaled agent.

Rebreathing

- Exhausted CO_2 absorber
- Malfunctioning valve
- Flows too low

That's a little easier.

SUMMARY

If there is one thing you need to drill on, it is this list. Because you know a vital sign aberration will appear on the exam, make sure you can recite chapter and verse on the following:

- Tachycardia
- Bradycardia
- Hypertension
- Hypotension
- Hypoxemia
- Hypercapnia

Vital signs are vital to your patient and to your board certification.

5

Without Further Ado, the Airway

Money and sex explain most things.

I am positive somebody said that, and as far as most anesthesiologists are concerned, the airway explains everything else. Chapter 4 looked at vital signs, which are certain to be on the test. We now jump to the next topic sure to be on the test: managing the airway. What is more important than the airway in the realm of anesthesiology? We are the airway people, and board examiners expect us to know this airway business up, down, and every which way. In this chapter, we consider the airway in the preoperative, intraoperative, and postoperative realms.

PREOPERATIVE APPROACH

The history and physical examination trump everything else during the preoperative period.

History

When obtaining the patient's medical history, ask whether he or she has had anesthesia. On rare occasions, you will get "the real deal" straight up:

> *"They told me I was hard to intubate."*

> *"They gave me this letter—something about a fiberoptic awake something."*

> *"Last time, they trached me in a big hurry."*

Responses such as these are rare in practice and unlikely to be handed to you on the oral board exam. You may get some indirect clues about the difficulty:

> *"They chipped my tooth."*

> *"My throat was real sore afterward."*

These responses indicate that someone was having a hell of a time getting that tube in.

It is great if you can get old anesthetic records. (On the boards, the examiners will probably say the old records are unavailable.) Even an old anesthetic record is not a guarantee of accurate information:

- The airway might have worsened since that anesthetic because of increasing obesity or worsening arthritis.
- The last anesthesiologist might have been the best laryngoscopist in the world.
- The last anesthesiologist might have had trouble but did not bother to write anything about the difficulty on the anesthetic record.

Specific conditions in the patient's medical history may cause you to suspect a bad airway:

- Pierre Robin syndrome
- Any of the mucopolysaccharidoses
- Trisomy 21
- Arthritis
- Scleroderma
- Obesity
- Pregnancy (i.e., much higher incidence of lost airways in parturients)
- Cervical disk disease and operations, especially fusions
- Neck injury (i.e., special care required to avoid worsening an injury)
- Irradiation of the neck
- Tumor or abscess in the airway (have a heart-to-heart talk with the ear, nose, and throat [ENT] surgeon)

Physical Examination

During the physical examination, look for the "usual suspects" that coexist with a bad airway:

- Large teeth
- Short thyromental distance
- Large tongue
- Mallampati glottic view of grade 3 or 4
- Head in a collar or a halo (unless you are good at bending steel)
- Radiation or surgical scars or masses (e.g., goiter) altering the airway

As you examine the patient, consider how hard it will be to ventilate the patient if you fail to intubate:

- Morbidly obese: difficult mask ventilation
- In a "jungle gym" orthopedic bed: hard to get at the airway
- On some burdensome radiology bed: hard to get the bed into reverse Trendelenburg so you can take weight off the diaphragm and aid oxygenation
- Full stomach: intubation better than mask ventilating a patient at risk for vomiting and aspiration
- Middle of the night, weekend, or holiday: lack of personnel to offer help (as in the movie *Aliens*, no one hears you scream)

INTRAOPERATIVE APPROACH

Here's my personal approach to the airway, which partly offers advice for the boards and partly for the real world.

The following points apply to awake intubation:

1. Have a low threshold for doing awake intubations. The more you do, the better you get at them, and the less you "fear doing it awake."
2. The biggest problem about doing an awake intubation is gathering all the stuff to do the topicalization, so get it together ahead of time.
3. What is the best sedation for awake intubation? Dexmedetomidine, hands down.

4. Because the patient has to be dry, get anti-sialagogue in early. Do not flounder in an ocean of saliva and local anesthetic.

5. Is the patient uncooperative? You will be amazed how they calm down with dexmedetomidine.

6. Is the patient extremely uncooperative? If you have someone who will not hold still (e.g., drunk car wreck guy, thrashing around and may pith himself), you really cannot do it awake.

7. Should you use a nasal or oral approach? Nasal gives you a better angle, and the tube can and sometimes does go in by itself. However, you risk hemorrhage, which is a potential disaster if you later give heparin (e.g., heart case). The oral approach does not provide as good an angle, but at least you do not risk nasal hemorrhage.

8. What do you do if you only see pink in the fiberoptic scope? Pull the tube back. Keep pulling back until you see a kind of cave, which means you will have enough room to look around, find that epiglottis, and go for it.

9. What if you are through the cords and cannot advance the tube? Do not force it. Rotate it, try again, and keep rotating until you eventually feel it "give."

10. Use oxygen in the suction port to blow secretions and blood away. Do not use suction. The hole is too small, and suction pulls fluid up to the end of the scope and obscures your view. By insufflating oxygen, you help with oxygenation.

The following points apply to regular intubation:

1. Be diligent about preoperative oxygenation. You are filling your "scuba tanks" before a dive into the unknown. The more reserve O_2 you have, the better in case you get in trouble (on the boards, the examiners are sure to get you in trouble).

2. Tilt the patient up a little. That takes the weight off the diaphragm, and it gives you a little extra functional residual capacity, a little easier time mask ventilating, and a little more time before desaturation.

3. Have all your goodies nearby: light wand, intubating bougie, fiberoptic scope, Bullard laryngoscope, laryngeal mask airway (LMA), and ENT surgeon with sharpened knife. You do not want to struggle to find them after you are in the heat of battle.

4. Before inducing, optimize the patient's head position. For obese patients, go around to the side and build up the shoulders and neck until you have the best possible first shot. It will be your best, so optimize it.

5. Succinylcholine (absent contraindications such as spinal cord injury, burn, muscular dystrophy, or prolonged immobilization) gives you the possibility of a quick return of muscle function in case you cannot intubate.

6. Do not reinforce failure if you get in trouble. Change blades, head positions, practitioners, or techniques—change *something* if one method does not work. Do not force the issue, tear up the airway, cause bleeding and swelling, and make things worse.

So you are taking the test. You have been diligent about your airway-oriented history and physical examination, but you still get into trouble in a "cannot intubate, can ventilate" situation or in its more sinister cousin, the "cannot intubate, cannot ventilate" situation.

1. Do not panic. This is part of the test, a question the examiners were going to get to eventually, so do not fight with them. Just go with it.
2. Know your American Society of Anesthesiologists (ASA) difficult airway algorithm.
3. You can answer, "At this point, I would follow the difficult airway algorithm." They may press you on this and may ask for more details, but that is a valid response.

A few key points from the algorithm may be helpful:

1. You do not have to intubate, but you have to ventilate. Take a break from intubation attempts to mask ventilate.
2. The intubating bougie is extremely effective at making that "little upward turn" on the anterior airway.
3. The LMA affords a good (not perfect) airway, and you can intubate through it.
4. Waking up the patient is often "the better part of valor."

We must address the most severe degree of trouble—cannot intubate, cannot ventilate:

1. If you must go surgical, then *go for it*. Do not hesitate if the only option is patient harm or death from hypoxemia.
2. It will be messy.
3. If the option is death, live with the mess.
4. Do not do a tracheotomy, because it is low and slow. Perform a cricotomy, which is high and fast.

POSTOPERATIVE APPROACH

After all the Sturm und Drang of a tough intubation, you may be asked this postoperative question on the oral boards: How and when do you extubate the person who gave you so much trouble during intubation?

Extubate only when the patient meets all extubation criteria:

1. Patient is maintaining adequate oxygenation and ventilation without need for ventilatory support (e.g., high positive end-expiratory pressure [PEEP], intermittent mandatory ventilation [IMV], high inspired O_2 fraction [FIO_2]).
2. Patient is hemodynamically stable.
3. Patient is neurologically able to protect the airway.
4. Patient passes clinical tests of adequate respiratory effort (e.g., respiratory rate, negative pressure generation).

Ensure that the airway is not in danger of collapsing on removal of the endotracheal tube:

1. Do a leak test, in which you let down the cuff and see if the patient can breathe around the tube.
2. On physical examination, the airway does not appear distorted or swollen. This is a common sense test to make sure you do not extubate someone whose head looks like a giant pumpkin.

Take other steps to ensure success:

1. Any spooky extubation should be done in the daytime, when there are lots of people around to help out if you get in trouble. Do not extubate a "toughie" in the middle of the night.

2. If you are really spooked, put a tube exchanger down the tube, pull out the tube, and keep the tube exchanger in the trachea as a "safety net" for a few minutes. It is surprising how well patients tolerate this.

APPROACHES TO COEXISTING PROBLEMS

Bad airways vex you the most when they are combined with another disease. The bad airway usually takes precedence over the other condition, and you should perform the intubation awake despite the other condition. Here are a few examples of the "do them all awake" rule.

For *asthma and a difficult airway*, the best approach is to optimize the asthmatic's status as best you can, including the use of steroids and β-adrenergic agents, before you start topicalizing. The approach is difficult because you want the topicalizing agent to get into the trachea to numb it, but the aerosolized particles can trigger asthma. Talk about a Catch-22 situation!

Another option is to keep the asthmatic breathing spontaneously. Use deep-breath inhalation induction with sevoflurane, and then place the fiberoptic scope in and do an "asleep fiberoptic" procedure. The patient must be a good candidate for an inhalation induction. If the patient is obese or has a full stomach, it is not a good idea.

For *heart disease and a difficult airway*, do not rush the procedure. Make sure the patient's hemodynamics are monitored closely while you are topicalizing and sedating. Do not proceed if the heart rate gets high or the ST segment is elevated. Stop! Tend to the hemodynamics (e.g., vasodilator, β-blocker), and proceed only when things are under control again. A well-conducted, well-sedated, well-topicalized, awake intubation can give you the most stable hemodynamics you have ever seen!

For an *open eye or increased intracranial pressure and difficult airway*, the airway takes precedence. Yes, the coughing and bucking can worsen the eye injury or cerebral injury, but a lost airway and hypoxemia will hurt *everything*, so the airway trumps all else.

It all boils back down to this: If you keep in good practice doing awake intubations, whatever other challenge is attached to it, you can still work a smooth induction, keep the patient comfortable, and minimize collateral damage to other organ systems as you secure the airway.

EXCEPTIONS TO AWAKE PROCEDURES

There comes a time when the awake fiberoptic procedure is just not possible. On the exam, the examiners can always give instructions that curtail your options:

- The fiberoptic is broken.
- The patient absolutely refuses.
- You try the fiberoptic approach but cannot get it.

There are other times when it is not an option:

- The patient is intoxicated and out of control and has a possible cervical injury. A thrashing battle could worsen the cervical injury.
- An adult is unable to cooperate because of mental challenges. You end up fighting someone bigger than you—a losing proposition!

- You can explain all you want to a 6-month-old child with Pierre Robin syndrome, but the kid is still not going to hold still for it.

Do the following if the patient is intoxicated and out of control:

- Follow the guidelines laid down by the Maryland Shock Trauma Center.
- Induce and maintain in-line stabilization.
- Take your best look, being careful not to extend the neck.
- If you cannot get it, cut the neck.

Do the following if the adult patient is unable to cooperate:

- Induce.
- Keep the head up to aid ventilation.
- Use an intubating LMA.

Do the following for children:

- Keep children breathing spontaneously.
- Use the fiberoptic approach when they are induced.
- Back out and ventilate between attempts.

CONTROVERSIAL POINTS ABOUT THE AIRWAY

Just like everything else in anesthesiology, controversies abound. Cricoid pressure and an unstable neck are two such topics.

In theory, cricoid pressure closes off the esophagus and prevents aspiration. Textbooks say to use cricoid pressure. They tell you to maintain cricoid pressure and ventilate when you run into the "cannot intubate, can ventilate" situation during a cesarean section with fetal distress. Cricoid pressure is here, there, everywhere!

There are, however, a few problems with cricoid pressure:

- It does not close off the esophagus; it pushes it to the side.
- It does not prevent aspiration, because the esophagus is still "open at the top."
- It has not been proved to prevent aspiration.
- Cricoid pressure does make it harder to mask ventilate and harder to intubate (Oh, that!).
- It is widely endorsed but rarely questioned.

How should you answer on the test? I would tell the examiners what I told you here.

There is no one way that is superior to another for managing an unstable neck, and every maneuver to protect the neck makes it harder to see. There is no hard and fast rule on how to handle the fractured neck. All reviews end with an anemic "secure the airway the best way you know how." *Ay caramba!* I *always* secure the airway the best way I know how.

The next chapter goes right to the heart of the matter.

6

Mending Broken Hearts

Honey, I got the winning lottery ticket! Fifty million dollars! Pack your bags!

Oh great! Where are we going? Paris? Tahiti?

I don't care where you're going.

I stole this joke from somewhere on the Internet. That jilted spouse needs cardiac mending, and some of you may need some cardiac mending.

People at the Board Stiff Live review course are forever asking us to review cardiac cases. Because few people "do hearts" after their training is done, this remains a weak point. This chapter looks at various cardiac issues and offers a lightning review of how to do a cardiac case. That should bring you up to speed. As with the airway chapter, we will address the preoperative, intraoperative, and postoperative questions likely to arise on the boards. The emphasis is on the intraoperative portion (intraoperative questions are emphasized during the boards, so what the heck), with attention paid to several thorny issues:

- Swan-Ganz catheter insertion: Is it as bad as some say or as good as others believe?
- Transesophageal echocardiography (TEE): You can no longer say, "Oh, I don't know anything about TEE."

WARNING, WARNING, WARNING, WARNING!

Most of anesthesia stays the same over the years, with a little adjustment here and there, as these examples demonstrate:

- Neuroanesthesia: Hyperventilation went out of style, but most everything else is the same.
- Preeclampsia: We used to say you could not do a spinal block for it, but turns out that you can. All other considerations remain the same.
- Vital signs: Look over the differential diagnosis for hypoxemia or hypotension. Has anything changed there? No.
- Airway: The laryngeal mask airway (amen) has entered the equation, and we get a new toy or gizmo every now and then, but there has not been extensive change in terms of managing a difficult airway.
- Pediatrics: The main things examiners are looking for on the boards have not changed much. Physiologic and anatomic differences between kids and adults are the same as they ever were.
- Thoracic anesthesia: Isolating a lung means a blocker or double-lumen tube. There have been no big changes in thinking in this area.
- Fluids: Colloid versus crystalloid remains the issue, and although no substantial differences have been shown, the debate drags on.

CHANGES ABOUND IN THE CARDIAC REALM!

If there is one area in anesthesia for which recommendations change all the time, it is cardiac procedures. Whatever I write in this chapter may be turned upside down by the next set of recommendations by the American College of Cardiology (ACC) or the next β-blocker review. You owe it to yourself to go to the latest American Society of Anesthesiologists (ASA) refresher course or to read the latest ACC guidelines (last updated in 2006) to make sure you are up to speed on current practices.

For the "hot button" topics addressed in this chapter, I describe the state of the art as I see it and then give my recommendation about what to say to the examiners. However, you should also look up these issues, wrestle with them, and come up with your own answers, which may be better than mine. Perhaps the best thing you will gain from this chapter is *seeing the problem points*. Make sure you think them through and have something to say about them on the big day.

Sure enough, this very thing happened! Between the time Elsevier got this manuscript and publication, everything has changed. Go to *Anesthesia and Analgesia*, Vol. 106, No. 3, March 2008. Plow through the ACC/AHA 2007 Guidelines on Perioperative Cardiovascular Evaluation and Care for Noncardiac Surgery: Executive Summary.

The recommendations are getting MORE vague as time goes on because no one can prove that finding and fixing a coronary blockage even makes a difference. So hell, you can read this chapter if you want, but you would be better off just grinding through that article.

The gist of the article, by the by, is this: unless you have the kind of thing that would grab your attention enough to merit an ER visit (MI happening, valvular disease making you decompensated), no one knows whether the whole pre-op workup (stress test, cath) does any good.

PREOPERATIVE CONSIDERATIONS

In Miami, one of my colleagues suggested we put a red phone on our desk to handle questions from the preoperative clinic. In the early days, we had an automatic recording that said, "Yes, go ahead and get the stress test, and give them a β-blocker." As time passed and recommendations changed, we changed the recording to say, "Do not get the stress test, and do not give them a β-blocker." With more time and updated recommendations, the recording said, "Get the stress test only if it is indicated, and give them the β-blocker only if it is indicated." We did not bother saying what those indications were, because we were not sure ourselves.

We should jump right into the sticky wickets likely to appear on the test. All of the controversial issues will reappear in the practice exams later on. I snipped out the clearest explanations from those tests and put them right here.

Blood Pressure: How High is Too High?

The dilemma is that the only study that looked at the upper limit of blood pressure is very old, it looked at only a few patients, and it predated our use of esmolol, labetalol, and other medications. So if you just say, "Cancel and bring him back when his pressure's under control," you are groping in the dark regarding many issues:

- How low does it need to go?
- How long does it need to be under control?

- Are you running the risk of cerebral ischemia because the patient has shifted his cerebral autoregulation curve to the right (we use this "shift to the right" concept all the time, not really knowing how far to the right it goes)?

On the other hand, you have to draw the line *somewhere*. In walks the man with a blood pressure of 220/130 mm Hg for a hernia repair. You would not say, "Oh the hell with it; let's rock!" So, the current best guess on this thorny and recurrent issue is as follows:

- If a patient for an elective procedure has a diastolic pressure greater than 110 mm Hg, she or he is at risk for end-organ damage and should have the procedure rescheduled.
- Blood pressure should be under control for at least 2 weeks before the procedure.

Neither of these recommendations is based on solid evidence. They are merely our current best thinking.

It is worth thinking through whether you "will proceed with the blood pressure XXX" because it is a recurrent question on the boards. You do not have to use *my* answer, but make sure you have *an* answer.

In the stem questions, there is a question about a patient undergoing carotid endarterectomy and how to manage his blood pressure. Here is a sneak peek at the answer to that one:

I would evaluate several different preoperative blood pressures from this patient from both arms to determine his blood pressure range. I would treat this patient's blood pressure only if it were higher than his preoperative normal values. Intraoperative goals are to maintain his blood pressure at the high-normal range of his predetermined preoperative range of blood pressures. In this particular surgery, it is better to maintain a higher rather than lower blood pressure to maintain cerebral perfusion through collateral flow (i.e., circle of Willis and vertebral arteries), during cross-clamping of the carotid artery. The brain's autoregulatory function is likely to be dysfunctional in a patient with sclerotic carotid arteries. The cerebral perfusion pressure will be low because of the stenosis at the level of the carotid arteries, and the cerebral vessels will already be maximally dilated, with no further autoregulatory ability. The perfusion of the brain will therefore be pressure dependent and not able to tolerate drops in systemic blood pressure.

You cannot beat that for an answer!

Who Needs the Big Preoperative Cardiac Workup?

In days of yore, we were the "ischemia bloodhounds," looking for anything that could in any way be ischemia and making sure everything possible was done to diagnose and treat that ischemia before anyone laid a finger on the patient. If the patient was seeking treatment for a hernia, and we thought there might be "something there," off he went for a stress test, catheterization, angioplasty, and coronary artery bypass grafting (CABG). After we "zapped the ischemia," we could safely do his hernia operation.

Time for a reality check. That zillion-dollar workup has its own set of problems: delay, money, complications during catheterization (e.g., vessel damage, dye hit to the kidneys, mortality rate), and complications during CABG (e.g., cerebral and cardiac adverse effects, hospitalization time, mortality rate).

Consider this not-too-far-fetched scenario. If we had just done the hernia, he would have done fine. Instead, we went ape doing the cardiac thing, and now he has had a stroke or even died!

What should we do instead of being zealous ischemia hunters? Enter the American College of Cardiology/American Heart Association (ACC/AHA) Task Force's guidelines (available on the Internet), which give us a logical, stepwise algorithm for applying common sense to this difficult issue. In the vast labyrinth of explanations are some common sense ideas:

- For a small procedure with little physiologic trespass, you do not need to do the big workup.
- For the big procedure in a patient for whom ischemia is a real threat, you do need to do the workup.

Let's jump ahead to an explanation given in one of the stem question answers. This is a case of a parturient with an ejection fraction (EF) of 30%, and the question is whether she should have the big workup. Because the recommendations draw on the 2002 ACC/AHA guidelines, review of the 2006 guidelines and see if there are any changes. You need to work when you read *Board Stiff Three*! Do not just sit back and take our word for it.

What are the ACC/AHA recommendations regarding preoperative cardiac evaluation in this patient?

At the time of the perioperative cardiac evaluation, according to the 2002 ACC/AHA guidelines, the patient is at intermediate cardiovascular risk when going for an intermediate-risk procedure.

Intermediate cardiovascular risk list (plucked straight from the guidelines) is determined by the following factors:

1. Mild angina pectoris
2. Prior myocardial infarction (MI) according to the history or Q-wave pattern
3. Heart failure (compensated or prior)
4. Diabetes mellitus (insulin-dependent form is more serious)
5. Renal insufficiency

Intermediate procedural risk is determined by the following factors:

1. Intraperitoneal or intrathoracic operation
2. Carotid endarterectomy
3. Head and neck surgery (what, the carotid is not in the neck?)
4. Orthopedic surgery
5. Prostate surgery

Now, reality check. The 2007 guidelines are considerably less specific.

During the test, it may be damned hard to dredge up these complete lists. In my humble opinion (and I don't have a humble opinion), you can say, "I would refer to the ACC/AHA guidelines to determine the level of risk to the patient" (available online or in your hand-held computer gizmo). You do not have to be an encyclopedia for the oral boards; you have to know how to make decisions, and looking up stuff is one of those decisions.

What about a patient undergoing an elective, noncardiac operation? It is unknown whether she has had coronary revascularization in past 5 years.

In this case, I would follow the algorithm, which involves asking whether there has been coronary vascularization in the past 5 years, whether symptoms have returned, and whether the coronaries have had "another look" to make sure the grafts are still patent. The point of these questions is to determine whether the patient is in optimal condition for the procedure.

The history continues, focusing on how much can the patient do. This is a toughie, because the patient has residual lower extremity weakness. If she reports moderate or excellent functional capacity (>4 metabolic equivalents of the task [METs]), she may proceed to the operating room given the intermediate risk of surgery.

If her functional capacity is poor or unknown, further noninvasive testing may be reasonable. Given the additional cardiac demands of pregnancy, an updated echocardiogram would be useful to assess cardiac function, especially with a pre-pregnant EF of only 30%. If the patient has not had a recent stress test (<2 years), a pharmacologic stress test (e.g., myocardial perfusion single-photon emission computed tomography [SPECT]) may be appropriate (2003 ACC/AHA Guidelines for the Use of Cardiac Radionuclide Imaging, pp. 1410-1411). It is unknown whether radionuclide testing is contraindicated in term pregnancy, but the contraindication is probably not absolute.

Something tells me that if you know this much, you will crush this question.

β-Blockade: Who Gets It, and Who Should Not Get It?

Deciding who gets β-blockade is another issue that has done triple backflips over the years. For a while, it seemed as if we should have crop dusters flying over our preoperative clinics and spraying metoprolol over everyone in the parking lot, just in case they were ever to going to get an operation ever in their lives. One whiff of a β-blocker would ensure they would live forever, or so it seemed.

A closer peek at the data revealed that β-blockade might not be the fountain of youth we thought it was, and the later recommendations are a little more snug. What the heck—let's go back to that stem question about the parturient with the poor EF and consider the β-blockade issue:

> Should β-blockade be instituted in the preoperative period? If so, how far in advance of surgery?

According to the 2006 ACC/AHA perioperative guideline on β-blocker therapy, the patient's status may be considered New York Heart Association (NYHA) class IIb (benefit = risk). The patient also should be counseled that although β-blockers have been safely used in pregnancy, fetal side effects could include bradycardia, hypoglycemia, respiratory depression, and intrauterine growth retardation. Infants whose mothers have been receiving β-blockade should be adequately monitored, and the risks and benefits of β-blockade in such patients must be carefully weighed.

You may not remember an entire citation during the exam, but it is worth keeping in your hip pocket, because it is the latest and greatest on β-blockade, and you are sure to have a β-blockade question on the test, and lest we forget we are in the business of taking care of patients, you are sure to have a β-blockade question in real life, too![1]

Add up the whole clinical picture, apply it to this patient, and you have a class IIb reason for giving this patient β-blockade. The 2006 ACC/AHA guidelines state, "Beta-blockers may be considered for patients who are undergoing intermediate- or high-risk procedures as defined in these guidelines, including vascular surgery, in whom perioperative assessment identifies cardiac risk as defined by the presence of a single clinical risk factor."

The Metoprolol CR/XL Randomized Intervention Trial in Congestive Heart Failure (MERIT-HF) showed that β-blockers were suitable and that they improved survival of patients with class II to IV heart failure and a left ventricular ejection fraction (LVEF) of 40% or less.

What about the revised Goldman cardiac risk index? Goldman lists six predictors of major cardiac complications:

1. High-risk surgery, such as intraperitoneal, intrathoracic, or suprainguinal vascular procedures
2. History of ischemic heart disease
3. History of heart failure
4. History of cerebrovascular disease
5. Insulin-dependent diabetes mellitus
6. Preoperative creatinine level greater than 2.0 mg/dL

This guy must have been an actuarial for a life insurance company, because he went on to quantify the risk of cardiac death, nonfatal MI, and nonfatal (but alarming) cardiac arrest according to the number of predictors:

- No risk factors: 0.4%
- One risk factor: 1.0%
- Two risk factors: 2.4%
- Three or more risk factors: 5.4%

Yikes! That "nonfatal cardiac arrest" is the one that scares the hell out of me as an anesthesiologist. Make sure the paddles are working, and make sure we paid the electric bill!

This is where Goldman and β-blockade get married, and this is where you really start to consider who should get β-blockade instead of following our earlier idea of putting β-blockers in the air conditioning system and piping it into every room in the hospital, including the cafeteria.

The rates of cardiac death and nonfatal MI, cardiac arrest or ventricular fibrillation, pulmonary edema, and complete heart block can be correlated with the number of predictors and the nonuse or use of β-blockers:

- No risk factors: 0.4% to 1.0% without versus less than 1% with β-blockers
- One or two risk factors: 2.2% to 6.6% without versus 0.8% to 1.6% with β-blockers
- Three or more risk factors: less than 9% without versus more than 3% with β-blockers

Important stuff! Go to the source on this one, and read it yourself.[2]

According to the Goldman cardiac risk index, the patient has three independent predictors of cardiac complications. Institution of β-blockers can reduce the risk for major cardiac complications. If the patient is not already on this medication, a β-blocker should be started up to 30 days before surgery by titrating to a target of 50 to 60 beats/min.

Management of Cardiac Risk for Noncardiac Surgery

The following material comes from stem question 16. It is the crown jewel of the stems, addressing the toughest questions. If you review one question before you take your test, review "sweet 16."

- The 2006 ACC/AHA guideline update on perioperative β-blocker therapy recommended β-blockers in patients already being treated with one of these drugs for some other indication and in patients at high cardiac risk when undergoing vascular surgery. β-Blockers also were considered reasonable in other selected patients at increased risk.
- A 2006 review by Auerbach and Goldman concluded that perioperative β-blocker therapy should be limited to patients at moderate to high risk. Among patients undergoing major noncardiac surgery, β-blockers should be started and titrated to a target heart rate of 60 to 65 beats/min before anesthesia is begun.
- In patients with heart failure not treated with a β-blocker or with preexisting bronchospastic lung disease, the possibility of exacerbating these conditions must be weighed against the potential benefit.
- There are insufficient data to support perioperative β-blocker therapy in patients at low to intermediate risk (e.g., Revised Cardiac Risk Index [RCRI] score of 0 or 1). However, given the risks of sudden cessation of β-blockers, therapy should be continued in such patients who are already taking a β-blocker.
- When a β-blocker is given, perioperative treatment with a β_1-selective agent is recommended. If possible, oral therapy should begin as an outpatient up to 30 days before surgery, titrating to a heart rate between 50 and 60 beats/min. Tight heart rate control may be an important determinant of efficacy.
- Long-acting β-blockers may be more effective than short-acting agents (e.g., atenolol versus metoprolol). Options include atenolol (50 to 100 mg/day orally) and bisoprolol (5 to 10 mg/day orally).
- If time does not permit, atenolol can be given intravenously (10 mg over 15 minutes) before surgery. Atenolol is then given intravenously (5 to 10 mg every 6 to 12 hours) in the immediate postoperative period until oral intake resumes. The previous dose of oral β-blocker should be restarted when the patient is able.
- There are no data about the duration of therapy. We suggest that β-blockers be continued for at least 1 month after surgery; they are usually continued indefinitely because most of these patients have underlying heart disease.

In the cardiac realm, the three biggest and toughest questions you will face are about blood pressure, ischemia "pursuit," and β-blockade. You now should have a good jump on answering these questions.

What do the 2007 guidelines say? On page 701, "Since publication of the ACC/AHA focused update on perioperative beta-blocker therapy, several randomized trials have been published that have not demonstrated the efficacy of these agents." Ay Caramba! What are you supposed to do? Hard to say.

INTRAOPERATIVE CONSIDERATIONS

We now review how to do a cardiac case from very beginning to very end because many people feel weak in the realm of doing a cardiac case. If you just trained and are confident about how to do a cardiac case, you may want to skip this section. If you have not done a heart in 6 years, you may want to go over this one a few times and make sure you have it down. There is some overlap of preoperative and postoperative considerations, but everything is kept together for coherence.

Preoperative Evaluation for Adults

Several things are important in the preoperative evaluation:

- Airway
- Airway
- Airway
- Ejection fraction
- Can we stick the neck (i.e., is there carotid stenosis that may incline us to stick the subclavians)?
- Other stuff

Often forgotten in the preoperative evaluation is a recurrent theme in cardiac anesthesia: *At the heart of a heart case is a regular old case.* Especially in the early part of the case, you can lose yourself in didactic, hemodynamic, echocardiographic, and inotropic reverie. Visions of multiple pumps going wide open and blood pressure backflips dance in your head, and you picture yourself winning the Nobel Prize in cardiac anesthesia. Then, you cannot intubate the patient, and kill him the old fashioned way: lost airway.

Examine the airway with even more meticulousness (meticularity? meticulitudinosity?) than other cases. A lost airway and hypoxemia in the patient with a bad heart disease will quickly get everyone's attention.

Most cardiac patients have an EF listed somewhere in the jumble of their charts. Try to smoke it out. An EF of 55% gives you some latitude in induction. An EF of 10% means you may have to open a bottle of etomidate in the back of the room and wave it around lest you cause a cardiac collapse.

We usually stick the neck for central lines. If the patient suffers from carotid disease, we may opt for a subclavian line. It is *advisable* to know what is going on in those carotids.

Other stuff includes chronic obstructive pulmonary disease (COPD), hypertension, renal failure, diabetes, and allergies. Yes, yes, a thousand times yes, you have to know all this stuff. Is esophageal pathology making TEE probe placement problematic? Is there a family history of malignant hyperthermia? Of course; I insult your intelligence.

If we can get the endotracheal tube in the right place, and if we can get the central lines in, we are at least off to a good start in the heart room. Recite the mantra: *At the heart of a heart case is a regular old case.*

Preoperative Medications and Devices

Make sure the patient gets all the regular medications, and be sure to write prescriptions for them individually:

"Patient to get usual AM meds." NO!
"At 6 AM, have patient take his atenolol, 25 mg PO, with a sip of water." YES!

Do beta blockers help? Very difficult to say.[3] Most of us would continue beta blocker therapy, that's about all you can say.

If a heparin drip is in place, the decision can be a toughie. Do you keep heparin going right up to and into the operation room (then you miss the arterial line or the central line, and you get a bloody mess), or do you turn it off 4 hours ahead of time (then a critical lesion in the left main develops a clot, and the patient codes)?

When you are stuck on the horns of a dilemma, talk with the surgeon. If the patient is truly hanging by a thread ("He has tight lesions all over the place. If two platelets even linger next to each other, this guy's a goner."), I would keep the heparin going. If the patient is not in such dire straits, I would stop the heparin a few hours preoperatively.

What about preoperative sedation? Sure. I would not want to be bright-eyed and bushy-tailed just before my heart operation.

What about a morning admission? It is damned complex to get patients sedated upstairs. You try to call upstairs, but no one is there yet. You beep a resident you think is there, but you get no response. It is aggravating, and you are trying to set up the room and get to grand rounds or Tuesday morning journal club or the Friday lecture. See patients when they come down, and sedate them in the holding area.

What about kids? Check with the individual attendings. Little bitty kiddies with complex problems and immature respiratory center responses require, pardon the pun, kid gloves with sedatives of any kind.

There is a lot to remember to give in a transplantation case. "Uh oh, I forgot to give the Solu-Medrol, I hope they don't notice," just does not fly. The patient will reject the heart, and everyone will notice! I make a list, go over it with the surgeon, cross things off the list as I give them, and double-check with the surgeon as I am giving them. Swallow your independent streak, and work with the surgeon to make sure the patient gets what he or she needs. It is better to appear the fool and get corrected than try to look slick and hurt the patient.

Antibiotics

All patients receive antibiotics for prophylaxis: cefazolin (Ancef), clindamycin, or vancomycin. TEE requires no additional or special antibiotics.

What should you do about a penicillin allergy? Ask the surgeons if they prefer vancomycin (give it slowly to avoid the red man syndrome) or clindamycin.

Give antibiotics before the skin incision.

Antibleeding Stuff

For off-pump cases, you do not need anything. For on-pump CABG cases, ask the surgeon if he or she wants to use Amicar (aminocaproic acid).

There are many different schedules for Amicar. I give 10 g by intravenous push and then run a drip of 1 g/hr.

What if you anticipate trouble? There is a long lag time between ordering yellow stuff (e.g., platelets, fresh-frozen plasma [FFP], cryo-poor plasma) and getting it. Order FFP early if you anticipate an antithrombin III deficiency (e.g., a patient who has been on heparin for a few days in the unit). If you have the FFP handy, you can solve the problem of an activated clotting time (ACT) that will not rise! Give the FFP. The patient now has antithrombin III, the heparin has its cofactor, and the ACT rises, and you can go on bypass.

If, in contrast, you wait, the following occurs. Give heparin. The ACT does not rise. Order FFP. Wait. Wait some more, and by now, the surgeon is screaming bloody murder. The FFP finally arrives, and you can proceed.

NOTE! PEOPLE TELL ME THIS IS A COMMON QUESTION ON THE BOARDS: "YOU GIVE THE HEPARIN BUT THE ACT DOESN'T RISE." MAKE SURE YOU KNOW THIS SEQUENCE!

Zapomatic Material

Make sure there is a defibrillator in the room. If it is a repeat procedure, put the external defibrillator pads on. Scarring is likely in a repeat procedure, making it hard to get into the chest in a hurry, and the external defibrillator pads allow you to defibrillate or pace.

Make sure that you have a pacemaker box in your grubby little mitts and that the stupid thing works. Have it by you at the beginning of the case. You may suddenly need it in the early part of the operation, and you will certainly want it when you are ready to come off bypass. Make it a habit to have that pacer at the head of the bed early.

Routine Case Sequence

For those who have not done a heart case in a long time, this may be the most useful section of this review because it refreshes you about what happens first, second, and third in a heart case.

CAVEAT!

Routine is a good and necessary thing, but you must keep in mind one important thing in cardiac cases: If a patient starts to crash, move! Consider the airway, breathing, and circulation (ABCs), but do not dawdle until things are "pretty and perfect." Get that patient in the room, secure the airway, get heparin in her, and crash on bypass. No time to waste! An emergency, by definition, is *not* routine.

- Check patient's name and number on the ID bracelet.
- Check that the consent form has been signed.
- Review laboratory results.
- Check blood availability (for a repeat procedure, have blood in the room and check it—the sternal saw can and has entered the heart).
- Make sure a perfusionist is near, ready, and coherent.
- Make sure there is a bed in the intensive care unit (ICU), which is always an issue.
- Check the catheter or echocardiographic results, and double-check the planned operation with the surgeons.
- Compare the recent electrocardiogram (ECG) to old ECGs.
- Make sure the room is ready.

Let the operating room nurse go through the nursing checklist. Rushing the nursing staff or blowing off their concerns is bad for the patient and bad for the work environment. We all work together. This is not some fluffy, New Age cliché. This is the truth, the whole truth, and nothing but the truth.

Do not be blind to things that can throw off the routine, such as the patient saying, "Doc, my chest hurts!" You must always be ready to leap into accelerated mode if something goes wrong.

Hi ho, hi ho, it's into the operating room you go. Once there, focus on the patient. This is no time to be setting up.

- Put the usual monitors on the patient.
- The pulse oximeter gives you the most information (saturation, rhythm, a sort of perfusion rate) in the least time, so put that on first.
- Make sure the intravenous line you have is good enough to get you through induction. If not, place the central line before induction.
- Make sure the computer is picking up the vital signs.
- Place the arterial line. You need beat-to-beat blood pressure monitoring during induction.

Induction

Every induction known to man has appeared in the heart room, from awake intubation to failed intubation with an immediate tracheostomy (stat trach—try to limit these) to rapid sequence to inhalation to intravenous induction with fentanyl or etomidate or pentathol or propofol—you name it!

It is not what you use; it is how you use it. Keep in mind the following principles:

1. Securing the airway takes precedence over everything else. Hypoxemia, hypercarbia, and their accompanying sympathetic thunderbolts are not good for anyone, especially at-risk patients.
2. In general, slow but sure wins the race. No matter what you use, watch the hemodynamics. You want to induce the patient but do not want the pressure too low (i.e., bad for perfusion across already stenosed coronaries) or too high (i.e., excessive stress on an already stressed heart).
3. If one rhythm is bad, bad, bad, it is a fast rhythm. Fast heart rates shorten diastole, when the heart is perfused, and make oxygen demands that a heart may not tolerate. During induction, mind the heart rate, and do not be shy with β-blockers. This approach is modified in the setting of a regurgitant valvular lesion, in which case you do not want a very slow rate, because it prolongs the time of regurgitation.

Maintenance

The days of mega-narcotics are gone. Use narcotics and relaxants judiciously, with the aim of an extubation in the operating room or in the ICU in a reasonable time frame (e.g., within 2 hours of arrival).

Through the Looking Glass

The following are considerations at each point along the way for a typical case after you have induced:
1. Thank the Lord that somehow the patient survived your induction.
2. If you hypercranked the head to achieve intubation, return the neck to a neutral position. Vertebral artery occlusion can occur in the hyperextended neck.
3. Do not turn the head hard left or hard right. Contralateral brachial plexus stretchosis can occur.
4. Place a nasal temperature probe.
5. Suck out the stomach.
6. Place the central line if you have not already done so.
   a. One way to prevent hitting "big red" is to draw an arterial sample from the arterial line for color comparison.
   b. After you have the wire in, slip the 18-gauge, blue-hubbed catheter down the wire, withdraw the wire, and look again for squirting. Hook up intravenous tubing to it, and do a poor man's central venous pressure (CVP) measurement to make sure you are in the right place. You can even go all the way and transduce or draw a blood sample and make blood gas measurements.
   c. Whatever you do to prevent placing a 9-French tube in the carotid is time well spent!
   d. If you do put the monster in the carotid, do not panic. Leave it in, and tell the surgeons. They may have to do an open repair.
7. Place the TEE equipment.
   a. Make sure it is unlocked.
   b. Give the probe a little anteflexion.

c. Grease it up good.

d. Place a bite block if the patient has teeth.

e. Do not force it; use the laryngoscope if you have any trouble.

f. TEE is most stimulating! Turn up the vapors or give some narcotics before you ram that puppy home.

8. Watch the intravenous volume.

a. For an on-pump case, run the patient as "dry" as is safe. The patient gets a ton of fluids from the pump prime.

b. For an off-pump case, be more generous with fluids; 1.5 to 2 liters is not uncommon. When the surgeons hike the heart up and the pressure drops, it is most often fluid related, so load the patient early.

c. Keep an eye on the CVP, TEE, and the heart itself to help guide the fluids. The fellow with an EF of 15% is not going to tolerate fluids as well as the patient with an EF of 55%.

9. Let down the lungs when the surgeon saws through the sternum. Remember to inflate the lungs afterward, because most patients are not facultative anaerobes.

10. Watch the blood pressure.

a. For on-pump cases, work the systolic blood pressure down to about 90 mm Hg for aortic cannulation. The cannulation site is just the thing to start an aortic dissection, so after the cannula is in, do not let the pressure leap up.

b. For off-pump cases, keep the systolic pressure at about 130 mm Hg. When the surgeon hikes the heart and you lose about 30 mm Hg, the systolic pressure will be at about 100 mm Hg. Do the math. If you *start* at 90 mm Hg, the pressure will be 60 mm Hg after the surgeon hikes the heart. Yikes!

11. Watch the ECG (I feel like a cardiologist!). While we are at it, avoid hypoxia and hypotension. We watch so many things that it is easy to forget the good old ECG. It is a sinking feeling when the surgeon looks up and asks, "How long have those ST segments been up?" You say, "Uhhhhhhhhhhhhhhh."

12. Get a baseline blood gas determination and ACT after the sternotomy. If something merits investigation, get a blood gas determination earlier. For example, an emergency patient who zoomed into the room needs a blood gas determination right away.

13. Give the heparin through a central line, and aspirate first to make sure that stuff gets in there. The perfusionist will tell you the dose.

14. Get an ACT 3 minutes after heparin administration.

15. During an off-pump case, you will work like a dog and sweat bullets.

a. There is no magical way to do these cases.

b. Keep glued to the vitals. Use fluid to keep the blood pressure up, and neo-synephrine if you must. It is a question of paying attention and reacting. Let the record go if you have to; you can always complete it later. Off-pump procedures are real nail-biters until the surgeon finally drops the heart the last time, and you can breathe a little easier.

c. You have to go on the pump if the patient cannot tolerate the hike in the heart rate, as shown by refractory hypotension, big wall motion abnormalities, rising pulmonary artery (PA) pressure (or, most often in our cases, CVP), and bad news rhythm trouble. Usually, it is obvious to all concerned that "this baby ain't flyin'."

d. The art is in discernment. Who is so bad that we need to go on pump, and who can limp along? In time, you will develop a sense about this, grasshopper.

16. If you do an on-pump case, follow several guidelines.
    a. If you have a PA catheter, pull it back 2 to 3 cm with the onset of cardiopulmonary bypass (CPB).
    b. When you go on pump, do not be in such a blazing hurry to turn off the ventilator. Wait until the perfusionist says, "Full flow," and everything is groovy.
    c. Turn off and disconnect the ventilator. If you keep it attached, you could set up a suction in the lungs, leading to negative-pressure pulmonary edema.
    d. Turn off your vapors.
    e. Make sure the perfusionist and surgeon are happy. Dark blood should be draining out, bright blood should be pumping in, and the heart should not be swelling up. Bizarre stuff can throw a wrench in the works— aortic dissection, hemodilution causing a big blood pressure drop, cannula reversal, arterial-pulmonary shunt, demonic possession, or an alien tractor beam.
    f. Make sure a good arrest occurs (unless you are doing a beating heart case). If the surgical team is attempting to arrest the heart and cannot, the heart is not getting good protection. Everyone will suffer later when you try to come off pump and the patient's heart just sits there.
17. Do some things while the pump is running.
    a. Monitor blood gases to keep track of everything.
    b. Keep the ACT above 400, lest the blood clot on the pump, and "Tha-bada-tha-thaaaaaaaaaaaaaaaaaaat's all folks!"
    c. Keep an eye on the CVP. If the cannulas are misplaced and the superior vena cava becomes obstructed, the CVP will rise, and the patient's head will get all swoll up.
    d. If you have a PA catheter, watch the pressure. If it rises, there may be inadequate left ventricular venting, and the heart may get all distended.
    e. Monitor mean arterial pressure. Volumes are written about what is correct, which proves no one really knows. Check with your attending to determine what is considered correct for the case.
    f. Follow urine output. If the flow creeps down, do not panic and douse the patient with tons of Lasix. Often, the kidneys do not get rolling again until you reestablish pulsatile flow. Just how long you should wait and how much you should pray that pulsatile flow gets things going again is a matter of debate (most of the stuff in the cardiac room is based on rumor, hearsay, voodoo, and institutional cerebral arthritis).
    g. There is a lot of down time on bypass. If you think the patient will need inotropes to leap off bypass, mix them now. My preference is to mix what I think is needed, run it through the pumps, hook it up to the patient, and run it at 1 mL/hr. With this approach, you can determine while the patient is on pump whether the infusion pump works or whether it has upstream occlusion, downstream occlusion, air, malfunction, an evil genie, malice aforethought, or a balky personality. If you fix the pump so everything is totally hunky dory, you will be pressing buttons when the patient comes off pump, rather than dealing with the stupid pump.
    h. If you do decide to mix up protamine while on pump, do it in a sealed compartment 10 miles from the hospital with an armed escort who will shoot you dead if you bring the protamine anywhere near the patient. I wait until the surgeon asks for it.

18. You can do several things while the patient is warming.
    a. Make sure the patient gets good and toasty, at least 36°C.
    b. Make sure all the metabolic bureaucracy pertaining to the patient is okay, including pH and potassium, magnesium, and hematocrit levels. Make sure the soup the heart is sitting in is *good* soup. If you are a metabolic mess, all the king's horses and all the king's inotropes will never get Humpty Dumpty off bypass again.
    c. Begin ventilation when the surgeon says it is okay. Do ask. There is no penalty for saying, "Okay if I ventilate now?"
    d. Watch carefully during the first puff, and make sure you do not rip the left internal mammary artery off when the lung reinflates. Make sure both lungs come up (you may discover a right mainstem at this time), and get all the atelectasis out of the way. If the lungs are stiff, fix it with appropriate position, suction, a bronchodilator, or fiberoptic scope (so you can clean out the lungs). If the lungs do not work, the heart will not work.
    e. If you have a Swan-Ganz catheter, do not go wedge hunting! If you inflate the balloon, you may cause a PA rupture, which is not a good thing. Live with the PA trace; it can give you all the information you need.
    f. When the cross-clamp comes off, the heart does not beat, and the surgeon throws you a pacing wire, it is not the time to say, "Hey, I need a pacemaker box." Remember the room setup? Have a pacing box from the start.
19. Leap off bypass by attending to the airway, metabolic bureaucracy, and circulation.
    a. Check the airway, and make sure the lungs go up and down.
    b. Make sure the patient is metabolically in tip-top shape—warmed and with good potassium, hematocrit, and pH levels.
    c. Circulation can be broken down into another threesome.
        i. Rhythm is important. Asystole and ventricular fibrillation are not helpful rhythms. Sinus is the best, followed by atrial pacing, atrioventricular pacing, and ventricular pacing. You want the rhythm to give you the most you can get, and the atrial kick is especially nice.
        ii. Heart rate is important. After revascularization, you can tolerate a little more tachycardia, although let's be reasonable.
        iii. Contractility is where the inotropes come into play.
            (1) Epinephrine makes blood pressure go up and cardiac output go up. It is good stuff.
            (2) Dobutamine makes blood pressure go down and cardiac output go up. It is good for the patient with pulmonary hypertension.
            (3) Milrinone makes blood pressure go down (have levosimendan ready to go) and cardiac output up. You can give a bolus and then chill with some levosimendan to pick the blood pressure off the floor. If ever a drug bailed my sorry butt out of some hemodynamic jams, it was milrinone.
20. Several tasks must be done after bypass. (Textbooks devote monster chapters to the great "separation from bypass" agony, and this summary only scratches the surface. It requires finesse and some science. When I am in trouble, I give everything wide open and pray.)
    a. Give the protamine slowly. Purists say to give it through a peripheral intravenous line. I always figure that the arms are tucked and all my peripheral intravenous lines are infiltrated, so I give it centrally. Mix a little calcium in with it—a little upper to counteract the downer.

    b. Recheck the ACT after the protamine is given. Obtain gas determinations, and make sure nothing is rotten in the state of Denmark (e.g., low hematocrit, low potassium level, acidosis). The pump introduces a lot of mannitol to the patient, so you can lose a lot of volume and potassium through the urine. Do not let the potassium level drop so low that you start getting ectopy. A little dysrhythmia can turn into a heap of trouble and undo the whole procedure.

21. Transport
    a. Transport is a spooky time. For the entire case, you have been glued to the patient's every hemodynamic nuance. Now, you are wrestling with lines, lugging pumps, and paying attention to everything but the patient. Be extra careful.
    b. Monitor blood pressure, ECG, and SaO_2 on all patients during transport.
    c. Make sure the oxygen cylinder is on, and make sure it has some O_2 in it!
    d. The Spirit of Hypovolemia Present will visit you during transport. During the case, you keep fluids going at a well-monitored but usually brisk clip. Then you mess with getting ready for transport for 20 minutes, and guess what, you are behind on volume. Keep a big intravenous line ready to go for transport. Trust me, boys and girls, you will get behind on volume during transport.
    e. If you have a lot of pumps, bring the whole intravenous line pole. It is easier than hooking them up individually on the ICU bed pole, and you will not throw out your back.
    f. Remove needles, switchblades, cat o' nine tails, and any other sharp instruments.
    g. Bring emergency drugs along. You will be amazed by what happens in the hallway.
    h. Bring along the mask. Heaven help you if the patient gets extubated in the hallway; you can at least mask ventilate until you get to the unit.
    i. Squeeze the bag while transporting. People can become overwhelmed by the whole drama and forget the basics, such as breathing.

22. In the ICU
    a. Give a snap doodle report to the staff.
    b. Make sure that the ventilator works and that the patient's chest goes up and down. Ventilators can and do fail. Go back to hand ventilation if anything appears screwy.
    c. Chill and decompress. Get your paperwork in order.
    d. After a while, come back, and double-check everything. You win a lot of points and are a good doctor if you hang around a little. Do not be in a big rush: "Here's the patient. Ciao! I'm off to Disneyland!"

23. Do I extubate in the room?
    a. Hospitals are fast-tracking people more today.
    b. If everything is okay, and especially if you did an off-pump case, you can make an argument for extubating right in the operating room, just like a noncardiac case.
    c. A conservative approach says there is nothing wrong with an hour or so on a ventilator. If nothing else, keeping the tube in for transport ensures the airway is secured during the delicate time of transport.
    d. You will see both methods and ways of thinking during your rotation.

Two Controversies

I address two controversial issues in this section: Swan-Ganz catheter versus CVP and the use of TEE.

Monitoring with Swan-Ganz Catheter or Central Venous Pressure Measurements

This topic has bounced around almost as long as the crystalloid versus colloid issue. In a heart case or any other case, this question can come up: Is it better to monitor the volume status of this patient with a PA catheter or a CVP measurement? The traditional thinking was echoed in earlier versions of this book. Read it (*Board Stiff*, p. 76) aloud, and notice how confident we were about our answer!

With an MI so recent and all the potential fluid absorption from a TURP, a Swan is mandatory to guide fluid management.

Mandatory! In *Board Stiff Too* (p. 75), we reconsidered our position:

Traditional wisdom says you need a Swan when right-sided pressures do not reflect left-sided function. So, if the patient has bad lungs and/or a bad LV, then you need a Swan. The advent and more common use of TEE may be causing some rethinking.

We continue to rethink. The world is now interested in outcomes, and outcome studies with Swan-Ganz catheters have shown us some interesting twists.

- Proven outcome benefits of the almighty Swan-Ganz catheter are just plain not there.
- People may be harmed by Swan-Ganz catheters? People seem to do worse with it!
- Different populations have different outcomes. Responses are all over the place!

What do you say when the question arises: Do you use a Swan-Ganz or a CVP measurement in this heart case (or any case that comes up on the boards)? You can give any answer you want, as long as you can defend it.

Here is my answer, which does not have to be your answer. To my way of thinking, the Swan-Ganz catheter is an unproven, expensive, distracting nuisance, which gives me little to no useful information, delays my care, and runs the risk of rhythm disturbances, PA rupture, and clutter. For central access, I put in a Cordis catheter to provide big access. If the ICU staff members feel they need the Swan-Ganz catheter, they can float it. To monitor intraoperatively, I use the CVP, respiratory variation on the arterial line, blood gas measurements, monitoring of fluid balance, common sense, being "tuned in" to what is happening in the field, and the TEE.

Transesophageal Echocardiography

The use of TEE is controversial in heart cases, but here is my take on how much you need to know.

I used to say, "I wouldn't use TEE because I do not know how to use it." Later, I said, "I would call in a colleague who knows about TEE to help me." Neither approach is acceptable in this day and age. We should all know the rudiments of TEE well enough to make the following calls:

1. Is the heart empty or full?
2. Is the heart working well or poorly?
3. Is there an effusion and therefore the possibility of tamponade?

I would argue that with TEE and a blood gas determination (TEE cannot tell you the PaO_2 is 40 or the hematocrit is 14), you should be able to figure out hemodynamic instability in anyone. TEE is so good at telling you in a few seconds what is really going on that we just plain need this technology.

I can imagine some plaintiff's attorney asking, "The patient was unstable, doctor, why didn't you put in a TEE probe?" When you reply, "I don't know anything about TEE," the attorney will say, "So the patient died because you never bothered to learn about TEE?" Then, what can you say? This scenario is scary and not too farfetched.

What should you know about TEE, and how do you become informed? There are tutorials available free on the Internet (just Google around a little). The tutorials are not hard. Medical students with no knowledge of TEE can see the images, and within a few minutes, they can recognize several conditions:

- Poor ventricular function (the walls do not move much)
- Empty ventricle (the walls "kiss")
- Tamponade (effusion around the heart; technically, tamponade is a clinical diagnosis supported by findings of effusion plus the requisite hemodynamics)

On the boards, you should be able to describe these conditions. Here is an amateur TEE-ologist's list of things you should know:

1. Indications: Evaluation of hemodynamic instability
2. Contraindications: Esophageal surgery, pouch, or any pathology in the way of placing the probe
3. Views: The four-chamber view gives you the best first look; the transgastric short-axis view gives you a good volume assessment view and shows you walls fed by all three of the coronary vessels.
4. Hypovolemia: The chamber gets small (i.e., kissing ventricle).
5. Poor ventricular function: It is like pornography—you know it when you see it.
6. Effusion or tamponade: A dark "ribbon" around the heart is the effusion fluid, which compresses the heart, impairs filling, and produces the whole tamponade scene.
7. Regional wall motion abnormality: If a wall's blood supply is interrupted, the wall does not move anymore. A clotted graft shows a new regional wall motion abnormality in the area fed by the graft.
8. Mitral valve and aortic valve: These valves are most often involved in cardiac pathology, and they are easier to see than the pulmonic and tricuspid valves, so you should be able to peg obvious stenosis or regurgitation with these. A few minutes of an online tutorial will allow you to see the obvious stuff.

Let me put in a plug for my own book, *Board Stiff TEE*. It is not as complete as most TEE textbooks, but it takes you from knowing nothing whatsoever to at least knowing the rudiments of TEE. At 185 pages, you can get through it at poolside with a margarita in hand during one afternoon. It provides that little dusting of TEE knowledge that may pay off at board time.

That is just about everything you ever wanted to know about cardiac cases and maybe even a little more than you needed. The next chapter looks at lung cases.

References

1. Fleisher L.A, Beckman JA, Brown KA, et al: ACC/AHA 2007 Guidelines on Perioperative Cardiovascular Evaluation and Care for Noncardiac Surgery: Executive Summary. Anesth Anal 2008; 106:685-712.
2. Auerbach A, Goldman L: Assessing and reducing the cardiac risk of noncardiac surgery. Circulation 2006;113:1361-1376.
3. Bangalore S Messerli FH, Kostis JB, Pepine CJ: Cardiovascular protection using beta-blockers: a critical review of the evidence. J Am Coll Cardiol 2007; 50:563-572.

7

Lung City

Open your mouth; your life depends on it.

CHRISTOPHER GALLAGHER

I said that just before I awakened and intubated a dying patient with Goodpasture's syndrome who was exsanguinating from his trachea. Lung cases are arguably the biggest stressor for us. There is something about facing bright red blood pouring from the thing that is supposed to be providing oxygenation. It is very unsettling.

I am happy to report that the Goodpasture guy made it. What follows is a preoperative, intraoperative, postoperative look at the most important issues in lung cases.

PREOPERATIVE CONSIDERATIONS

All the routine preoperative concerns occur in lung cases because the patients often have concomitant cardiovascular disease. The main question about lungs on the oral boards concerns pulmonary function tests (PFTs). Who needs them? Who does not?

For any lung resection, PFTs are needed to know how much will be left after the procedure. The surgeon may say it is only going to be a wedge or a lobe resection, but patients do not always read the book! Tumor extension, surgical misfortune, and unanticipated bleeding can turn a lung case into the nightmare of a pneumonectomy. You have not lived until you hear the surgeon say, "Damn! I just cut the pulmonary artery."

You want to know how much tissue and function will be left, because you want to be sure the patient can survive without ventilator dependence. If the PFT results are close to 50% of predicted values, the patient may not have enough lung tissue left after resection to survive with a ventilator.

Other than the PFTs, the rest of the preoperative focus is clinical, and the big question is whether the patient is about as good as he or she can be. The patient with chronic obstructive pulmonary disease (COPD) is never going to be great. Those days are just plain gone, and the history and physical examination should center on anything new or problematic that would make you "wait until this guy is really ready" for an elective procedure. Look for the kinds of things that need "tuning up" preoperatively:

- Fever
- Change in sputum production
- Worse symptoms than usual

Because these patients often have cardiac disease, you need to address all the issues in Chapter 6:

- How is the patient's blood pressure control?
- Does he need the million dollar cardiac workup?
- Are β-blockers a good idea?

The last one can be a toughie, because you have a desire for β-blockade for cardiac benefit but a desire for a β-adrenergic agent for pulmonary benefit. Opinion seems to favor using a β-blocker, even in COPD patients, as long as it does not trigger bronchospasm, but even that is controversial.

INTRAOPERATIVE CONSIDERATIONS

To epiduralize or not to epiduralize—that is the question. For an open thoracotomy, place a thoracic epidural. Check the coagulation parameters before you stick the patient's back! When you run a case with a local anesthetic, keep in mind that sympathectomy can drop the pressure. During a lung case, the surgeon is grabbing, twisting, and cutting off venous return, tickling the heart and producing all kinds of problems. The sympathectomy from the epidural can cloud the reason for low blood pressure. I administer the epidural only when the surgeon is starting to close to keep the blood pressure picture a little cleaner.

Should you use a double-lumen endotracheal tube or Univent (bronchial blocker) tube? This is a topic of active debate. A double-lumen tube is big and clunky and less likely to go in easily if there is a difficult airway. However, after a double-lumen tube is in place, it tends to stay put and behave. A Univent tube is better for the difficult intubation situation. You can place the Univent tube with the patient awake, or you can place a regular tube with the patient awake, put down a tube changer, and get a Univent tube in over the changer. However, because Univent tubes tend to pop out of place more with surgical manipulation, you will be dealing with them more in the middle of the case.

What if the damned lung will not go down? Think through the lung deflation sequence ahead of time. Are you too high, and air is sneaking across? The key in positioning is always this: *You must get a nice view of the carina!* Without that, you will never figure it out. The trachea has regular rings and a linear muscular band posteriorly. If you are "one branch too deep," you will be looking at a fake carina. You will not see the regular rings of the trachea and the muscular band posteriorly. If in doubt, pull back until you see the trachea clearly.

Does oxygen desaturation occur when the lung is deflated? Never kill the patient to prove you can get a lung down. If the saturation level plummets, go to 100% oxygen (duh!), and inflate both lungs. It is better to delay surgery while you figure things out than to let the saturation level go to hell in a hand-basket. After you have gotten the patient out of the death zone and have time to think, use this approach to the "one lung and we cannot keep the saturation up" problem:

- Make sure you are in the right place. Confirm with the fiberoptic scope.
- The best first approach is to give continuous positive airway pressure (CPAP). You do not need to say, "CPAP to the nonventilating lung," because CPAP implies you are not doing positive-pressure ventilation. The idea is that the nonventilated lung is a poor shunt. Blood is going through, but no oxygen is there for the blood to pick up. Providing a little CPAP (not so much that the lungs blow up in the surgeon's face) changes that shunt to not-a-shunt and should improve oxygenation.
- You can give positive end-expiratory pressure (PEEP). You do not have to say, "PEEP to the ventilated lung," because PEEP implies you are ventilating that lung. However, this is better as a second maneuver than as a first, because you can push some blood to the other side (i.e., non-ventilated lung) with PEEP and worsen the shunt.

- Tilt the patient's head up. Just as in the awake patient, this takes a little weight off the diaphragm, improves the functional residual capacity (FRC), and may help the saturation level a little.
- Switch to total intravenous anesthesia (TIVA). Because potent inhaled anesthetics impair hypoxic pulmonary vasoconstriction, TIVA instead of using a vapor-based anesthetic may do the trick.

POSTOPERATIVE CONSIDERATIONS

Do you extubate or keep the specialized (double-lumen or Univent) tube in? This is the most important question you will face at the end of a lung case.

If blood loss has been extensive or fluids were given generously (e.g., during an esophagectomy), the head and airway may be alarmingly swollen. If in doubt, keep the patient intubated, and do not even change the tube! Respiratory technicians and nurses may freak a little when they see the double-lumen tube, but you can always give them a little in-service and explain to them how to ventilate through a Univent or double-lumen tube.

This situation is manageable. Trust me. I have done it a hundred times. Sit the patient up, let the swelling go down, and later, when the airway is less perilous, you can change to another tube, or better yet, you can extubate if the patient is ready.

There are several thrillers in the stem questions regarding thoracic cases. You will thank your lucky stars you were not in the room when they happened!

8

Obstetrics Means Preeclampsia

You're pregnant! How did that happen?

A COMMON EXPRESSION

When preparing for your oral board exam, you should go directly to the topic of preeclampsia when studying for the obstetrics question. Someone who took the past week's exam told me his second stem question was (what else?) preeclampsia.

This is good news for you. The examiners almost always ask about preeclampsia, and if you know it cold, you are sure to nail this part of the test. You know this challenge is coming, so it is time to prepare!

PREECLAMPSIA CONSIDERATIONS

Physiologic Changes of Pregnancy

Cardiac Changes

- Increased intravascular volume
- Increased cardiac output
- Dilutional anemia (i.e., more volume than red cell mass)
- Supine hypotension (remember left uterine displacement!)

Pulmonary Changes

- Increased minute ventilation and oxygen consumption
- Decreased functional residual capacity and residual volume
- The first two account for quicker desaturation in the parturient
- Swollen upper airway and friable mucosa

Airway Changes

- Lung and airway changes constitute the number one concern in obstetrics: losing the airway and death.
- Cesarean sections under general anesthesia are 16 times more likely to be deadly than under regional anesthesia.

Gastrointestinal Changes

- Decreased gastric emptying
- Increased gastric volume and pressure (even if receiving no oral intake, patients are considered to have full stomachs)
- Progesterone relaxes the gastroesophageal junction.
- After the first trimester, patients are considered to have full stomachs.

Neurologic Changes

- Engorged epidural vessels
- Decreased local anesthetic needed for spinal and epidural compared with nonpregnant patients

Preeclamptic Complications of Pregnancy

Cardiac Changes

- Volume management is problematic because patients are volume depleted but can have left ventricular dysfunction, making it easy to overload them.
- Preeclampsia should be considered a panvasculopathy, because it affects all vascular beds.

Pulmonary Changes

- Patients can have leaky capillaries, leading to pulmonary edema.
- Coupled with cardiac and renal problems, pulmonary problems can paint you into a corner.

Cerebral Changes

- Visual disturbances, headache, seizures (i.e., eclampsia), and intracranial bleeding may occur.
- If you use a general anesthetic and do not control the response to intubation, the patient may have very high blood pressure, leading to an intracranial bleed.

Airway Changes

- Even more edema compared with a normal pregnancy
- Trouble intubating compared with the healthy parturient

Hepatic Changes

- Rupture of Glisson's capsule
- A tsunami of blood loss

Renal Changes

- Oliguria and proteinuria (one criterion for preeclampsia)
- Can progress to renal failure

If the patient has lost much protein, and her kidneys are not working well, the addition of poor left ventricular function and leaky capillaries in the lungs can create a real nightmare of fluid management.

Uteroplacental Insufficiency

- Vasculopathy in the mother is a panvasculopathy, which also affects the uteroplacental unit.
- Dropping the blood pressure in this "diseased" organ can lead to insufficient flow.

Blood Changes

- Coagulopathy, specifically a low platelet count, is the main concern.
- How low do you go before you cannot use a regional anesthetic?

My approach to this sticky question is basically unchanged since written in *Board Stiff Too*. If you take the high and mighty road and say, "No way will I place an epidural if the platelet count drops below 100,000!" (the concern is an epidural hematoma), you are stuck managing some preeclamptic woman's pain with . . . what? Fentanyl? Demerol? Now the pain relief is inadequate, and her pressure goes up further.

Will you use general anesthesia if the procedure becomes a cesarean section? What about that swollen upper airway? Do not forget about the possibility of intracranial bleeding if you get a hyperdynamic response to intubation.

Oh, you lost the airway! Who is going to do the cricotracheotomy—the obstetrician?

Some obstetric anesthesiologists consider an epidural down to 50,000 platelets with close neurologic monitoring. You could also do a spinal. But wait—can you do a spinal in a preeclamptic woman? Isn't that sympathectomy "too much too fast"? We used to think so, but no more. You can safely place a spinal in a preeclamptic woman. You do not have to place an epidural and bring the level up very slowly.

OTHER ISSUES

We now shift gears to go over other common questions that show up year after year on the oral board exam.

Monitors

What monitors would you place in a preeclamptic woman? If preeclampsia is severe (systolic greater than 160 mm Hg), place an arterial line. If you are doing a cesarean section under general anesthesia (hope not!), your biggest concern will be an intracranial bleed, and you need a beat-to-beat blood pressure measurement in that case.

Should you use a central line? Yes, if the patient's oliguria is unresponsive to standard fluid maneuvers and if there is evidence of congestive heart failure or pulmonary edema.

Should you use a Swan-Ganz catheter? See Chapter 6 for information about this controversial issue. You may like one; I would not.

Cesarean Section

Do you take the time to do a regional in a stat cesarean section? This is a toughie, because it depends on how immediate stat is. Because the mortality rate is 16 times greater with a general anesthetic, if you do have some time, get the patient on her side, and put in a spinal anesthetic. (Use a 22 gauge. Who cares about the spinal headache? You have a life to save here!) However, if there truly is not time, your hand is forced.

Awake Intubation

Can you do an awake intubation? Sure. If you need to give sedation, give it, and tell the pediatrician you will need to support ventilation for a while.

Intubate through the mouth. If you go through the nose, the patient will bleed all over creation.

Placenta Previa

What are the considerations for placenta previa? Access, access, access. Anticipate a big blood loss. This case may need a general anesthetic, because you cannot afford the sympathectomy.

Intubation and Ventilation

What happens if you cannot intubate but can ventilate? Wake the patient up, and do an awake intubation. If the baby is in trouble, you have a real beastie here, because it is hard to ignore the fetal distress and say, "Mom is more important; let the baby go while I wake her up and get the fiberoptic scope." Cesarean sections have been done under mask general anesthesia and are now done with laryngeal mask airways. There is the risk for aspiration. Textbooks say do this procedure while maintaining cricoid pressure, but I hope my earlier diatribe on the uselessness of cricoid pressure persuaded you that this is not a good idea.

What happens if you cannot intubate and cannot ventilate? Do a cricothyrotomy. You could wake her up and do it under local anesthesia, but Holy Moley, you better hope she is stoic as hell! This is the ultimate in toughness as far as obstetrics questions go, so make sure you can answer it! You can use what I have said, but you may have something better.

Wet Tap

What happens if you get a wet tap? Place the catheter—and label the living hell out of it—or go to a different space, and place another one.

Spinal Headache

How do you handle the patient' spinal headache? Make sure it really is a spinal headache and not something more sinister. Consider the patient's history and physical examination results and whether there is any concern that there is a bleed in the back or the head.

After you have determined it is a spinal headache, offer a blood patch. Conservative treatment and caffeine do not work. Do the patch, make the patient better, do not be a weenie about it.

On to the result of all this obstetric effort, the issue of our loins: kids.

9

Adults without Intravenous Lines: Pediatrics

What is a kid in the OR? A kid is an adult without an IV.

PEDIATRIC ANESTHESIOLOGY SAYING

This chapter offers a system-by-system rundown of important kiddie considerations. Emphasis is on the pertinent anatomy, physiology, and (why we are here!) the questions that keep appearing on the oral board exams through the years.

AIRWAY CONSIDERATIONS

The newborn takes a 3-mm, the 1-year-old child takes a 4-mm, and the 2-year-old child takes a 5-mm endotracheal tube (ETT). For kids, always have a half-size bigger and a half-size smaller ETT available because there is variation. A newborn should have the tube to about 10 cm at the gums, a 1-year-old child at 11 cm, and a 2-year-old child at 12 cm. As the child gets older, use this formula to estimate the size: (16 + age)/4.

You can measure the kid's pinky to get a feel for how big the trachea is. The narrowest part of a kids' airway is subglottic, so use uncuffed tubes until they reach the age of—this is controversial and being actively debated. Textbooks recommend using uncuffed tubes until age 5 years. You can always put in a cuffed tube and not inflate the cuff. The main thing is to appreciate that the trachea is small, and your tube should not be so tight that it causes edema. Whatever you use, make sure there is a leak at about 20 cm H_2O.

You have less room for error in smaller kids. Extending the neck can pull the tube out, and flexing the head can move the tube to an endobronchial location. Listen closely to your patient, and maintain vigilance for tube misplacement.

A child's epiglottis is small, stiff, and hard to lift. Most often, we use a straight blade to get in there and see the cords.

In adults, a difficult airway is often an acquired complication (e.g., obesity, arthritis, cervical injury), whereas most difficult airways in children are congenital problems (e.g., Treacher Collins syndrome, Pierre Robin syndrome, glycogen storage disease, trisomy 21). Unlike adults, kids do not tolerate the awake intubation option, and you are left with breathing them down and using specialized equipment under general anesthesia. A tracheotomy is sometimes done (you do what you have to do), but it is tempered by the concern that it can lead to tracheal stenosis in a very small child and lifelong airway troubles.

INTRAVENOUS LINES

Kids usually do not have intravenous lines. Unless the case is an emergency and involves a full stomach, you usually breathe a kid down, and place the intravenous line after induction. If you do need to put in a line while the kid is awake, try EMLA cream (give it time to work), and put it in two locations, in case you miss the first one.

A none-too-trivial question comes up about the patient with the bleeding tonsil who comes back, and no one can get an intravenous line in him or her. Will you breathe down a kid with a full stomach and tenuous volume status? Are you going to stick and stick, with the kid thrashing around and screaming, making the blood loss worse?

Among few good options, one is placing a femoral line with people holding the kid down or placing an intraosseous line (yes, they do run fast!). You can also give intramuscular ketamine to get the kid to hold still until you can place that all-important line for resuscitation.

Do you use glucose in a pediatric intravenous solution? No, except if the child has absolutely no glucose reserves (e.g., micropremie) or is at special risk for hypoglycemia (e.g., on hyperalimentation that stopped).

CARDIAC CONSIDERATIONS

You need no β-blockers for children! They have not gummed up their coronaries with Pall Malls and BLTs with extra mayonnaise.

Kids have a cardiac output that depends on heart rate. Because their hearts are relatively stiff, bradycardia means low cardiac output, and it can be an ominous sign. Premature infants especially have a maladaptive response to stress—the spooky apnea-bradycardia I saw a thousand times in the neonatal intensive care unit. It scared hell out of me every time!

A newborn's heart is about the size of a walnut, and you cannot just pound that first liter of lactated Ringer's solution in there. You must do your homework ahead of time and calculate to the milliliter how much fluid you will give.

What about the kid with congenital heart disease? (They asked one of my colleagues about a kid with tetralogy of Fallot last week!) These cases can be baffling, especially when the child has had an operation including a *baffle*.

Get it? I kill myself sometimes with these jokes!

You cannot expect to be a pediatric cardiologist, but you can at least remember these broad ideas to keep kiddies with congenital heart disease happy:

- Get a note from the cardiologist detailing exactly the nature of their heart disease.
- In general, bad conditions, such as hypoxemia, hypercarbia, or hypothermia, can be expected to make whatever they have worse.
- A definitive procedure (e.g., closing a patent ductus arteriosus, closing an atrial septal defect) means the kid should be okay from then on. Subacute bacterial endocarditis prophylaxis should always be considered.
- A palliative procedure (e.g., complicated repair of a single ventricle) means the kid likely will undergo heart transplantation some day. Congestive heart failure is always a possibility. Any kid with a complex history should probably be operated on at a specialized hospital with real pediatric expertise.

NEUROLOGIC CONSIDERATIONS

All of the kid's systems (e.g., liver, kidney) are immature at birth, but one aspect of the kid's neurologic system needs special consideration: the eyes. Because preemies are at risk for retinopathy of immaturity, keep the level of inspired oxygen low enough so that their eyes are not affected. How low is low enough? It should be enough to keep the Po_2 at about 80 mm Hg and the oxygen saturation level at about 94%. That can be tough, because the very kid you want to avoid giving oxygen to (i.e., concern about the eyes) is the one you need to give oxygen to (i.e., poor lung function).

PULMONARY CONSIDERATIONS

The ratio of functional residual capacity (FRC) to cardiac output and oxygen metabolism requirements are lower in kids than adults. Kids desaturate in the blink of an eye, get blue as your surgical scrubs, and make you so scared you nearly defecate a cinder block when you see it.

An arrest in a newborn is almost always respiratory in origin. The other leading causes of a newborn arrest are respiratory and respiratory, respectively. Before you "go to drugs," make sure you have established adequate ventilation.

Meconium

Meconium is fecal material expelled by the fetus in response to distress. Aspiration of meconium can lead to severe and prolonged respiratory troubles, so a few moments' work in the delivery room can make all the difference to a kid:

- Suction the mouth like mad.
- Intubate.
- Suction as you pull the endotracheal tube out.
- Then intubate.

This is a lot easier said than done, because you want to mask the kid. However, if you succumb to that temptation, you can push the meconium down into the lungs, and you have blown it.

Choanal Atresia

Choanal atresia is easy to fix *if you think of it*. The nasal route to breathing is obstructed. An oral airway "props everything open" and allows air exchange. Because kids are obligate nasal breathers, choanal atresia can be a serious problem.

Diaphragmatic Hernia

You should remember a few things when addressing a congenital diaphragmatic hernia:

- The intestines enter (85% of the time) the left chest, and the left lung never develops properly.
- You need to decompress the gastrointestinal tract first with a gastric tube.

- Mask ventilation can further inflate the loops of bowel and worsen the respiratory situation.
- Keep your arterial line or pulse oximeter on the right side.
- The left side may be seeing desaturated blood coming through persistent fetal circulation.
- Hypoxemia, hypercarbia, crying, acidosis, and hypothermia increase pulmonary vascular resistance and can worsen the shunt, so avoid all of these situations (if only life were that easy).
- Do not try to inflate the bad lung. You will cause a pneumothorax in the good lung!

Epiglottitis

Follow a few guidelines:

- Keep everyone (especially you) calm.
- Do not send the kid off to radiology; go straight to the operating room.
- Do not place an intravenous line, because it will freak the kid.
- Breathe down with the ear, nose, and throat specialist nearby to do a tracheotomy if you lose the airway.
- Do not lift the epiglottis, because if you touch it, it may bleed all over the place.

NEUROMUSCULAR CONSIDERATIONS

Kids may have an undiagnosed myopathy, and sux can trigger a hyperkalemic disaster. For this reason, sux is usually avoided in pediatric anesthesia.

In adult intubations, neuromuscular blockers typically are used, but this is not the case for kids. You usually can induce a kid deeply and intubate without the need for paralysis.

METABOLIC CONSIDERATIONS

This is a good place to touch on the last two "big guys" that happen to the "small guys."

Pyloric Stenosis

The most important thing to remember is that pyloric stenosis is a *medical emergency*, not a surgical emergency. These kids have been vomiting, losing volume and acid, and have a hypochloremic, hypokalemic metabolic alkalosis. They need volume and electrolyte resuscitation. After they are stable, they can proceed to surgery.

Malignant Hyperthermia

Although not limited to kids, malignant hyperthermia (MH) is a disease we need to know about. Consider these guidelines:

- The condition is familial, so get a personal and family history.
- Triggers are potent vapors or sux.

- Trigger-free anesthetics are easy to do with propofol.
- Think of MH as a metabolic supernova; you will see tachycardia (often the first sign), increased oxygen consumption, increased carbon dioxide production (amazingly high at times), a metabolic and respiratory acidosis (in case of doubt, get a blood gas!), muscle rigidity, and hyperthermia (a late sign).
- Treatment consists of stopping the operation, switching to total intravenous anesthesia (TIVA) if the case cannot be stopped, dantrolene, cooling measures, and renal and hemodynamic support. You will need extra hands for this.

There are some nettlesome questions about MH. For instance, what does masseter spasm mean? Although it is not a certain sign of MH, it *may* be a sign; if you see it, assume the worst. Who should get a muscle biopsy? The biopsy is expensive, painful, exposes the patient to another procedure, is done in only a few specialized places, and is not perfect! In my opinion, no one should get a muscle biopsy. If you suspect something, treat the patient as if he or she has MH, and get a Medic Alert bracelet in case the child is in a car wreck some day and cannot tell the doctors about being susceptible to MH.

SCOPE OF PEDIATRIC ANESTHESIA

Before we sign off on pediatric anesthesia, it is worth reminding you that this pediatric section is less than five pages. Entire fellowships are dedicated to pediatric anesthesia, and entire textbooks are written on the myriad implications and subtleties of this demanding subspecialty. This chapter covers only the most common questions that tend to pop up on the oral boards regarding pediatric anesthesiology. It is laughable to think of this as even a review.

As I said at the beginning of this book, do lots of practice tests aloud, and fill in the gaps by reading in the real textbooks. Do not depend on only these small chapters for your knowledge base.

Now it is on to the last review section. Then it is time to roll up your sleeves and jump into the real meat of this book—the practice tests!

10

Oh, the Things You'll See!

Look, up in the sky! It's a bird. It's a plane.

Superman was a common sight up there, flying around the *Daily Planet* building. You are going to hear a few common questions flying around in the oral board exam. None of them merits its own chapter, but each deserves a section in this one, which is the last of the review chapters. You are bound to hear at least one or two of these items.

INTENSIVE CARE UNIT

The oral exam is not about board certification in ICUology, and you do not need to know superweird stuff understood only by the critical care gurus. You will be expected to know the generic stuff that all anesthesiologists should know.

The best way to approach any intensive care unit (ICU) question is to remember that the ICU is the operating room (OR) in slow motion plus antibiotics and hyperalimentation. Voila!

Airway, Breathing, and Circulation

Any ICU question, like any OR question, starts with an evaluation at the bedside of the adequacy of airway, breathing, and circulation (ABC). Here is an example that happened to me:

I was called to the ICU to sedate a patient with atrial fibrillation for a cardioversion. On arrival, I noticed the patient had just arrived from a *Braveheart* re-enactment and still had blue paint on his face or was hypoxemic. Turns out that the guy was not a big Mel Gibson fan and that he was turning into a facultative anaerobe right in front of my eyes. "May I be so bold as to suggest," I offered, "that I intubate him and that we ensure he is well oxygenated before our little electrical adventure?" The assembled masses nodded appreciatively at this novel idea. To all appearances, they seemed impressed by my observation that, with the exception of blue-green algae and some bacteria that live off sulfur bonds, most terrestrial forms of life require oxygen.

What to our wondering eyes appeared after he was oxygenated? Sinus rhythm! Amazing! Sheath those paddles; there is no need to shock someone out of a dangerous rhythm. By fixing his ABCs, I fixed the problem.

Lines

All the central venous pressure (CVP) versus Swan-Ganz catheter battles are fought again in the ICU! Whatever arguments you use in the OR reappear in the ICU setting:

- You need all the information that a Swan provides to be able to guide fluid and inotropic support. Without it, you are flying blind.
- The Swan causes more complications and distraction than it is worth. And while we are at it, it is not worth anything!

Maybe you believe the first statement. Fine. Defend it. Maybe you believe the second statement. Fine. Defend it.

Advanced Cardiac Life Support

Were you called to the ICU to manage a code? That is a reasonable expectation. People code in the unit all the time. Brush up on your advanced cardiac life support (ACLS) guidelines (yes, they asked it during the April tests). Remember the new highlights of ACLS guidelines:

- "Hard and fast" chest compressions are emphasized.
- Use one shock at 200 J biphasic or 360 J monophasic settings, and then resume compressions immediately.
- Use epinephrine or vasopressin.
- Shock right away if it is a shockable rhythm. Do not delay in securing the airway.
- After the airway is secured, do not hyperventilate the patient! It decreases venous return and worsens everything.

Management of Acute Respiratory Distress Syndrome

Any patient can develop acute respiratory distress syndrome (ARDS) on the boards (and, unfortunately, in real life), including the healthy muscular guy who has an obstruction after extubation and develops negative-pressure pulmonary edema or the patient who aspirates. ARDS can result from transfusion-related lung injury, from sepsis, from congestive heart failure, or from anything in the world, if you think about it. How do you approach this? It is mainly common sense stuff, such as making sure the tube is in the right place.

The main remedy for ARDS is treating the instigating cause. Use appropriate antibiotics for infection, drain the abscess causing the sepsis, and do not forget the primary treatment. Medical treatment of asthma (e.g., steroids, β-adrenergic agents, the usual suspects) is appropriate if that is part of the picture.

The rest is supportive care and hoping against hope that the body can take care of the insult. Negative-pressure pulmonary edema resolves in a day or so without treatment, but a double-lung transplant in acute rejection is going to be a longer haul!

As soon as possible, try to get the patient out of the "toxic range" of FiO_2. Anything higher than 50% causes lung damage, so use positive end-expiratory pressure (PEEP) or other measures (e.g., drying out the lungs with diuresis) to get to a level of 50% or lower.

The best PEEP is an important concept. You want the best PEEP that optimizes oxygen delivery. With too little PEEP, you cannot oxygenate. With too much

PEEP, you cut off venous return, decrease cardiac output, and ultimately impair oxygen delivery. So you have to find that right level.

Use clever ventilator settings. People with obstructive disease need prolonged expiration to let the air out. I have seen the use of every different kind of ventilator setting, with all sorts of exotic names. If you have to get extremely clever in your "trick ventilator" settings, this usually heralds a poor prognosis for the patient.

The lungs and kidneys have different treatment demands, producing a common tug o' war in the ICU. You want to "dry out the lungs as much as possible" by vigorous diuresis. That improves oxygenation, but too much diuresis, and the kidneys start to protest (the creatinine rises—you have overdone it!). You give more fluids, and the kidneys like it, but you have overloaded the lungs. You dry them out, you rehydrate, you dry them out, and you rehydrate because they are too wet, too dry, too wet, and too dry. The worse the "oxygenation triad" for lungs, kidneys, and heart, the harder it is to find the perfect balance of needs.

The main take-home lesson for ARDS is this: If they get better, take the credit for your brilliant ICU management. If they do not get better, dodge the blame by saying, "There was nothing anyone could have done."

Ventilators

This is where the ICU guys run rings around us, but for us ICU amateurs (the examiners are most likely ICU amateurs, too), there are a few basics about ventilation we can lean on.

Never trust a ventilator completely. If something seems wrong, disconnect it, and hand ventilate. This is a true story from my long list of misadventures:

I finish a beastly heart procedure, drop off the patient in the ICU, and hook up the ventilator. As I am doing the paperwork, I glance up and see that the pressure is plummeting and the chest seems overinflated. I reach up, disconnect, and hear a huge whoosh as the pressure comes back. The ventilator had been inspiring but not bothering to expire, so the breaths stacked up.

Lots of people (me included) get handed an arterial blood gas measurement during their oral exam and are asked to interpret it—respiratory acidosis, A-a gradient, and all that good stuff. Here is a rule of thumb in case you forgot the real live A-a gradient question from written board days:

For every 1% of oxygen, you should get about 4 or 5 mm Hg on your Pa_{O_2} reading. At room air (21% oxygen), you are about 80 or 90 mm Hg, and a patient on 100% oxygen should be about 400 or 500 mm Hg. If the patient's blood gas determination shows a Pa_{O_2} of 80 mm Hg on 100% oxygen, you have an A-a gradient of about 320 to 420 mm Hg, and that is high! This quick and dirty method is easy to remember and gives you some idea about the A-a gradient. You are not looking for incredible accuracy; you just want to know whether it is wrong or is improving.

Urine Output

What do you do when the urine output decreases? This question is always on the test; I guarantee it. This issue may appear with any intraoperative question, because in just about any case, the urine output can decrease. The examiners often ask it in the context of aortic aneurysm cases, other big intra-abdominal cases, or cases in which the ureters are in danger (e.g., hysterectomies, renal transplants). I include it in this section because the "what do you do when the urine output decreases " question can be asked about ICU patients.

YOU HOPE THEY ASK THIS QUESTION, BECAUSE YOU SHOULD CRUSH IT!

Approach the case by looking at the prerenal, post-renal, and renal causes. The easiest to diagnose is the post-renal possibility (e.g., kink, clot, misplacement of the Foley catheter, need to irrigate it). Special consideration is needed for an internal post-renal cause, such as cut ureters (e.g., hysterectomy) or kinked ureters (e.g., renal transplantation gone awry).

Next on the list of possibilities is prerenal oliguria. Review the fluid balance, ensure the patient is well hydrated, and use a CVP or transesophageal echocardiography (TEE) catheter to make sure the heart is getting what it needs. An extremely subtle but common internal prerenal cause is tamponade.

Because I do hearts, I have seen tamponade many times, but it escapes a lot of people. A few days out from a heart procedure, everything seems fine. The fluid balance is okay, and the Foley catheter is working. The urine output is down, but it can be corrected with a little more fluid. However, it is still down. BOOM! The patient crashes from tamponade. The patient was hypovolemic but "internally hypovolemic," and the heart could not fill because it was getting squished. Because the heart could not fill, the kidneys were not getting their "fair share," and urine output was the first signal that tamponade was starting.

Renal oliguria is a diagnosis of exclusion. What do you do about it?

- Post-renal: Fix the kink or clog.
- Prerenal: Replace volume.
- Renal: Dialysis may be necessary.

What about all the other stuff? Use mannitol? No, because it does not do any good. Use dopamine? No, because it has been proved to be a myth. Use Lasix? No, because it just worsens things.

You can do some things that make physiologic sense:

- Do what you can to improve venous return, such as lessen the PEEP if the patient can tolerate it.
- Have the patient breathe spontaneously, rather than paralyze him and put him on positive-pressure ventilation (if circumstances allow it). That approach allows the thoracic pump work a little and may help the kidneys.
- Review the myriad drugs the patient is on. There may be some nephrotoxic agents hiding in the list.
- Do not let vasoconstrictors do what volume should. Should you get the blood pressure up with high-dose norepinephrine or give another unit of blood? That is a tough one. I wonder which is better for the kidneys?

PAIN MANAGEMENT

The oral exam is not for board certification in pain management. It is designed to test you about the amount of pain management that an anesthesiologist should know. The board examiners sitting in the hotel room are most likely not practicing pain specialists. They probably throw people on patient-controlled analgesia (PCA) devices all the time, just like you do.

People report that the questions on the oral exam were at a basic level. One of my contributing authors, Brian Durkin, is a pain specialist, and he gave me a bunch of the grab bags on pain you will see later in the book.

The following material—from a non–pain specialist—covers the things we should all know. This is a good place to jump to the latest American Society of Anesthesiologists (ASA) refresher course lectures, because they always have the latest in pain management for non–pain specialists in there.

Acute Pain

The questions on acute pain usually are like this one: "What would you do for pain management for this patient having a thoracotomy or radical prostatectomy or cesarean section?" You will be asked about epidural or spinal narcotics, which you can pick or choose as you see fit.

Check the patient's coagulation status. In this day and age, when everyone has a stent or two, make sure the patient is off anticoagulants. Look for clinical signs (i.e., easy bruising and bleeding) that indicate a problem with the clotting system. A serious problem has arisen with the new drug-eluting stents. These patients need to be on Plavix, possibly indefinitely. Take them off the drug for the appropriate time preoperatively, and they may clot the coronary artery and have a myocardial infarction The jury is still out on that issue, but for pain question purposes, the main thing is to make sure the coagulation situation is okay before placing a neuraxial block.

Because respiratory depression is a possibility, staff must be trained to look for signs of respiratory depression and should have standing orders for responding. Intrathecal or epidural narcotics in the face of obstructive sleep apnea (OSA) requires even more vigilance because patients are more susceptible to problems in this realm (think "monitored bed").

Do you use infusions with local anesthetics? They are great for pain relief, but you should be aware of the sympathectomy and subsequent hypotension. Whenever a local anesthetic enters the equation, be prepared to respond to a local anesthetic becoming intravascular.

- Stop the infusion of the local anesthetic.
- Address the patient's ABCs.
- Use prolonged cardiopulmonary resuscitation (CPR)—all the way to cardiopulmonary bypass if bupivacaine (fast in, slow out, highly cardiotoxic) is injected.
- Use lipid emulsion solution. This has saved the day a number of times, so make sure you know about lipid emulsions! (Plus, make sure some lipid emulsion is on your block cart at your place.)

Effective pain relief provides a host of benefits, including decreased splinting, improved oxygenation, and decreased stress response (handy for the cardiac crowd).

Should you perform placement under echo guidance for peripheral blocks? Yes, indeed! Why go blind when you can see? My colleagues and I stopped doing blind intubations (we use a fiberoptic scope now), blind pain procedures (we use a C-arm), and blind hemodynamic management (we use a TEE probe). Pain management is jumping on the "see what we're doing" bandwagon, and physicians are placing blocks and catheters under echocardiographic vision.

Can you use adjuvant drugs to decrease need for narcotics? Clonidine shows promise as a preoperative medication to decrease anesthetic needs while providing sedation and sympathomimetic blunting. It acts as a kind of oral dexmedetomidine.

Chronic Pain

More and more, I hear about people having chronic pain on their exam. However, we need to know only about the basic stuff, nothing too esoteric.

Chronic pain is like every other facet of anesthesia, and you start with a thorough history and physical examination. Throwing steroids at neck pain or a facet block at lower back pain is a shot in the dark. The patient may have an unrecognized fracture or tumor. Make sure what you are treating is something amenable to pain treatment, not some pathology that needs definitive treatment.

The pain specialist is not a "needle jockey," although that is part of the treatment we are most involved in. Treatment should be multimodal, with psychology, physical therapy, and medical treatment (antidepressants perhaps) all part of a holistic approach.

Blocks often require a series to be effective. Complex regional pain syndrome in the arm requires stellate ganglion blocks. Complex regional pain syndrome in the leg requires lumbar sympathetic blocks. These blocks are done under fluoroscopic guidance to make sure they target the right place.

Ambulatory care should strive to get the patient back to normal functioning, even if complete absence of pain is not a realistic expectation. Palliative care for cancer patients with a limited life span should be aggressive, with every attempt employed to make them comfortable. Concerns about dependency are not applicable for this patient group.

TRAUMA

The exams include a bunch of good traumas. This material covers the main ideas you want to bring into any trauma case discussion.

Trauma means dealing with the patient's ABCs at warp speed. You may have to secure the airway before you have a cleared cervical spine, before you have a history, and before you know anything about this train wreck that rolled through the door with EMT helicopter pilots doing CPR. Hypoxemia worsens every injury (spinal cord, brain, heart—name an organ that likes hypoxemia!). You have to do a lightning assessment of what is making the trauma patient hypoxemic:

- Aspiration? The patient cannot protect her airway if she loses consciousness.
- Pneumothorax? The motor vehicle accident, gunshot wound, stab wound, and crush injury can all break a rib and poke the lung.
- Blood loss? Blood losses can happen before you see them (spilled in the street); occur as you are seeing them (spilling on your shoes); or be hidden (spilling into their thigh, their abdomen, their chest).

Trauma means associated injuries:

- Fell out of a tree and broke the arm? That is not all that hit the ground, so look for splenic laceration, chest trauma, and head and neck trauma.

- Neck injury? The whiplike movement that hurt the neck might have torn vessels in the head, so consider a brain injury.
- Brain injury? The same bash that hurt the skull and brain might have snapped and injured the neck.

When the neck is hurt, look at the head. When the head is hurt, look at the neck.

Look patients over from head to toe. As we were intubating a guy for an abdominal exploration, we noticed he was bleeding from the top of his head onto the front of our shirts. He was bleeding from *another* gunshot wound that happened to be in his head. This leads to a lesson in interpersonal relationships: If someone dislikes you enough to shoot you once, he may shoot you again, so be extremely circumspect in your choice of friends.

Gunshot wounds and electrical injuries merit special consideration. Both can do a lot more damage than it looks like on the surface. A bullet has a large shockwave of energy when it hits, and it can blow apart things far away from the path of the bullet. The bullet can bounce all over the place. Electrical injuries can look like small entrance and exit wounds, but a lot of internal searing and damage can occur along the path. The same holds for paint guns. There is a little entry hole, but the paint shoots inside a mile, gumming up a lot of tissue.

OBESITY

The standard questions on obesity are not too tough, but they are likely to appear on the oral exam. The toughie is management of the patient with OSA (a big topic at meetings because people from all over wrestle with it).

Obesity affects anesthetic care:

- Airway: Excess soft tissue, a large tongue, large breasts, and a thick neck add up to a difficult mask application and difficult intubation.
- Pulmonary effects: Decreased functional residual capacity and high oxygen consumption produce quick desaturation.
- Cardiac effects: Prolonged hypoxemia can lead to cor pulmonale and right heart failure from looking at "too-high pulmonary pressure" for a long time.
- Gastrointestinal effects: The patient is at risk for aspiration.
- Lines: The catheters can be forbidding.
- Monitors: It may be difficult to get a cuff to work, and you may need an arterial line just to get a blood pressure reading.

All of this means obesity presents a lot of challenges. You can make a solid argument for intubating the patient awake if you have any concern whatsoever about securing the airway.

Management of the patient with OSA is difficult. You wish you could send every single one of them to the ICU postoperatively, because they are susceptible to respiratory depression postoperatively. You have heard the horror stories about the guy who was asking for pain medication, got "just a little," and at shift change (or at home), was found dead the next morning, presumably from respiratory depression that went unrecognized.

God forbid that should happen to me! To the ICU with all of them! Oh, wait—that is impractical, or wait—I work in an outpatient center. I cannot send all of them to the ICU. Now what?

Because this is a tough and common situation, I am going to take the recommendations from the discussion section of one of the later stem questions (no. 32). These recommendations are worth seeing more than once. You should first read the Full Monty on this issue.[1]

OSA is a syndrome characterized by recurrent episodes of partial or complete obstruction of the upper airway during sleep. OSA is strictly defined as cessation of airflow for more than 10 seconds despite ventilatory effort for five or more times per hour, and it is usually associated with a decrease in arterial oxygen saturation of more than 4%. Obstructive sleep hypopnea (OSH) is defined as a reduction in airflow of more than 50% for more than 10 seconds for 15 or more times per hour of sleep, and it may be associated with a decrease in oxygen saturation of more than 4%. Both disrupt sleep, alter cardiopulmonary function, and may cause daytime sleepiness.

According to the ASA practice guidelines, predisposing physical characteristics include a body mass index greater than 35, neck circumference of at least 17 inches in men and 16 inches in women, craniofacial abnormalities, anatomic nasal obstruction, and tonsils almost touching in the midline. Symptoms associated with OSA include snoring, observed pauses in breathing during sleep, awakening from sleep or frequent arousals, and daytime somnolence or fatigue. The estimated prevalence of OSA is 2% among women and 4% among men. However, 60% to 80% of patients at risk for OSA remain undiagnosed. These patients are at increased risk for adverse outcomes when they receive sedation, analgesia, or anesthesia, and their risk increases as the severity of OSA increases.

A presumptive diagnosis of OSA may be made on the basis of symptoms, but a definitive diagnosis is made on the basis of a sleep study. It consists of monitoring the electroencephalogram (EEG), electro-oculogram (EOG), oral and nasal sensors for movement of air, electromyogram (EMG), end-tidal carbon dioxide level, pulse oximetry, noninvasive blood pressure, and electrocardiogram (ECG). Pulse oximetry desaturation data, ECG patterns, and changes in vital signs are reported. The total number of apnea and hypopnea events per hour is called the apnea-hypopnea index (AHI). The AHI is used quantitatively to classify the severity of OSA. Mild OSA is considered to have a value between 6 and 20, moderate OSA has a value between 21 and 40, and severe OSA has a value greater than 40. The total number of arousals per hour is reported as a total arousal index (AI). According to the ASA practice guidelines, the literature supports the efficacy of continuous positive airway pressure (CPAP) in improving the AHI and oxygen saturation levels in the nonperioperative setting. There are insufficient data to evaluate the impact of preoperative use of CPAP on perioperative outcomes, but the consultants agree that preoperative use of CPAP or nasal intermittent positive-pressure ventilation (NIPPV) may improve the preoperative condition.

The literature contains insufficient data to guide the decision about inpatient versus outpatient management or to determine the appropriate time for discharge. However, the consultants involved in formulating the ASA practice guidelines agree that procedures normally performed on an outpatient basis on non-OSA patients may be performed on an outpatient basis on OSA patients when local or regional anesthesia is administered. The ASA consultants are equivocal about performing superficial surgery or gynecologic laparoscopy under general anesthesia on an outpatient basis on these patients. They agree that for patients at increased risk, the outpatient facility should have the availability of difficult airway equipment, respiratory equipment, radiology and laboratory facilities, and a plan in place for transfer to an inpatient facility. Upper abdominal laparoscopy, airway surgery, and tonsillectomy in patients with OSA who are younger than 3 years should not be performed in an outpatient setting. Similarly, OSA patients with a severity score of 5 or greater should not have surgery in an outpatient center.

Supplemental oxygen should be administered until the patient can maintain her baseline oxygen saturation on room air. (If the patient had been treated with CPAP or NIPPV preoperatively, this should be administered in the recovery period). She should be maintained in the semiupright position. The goal is to have no episodes of desaturation or obstruction when left undisturbed. The ASA task force consultants recommend that patients with OSA be monitored for a median of 3 hours longer than non-OSA patients but 7 hours longer than the last episode of hypoxemia or obstruction on room air. The patient in stem question 32 was monitored in the postanesthesia care unit (PACU) for 7 hours and was eventually discharged from the ambulatory surgery center. Her subsequent postoperative course was uneventful.

She should be treated with nonsteroidal anti-inflammatory drugs and perhaps low-dose oral opiates to minimize sedative effects and the risk of airway obstruction. If her pain remained uncontrolled, she would be transferred to the inpatient facility to manage her pain in a monitored setting.

NEUROANESTHESIA

Neuroanesthesia people will go nuts to see that this entire subspecialty is reduced to a few comments. I mean no disrespect to the neuro crowd, but this is an oral board review book, and the comments are about the neuroanesthesia considerations that appear on the exams year after year and decade after decade.

Preoperative Considerations

How do you determine if there is increased intracranial pressure? The history and physical examination come to the rescue, as is often the case. Look over the chart and see if there is something *in* the head (e.g., tumor, leaking aneurysms, subdural hematoma, meat cleaver). The cranium is pretty stingy about yielding real estate. As the head becomes more crowded, intracranial pressure increases, decreasing cerebral perfusion. The body responds by increasing blood pressure, and a reflex bradycardia can set in (i.e., Cushing's triad, which scares hell out of you when you see it!).

Examine the patient. Is he nauseated or lethargic? Are there focal signs or a blown pupil (get a move on, because he is about to herniate!). All these features point to increased intracranial pressure.

Aneurysms deserve special consideration. As you plan ahead, make sure you do not increase the possibility of a rupture by altering the pressure balance (i.e., transmural pressure) in the aneurysm. If you increase the blood pressure, the aneurysm may pop (i.e., more transmural pressure pushing outward on the wall). If you hyperventilate and decrease the intracranial pressure, the aneurysm may pop (i.e., less transmural pressure pushing back from the outside). If you "increase the inside" or "decrease the outside," you can pop the bastard, and that's that.

Beat-to-beat blood pressure measurement is crucial in these cases. If the aneurysm does rupture, will you have adequate access? You want to find that out ahead of time, not when the disaster strikes.

Perform a preoperative neurological examination. This is one time when you want to document "what was there before." If the patient wakes up with one side not moving, you had damn well better know whether it was moving before!

Discussion about the risk of optic nerve ischemia is extremely tough! Long, prone cases run the risk of optic nerve ischemia and blindness. After extensive snooping around, only two things seem to correlate with optic nerve ischemia:

- Prolonged cases (6 hours or more)
- Blood loss more than 1 liter

Surprisingly, blindness does not seem to correlate with controlled hypotension or with any particular hematocrit!

This is a difficult situation. Do you tell a patient who is going to be prone for a 9-hour scoliosis procedure that he may wake up blind despite appropriate positioning, no pressure on the eyes, and doing "everything right"?

Intraoperative Considerations

Brain Swelling

A few questions come up all the time, especially the "tight brain" one, so we start with it: "Hey, the brain is tight," the surgeon yells. What do you do about it?

You first ensure adequate oxygenation and appropriate ventilation. Hypoxemia and hypercarbia will increase cerebral blood flow, increase the intracranial pressure, and "tighten things up" for the surgeon. Second, you make sure that the head is positioned appropriately and that you have good venous drainage. (This is my take on central lines, although I do not see many textbooks backing me on it. If I put in a central line, I put in a femoral line. It provides access, lets me get at it, and does not interfere with venous drainage.)

Mannitol and Lasix can decrease brain swelling, although this approach can be tricky. Mannitol requires an intact blood-brain barrier, but the surgeon is cutting in the brain—talk about a nonintact blood-brain barrier! Because these agents decrease "brain water," they also cause hypovolemia, which drops the cerebral perfusion pressure. You give more fluid to raise cerebral perfusion pressure, and you soon are going around in circles! I ask neuroanesthesia guys about this all the time, and they always say, "That's right. Hmm. Well, we do it anyway."

Make sure you are not above 0.5 minimum alveolar concentration (MAC) for a potent inhaled agent. This may increase cerebral blood flow. Lean on your intravenous agents.

To hyperventilate or not to hyperventilate—that is the question. We used to recommend hyperventilation, but no longer do. It can decrease cerebral blood flow *too much* and lead to cerebral ischemia. Instead, we recommend normocarbia. In the short term, if you are in a jam and need the cerebral blood flow down for just a little while and if the surgeon is completely stuck with the brain swelling too much, you do what you have to do.

Spinal Cord Monitoring

Somatosensory evoked potentials cover the sensory portion of the spinal cord but not the motor portion. (Some places do motor evoked potentials.) Ensure there is no damage to the spinal cord. You may have to do a wake-up test to ensure the motor tracts are intact.

If, during the course of a case, the potentials show decreased amplitude or increased latency, let the surgeon know. On your end, make sure you are not doing anything anesthetic (too much potent inhaled agent can interfere with the signals) or physiologic (hypothermia can interfere with signals).

Carotid Procedures

Should carotid procedures be done with the patient awake or under general anesthesia? The awake approach has the potential advantage of giving you real-time cerebral function (squeeze the ball!) during the case, but if the patient weirds out, you may have to switch to a general anesthetic with the neck open. Intubating at that point can be painful to *you*.

General anesthesia has the none-too-trivial advantage of a secure airway, but you cannot get a great picture of what is going on cerebrally. Bispectral (BIS) index monitoring is too global and will not give you hemispheric information. An EEG with an attached EEG technician is a good idea, but that presupposes that you have the machine and the technician. Many times, you do these procedures under the "go fast and hope nothing bad happens" rules of engagement. Neither the awaken nor the general anesthesia approach has been shown to be superior.

Sitting Craniotomy

Can you guess the question? You got it: venous air embolism. Thank the good Lord that most craniotomies are not done with the patient in the sitting position, but the question still appears on the boards. What should you do about a venous air embolism?

- Best monitor? Use precordial Doppler, and listen for the millwheel murmur.
- Nitrous oxide? Do not use it in the first place, or turn it off when the venous air embolism happens.
- Lines? Aspirate the central line you placed at the junction of the superior vena cava and the atrium. (This may or may not do any good, by the way.)
- Pressure drop? You may see a drop in end-tidal CO_2 (as with any embolism) and then instability as the "airlock" hits the right heart. Use CPR, get the patient flat, flood the field to stop further entrainment, and apply ACLS guidelines.

Postoperative Considerations

The big neuroanesthesia postoperative question is very much like the big oliguria question. You are going to get this question, the answer is broken into three parts, and you hope the examiners ask it because you are going to crush it.

At the end of the neurologic case (or any case), the patient fails to awaken. You must rule out three big causes: pharmacologic, physiologic, and neurologic.

The pharmacologic causes are anything that I, the anesthesiologist, gave or that the patient gave himself. The more common cause is what I gave the patient, and I would make sure my potent agents are off, the patient is not overnarcotized or sedated, and the neuromuscular agents are reversed. The less common cause is some pharmacologic surprise the patient took ahead of time, perhaps Valium at home or a street drug before coming into the trauma bay.

Physiologic causes include death (Oh, that!). I first check the ABCs and make sure the patient is stable and had enough "vital signs to be vital." (If I fail to notice a dead patient, you can flunk me right now.) I then go over the common physiologic aberrations that may explain a failure to awaken, such as hypoglycemia, hypoxemia, hypercarbia, hypothermia, and hyponatremia.

Neurologic causes often require a trip to the computed tomography (CT) scanner to see whether there is a bleed or some other pathology.

I AM TELLING YOU THAT THEY ASK THIS QUESTION, AND EVERYONE THAT HAS USED THIS APPROACH TO ANSWERING THE QUESTION FEELS CONFIDENT ABOUT THE ANSWER. IT IS, AFTER ALL, WHAT WE SHOULD DO IN REAL LIFE. NO WONDER THIS ANSWER HAS DONE SO WELL THROUGH THE YEARS.

LIVER OPERATIONS

Would the examiners ask you about a liver transplantation? I hate to say this, but yes, I do hear about people being asked about liver transplantation during the oral boards. Fear not! Your institution may not perform them (only a few places do), but guess what? The examiner does not do them either and therefore knows no more than you do!

You can review the basics of liver stuff. That is all you can reasonably be expected to do. You also can go back to the mantra of the cardiac chapter: *At the heart of a heart case is a regular case.* If you are asked about liver transplantation, think the same way: *At the heart of a liver case is a regular case.*

Preoperative Considerations

You do take the patient's history and perform the physical examination, keeping your eyes peeled for the special problems associated with liver failure. This stuff also will help you if you are asked a question about a patient with liver failure undergoing an operation for something other than liver transplantation.

Coagulation Disorders
The prothrombin time can be out of whack, and the platelet count can be low. Thrombopoietin is made in the liver, and just as renal failure patients have low blood cell counts (no erythropoietin from the kidneys), liver failure patients can have low platelet counts (no thrombopoietin from the liver). Bet you did not know that about thrombopoietin!

Respiratory and Pulmonary Problems
Little arteriovenous fistulas around the cirrhotic liver can lead to shunting that is refractory to oxygen therapy. Ascites can lead to a restrictive respiratory picture, but draining the ascites (reserved for such severe restriction that respiratory insufficiency is a threat to life) is only a temporary fix, because the forces that made the ascites in the first place are still there, and the ascites reforms—and then the patient is hypovolemic!

Pulmonary hypertension happens in some liver disease patients. It is always a concern in the transplantation patients.

Neurologic and Gastrointestinal Problems

In advanced liver disease, the patient can become encephalopathic. Ascites can lead to aspiration risk. Top that off with esophageal varices that can bleed at any moment, and you have got a lot of gastrointestinal headaches.

Intraoperative Considerations

What do you answer when they ask how you would do this liver transplantation? *At the heart of a liver case is a regular case.* Ah, a guiding voice!

To address the airway, I would do an appropriate evaluation, keeping in mind that this patient is probably at risk for aspiration because of his ascites. I would perform an awake intubation (if he appeared difficult) or a rapid sequence induction. Given the poor coagulation status, I would avoid instrumenting the nose.

Lines and monitors are the next issue. This case requires, shall we say, generous access. Because I do not handle these cases often (yes, you can say that), I would check with a colleague more experienced in liver procedures. However, I would likely need two arterial lines and a central line. Because varices are not a contraindication to TEE, I would use TEE to guide volume and inotropic therapy.

The phases of the case should be considered. During the anhepatic phase, I would expect vigorous blood loss, and I would take care to keep up and have at least one extra person around to help me pour blood into the rapid infuser. During the reperfusion phase, I would be aware that a big myocardial "hit" is coming my way (e.g., acid, potassium), and I would be prepared for resuscitative action, including volume, pressor (e.g., epinephrine), and bicarbonate issues. At the end of the case, I would keep the patient intubated, because the extensive volume resuscitation would have made the airway swollen.

HEY, THAT WASN'T THAT BAD!

See? If you just pay attention to the basics and know a little bit about the various phases of the case (read up about it), you can handle this question if it comes up!

EQUIPMENT

I do not hear a lot of questions about equipment, but you should brush up on this topic a little bit.

What are the mechanical features in the machine that make sure we are delivering oxygen?

1. Diameter-indexed safety system in the wall connections
2. Pin-indexed safety system with the cylinders
3. Color coding of lines and tanks
4. Oxygen on the far right of the manifold
5. Disconnect alarm on the ventilator
6. Oxygen analyzer (the only thing that makes sure you are giving oxygen!)
7. Oxygen ratio monitor controller to make sure you do not give too much nitrous oxide
8. Oxygen powering the bellows (in case there is a hole in the bellows)
9. Oxygen designated by a fluted handle; nitrous oxide and air designated by sintered handles

What is the fallback if the machine fails? To hell with the machine; get an Ambu bag and oxygen tank.

What are the functions of grounding, line isolation monitors, and the like? Macroshock hazard occurs if a machine has a grounding fault. The patient becomes the way to the ground and can get shocked. Microshock is much more sinister and happens at much lower currents. With as little as 50 microamps and a saline-filled line to the heart (good conductor), you can fibrillate the heart.

The line isolation monitor (they are not in all ORs) tells you that the electrical system in your OR is not grounded. The electrical supply from the power plant comes to the OR, the wiring system for the OR is put right next to the power plant wires, and *induction* causes a current to flow in the OR wiring system. If the line isolation monitor goes off, it indicates there is a leak of 2 to 3 milliamps. The line isolation monitor detects 2 to 3 *milli*amps, far more than the 50 *micro*amps that can cause a microshock hazard. The line isolation monitor is no protection against microshock.

Do not worry too much about the equipment. Even if you blow it, it probably will not be a big part of your exam.

It is time to ditch this review section and jump right into the practice tests, which are the meat of this book.

Reference

1. Gross JB, Bachenberg KL, Benumof JL, et al: Practice guidelines for the perioperative management of patients with obstructive sleep apnea: A report by the American Society of Anesthesiologists Task Force on Perioperative Management of patients with obstructive sleep apnea. Anesthesiology 2006;104:1081-1093.

Part II

Cases from Real Life

11

Stem Questions

CASE 1: YOU CRACK ME UP

Chris Gallagher

A 44-year-old denizen of Miami's mean streets presents with a nagging cough. Wise counsel dictates a chest radiograph to shed light on this malady. What appears next makes all and sundry gaze in wonder. Lying in the right main stem bronchus is a 6-cm-long, narrow, hollow, pipelike object that extends up into the trachea. It resembles, for lack of a more scientific term, the glass stem of a crack cocaine pipe!

Between coughs (the object is resting against the somewhat richly innervated carina), the patient admits that, well, yes, he does smoke crack on a more or less constant basis, taking time out from said activity to sleep, eat, and commit crimes to buy the crack.

Two days ago, while inhaling with gusto, he heard the glass stem of his crack pipe snap, felt something go down his throat, and started coughing heavily. All the king's horses and all the king's Robitussin had been unable to quell the coughing. The rest of his history is significant for no aversion to other sins of the flesh, with a positive result for the Venereal Disease Research Laboratory (VDRL), a toxicology screen that lit up like the millennial fireworks displays, and elevated liver enzyme levels consistent with a liquid diet unfettered by nonalcoholic beverages. Our surgical brethren assure us that time is of the essence because if the glass pipe breaks up, the shower of glass into the far nether regions of the lung would have a suboptimal effect on this young man's pulmonary status.

The patient has had no oral intake (NPO) for the past 12 hours. The physical examination is remarkable for a large beard, a Mallampati 2 airway score (edging toward 3), and a curious calliope-like sound with some of his coughs, which lends a carnival-ride atmosphere to the operating room (OR).

The surgeon plans a flexible bronchoscopy to remove the crack pipe from the trachea and right main stem bronchus. If that fails, he will perform rigid bronchoscopy. The procedure will be followed by a stern lecture about the evils of amateur pharmacology. If that fails, a discussion about how to inhale crack more safely in the future will have to suffice.

Intraoperative Questions

1. Besides the usual monitors recommended by the American Society of Anesthesiologists (ASA), what additional monitors would you place?
2. Does induction for a fiberoptic bronchoscopy differ from induction for a rigid bronchoscopy? If so, how? How are the goals different?
3. Does placement of the endotracheal tube (ETT) pose a potential threat to the placement of the foreign body? What if the foreign body were a peanut?
4. You induce and attempt to mask ventilate, but the heavy beard and mustache impede effective gas exchange. How do you modify your technique?

5. You attempt to place an 8.0-French ETT, but as sometimes happens, you cannot get a big tube in, and you are able to place a 7.0-French ETT. The surgeon says, "I cannot do this through a 7.0!" How do you help the surgeon?

6. Fiberoptic bronchoscopy fails. How do you conduct your anesthetic to allow for rigid bronchoscopy?

7. The surgeon has a hard time getting a big rigid bronchoscope into the trachea, and the patient desaturates to the mid-80s. He is still attempting to get the scope in. What do you do?

8. With the rigid bronchoscope in, the surgeon attempts to grasp the glass stem of the crack pipe, but it keeps "crumbling" every time he grabs it. What can you do to help?

9. The determination for a blood gas sample sent for evaluation in the middle of this epic struggle shows a pH of 7.23, P_{O_2} of 65 mm Hg, and P_{CO_2} of 69 mm Hg. What is your interpretation, and how do you intend to improve the patient's status?

10. After several attempts, the surgeon says, "Maybe we should wake him up and cancel this?" Are there any other alternatives?

Postoperative Questions

1. On the way to the postanesthesia care unit (PACU) the Foley catheter falls under a gurney wheel and snaps off. The end of it is not on the floor, but you cannot see anything on examining the patient. What do you do?

2. The glass stem is out, but the patient continues to cough violently. Is there anything else on the differential diagnosis for severe coughing? Is there anything you can do to alleviate this patient's distress?

3. A persistent sinus tachycardia of 120 beats/min gets the PACU nurse's attention. How do you evaluate this? Is it a concern in a 44-year-old man?

CASE 2: EXCEDRIN HEADACHE

Zvi Jacob

An 8-year-old, 37-kg girl is scheduled for a craniotomy because of a mass lesion. During the past 4 days, her parents noticed she was lethargic, complained about headaches, and had nausea. The girl's medical history identified no prior hospital admissions, and the workup for complaints of dizziness 6 months ago showed no pathology.

She has no known drug or food allergies. On examination, she was found to have a blood pressure of 128/50 mm Hg, heart rate 68 beats/min, and hemoglobin level of 13 g/dL. She had vomited three times a few hours ago. Yesterday's electrocardiogram (ECG) showed a normal sinus rhythm at 100 beats/min.

Preoperative Questions

1. What would be your neurologic examination of this patient?
2. What would be the anesthetic relevance?
3. How will you assess elevated intracranial pressure (ICP)?
4. Is magnetic resonance imaging (MRI) necessary? Is other imaging needed?
5. What laboratory studies will be helpful?
6. How will your findings affect your plan for premedication?

7. How will you assess the patient's volume status?
8. What type of fluid will you use for this case?
9. Will you add dextrose-containing solutions? Explain why or why not.
10. What monitors will you use? When a central venous pressure (CVP) monitor is indicated, how will you place it?
11. Will you include a precordial Doppler monitor?
12. What blood products should be available?

Intraoperative Questions

1. Describe your anesthetic plan for induction, maintenance, and emergence.
2. Please explain your anesthetic goals for this case. Are they different from those for adult patient management?
3. What are the risks during induction?
4. Discuss ways of controlling ICP during anesthesia.
5. During intracranial dissection, the patient suddenly becomes hypotensive and tachycardic. What is the differential diagnosis? If there is venous air embolism (VAE), what are the potential risks?
6. What methods are used to make the diagnosis? Which is the most sensitive?
7. What is your management plan for VAE?
8. Will you extubate this patient?

CASE 3: CT AND A BAG OF CHIPS

Chris Gallagher

A 5-foot 7-inch, 330-pound man is scheduled for cryoablation of a recurrent right posterior lung tumor under computed tomography (CT) guidance. His medical history is remarkable for an automatic implantable cardioverter defibrillator (AICD) placement, cardiomyopathy with an ejection fraction (EF) of 30%, and such poor pulmonary function that no surgeon is comfortable operating on him. The case is scheduled for general anesthesia and prone positioning in the CT scanner. He was operated on last year, and the surgeon smirks at you when he says, "They had a time of it last year."

Preoperative Questions

1. How can you honorably get the hell out of doing this case without dumping it on some unsuspecting colleague and incurring his or her eternal wrath?
2. What possible horrors are associated with the surgeon's comment, "They had a time of it last year"?
3. How will you determine the degree of the patient's pulmonary compromise?
4. Cryoablation will be done, but no cautery will be used. How do you manage the AICD? Is this different from "a regular case"?
5. How do you explain the risks of general anesthesia in these circumstances to this patient?
6. The surgeon and interventional radiologist concur that this is the only way to get the tumor. Do you need any further workup or laboratory studies? The patient has had a chest radiograph, electrocardiogram (ECG), and hematocrit determination.
7. The patient's rhythm is entirely paced. Discuss how this affects your assessment of the patient and the plan for your anesthetic. Does a magnet have any place here?

Intraoperative Questions

1. Physical examination shows a large tongue, thick neck, and an inability to lie down flat for any length of time. How will you secure the airway, keeping in mind you are "off site"?
2. As you are topicalizing and sedating for an awake intubation, the surgeon says, "They did not do this last year when they operated on him." Does this change your management plan? What do you say to the surgeon?
3. How do you manage sedation for this patient? How do you manage if a baseline arterial blood gas (ABG) determination puts the patient in the 60/60 club?
4. Do you need additional monitors other than the ASA standards?
5. You intubate successfully and move the patient to a prone position. Inspiratory pressures go up, and you are delivering only about 200 mL of tidal volume. What do you do?
6. After several ventilator adjustments, the end-tidal CO_2 level persistently remains at 75. Do you adjust the ventilator again? How? Do you cancel the case? What are the risks of a high CO_2 level?
7. Oxygen saturation drops to 89% when the patient is fully inside the CT scanner. What do you do?
8. How do you maintain anesthesia? Do you need muscle relaxants? If so, which muscle relaxants do you use?
9. At the end of the case, describe how you will ascertain this patient's readiness for extubation. Do you take any special precautions regarding the hypoxemic drive to breathe? Do you give any special considerations to the preoperative baseline CO_2 level?
10. Immediately on extubation, the patient breathes 40 times per minute, says he is short of breath, and keeps insisting you let him hang his feet down. What is your diagnosis? What is the treatment? Do you let him hang his feet down?

CASE 4: SOMETHING IS DISAGREEING WITH MY STOMACH

Chris Gallagher

A 36-year-old, mentally impaired woman (i.e., she can say a few things but cannot process anything you say to her) is scheduled for an exploratory laparotomy for a possible intra-abdominal abscess. She had congenital heart problems leading to an aortic valve replacement (AVR) and coronary artery bypass grafting (CABG) 4 years earlier. Her ejection fraction (EF) is now in the 20% range, and further surgery or stents are not practical because diffuse disease has recurred. She is having an infarction now, with troponin levels up and hemodynamic parameters consistent with sepsis. Her blood pressure is 90/60 mm Hg, heart rate is 145 beats/min (you double check, and it is 145), and temperature is 38.5°C. She has a red, sweaty face and flushed appearance. The surgeon says that without the operation, she will succumb soon. Her laboratory test results are remarkable for a hematocrit of 28% and the troponin levels. The ECG shows sinus tachycardia with ST-segment depression.

Intraoperative Questions

1. Invasive monitors are part of your plan, but the patient's mental status presents challenges. Which invasive monitors will you use, and how will you get them in, given these circumstances?

2. Describe the hemodynamic response to sepsis and how this plays against a background of evolving myocardial infarction (MI)?

3. Bleeding may be a concern. Should you use ε-aminocaproic acid? What is it, and how does it work?

4. This patient has a full stomach and an intra-abdominal abscess. How will you induce? Which induction agent will you use? Which muscle relaxant will you use? What are the potential complications associated with muscle relaxants?

5. The patient has buckteeth, and she holds her head off to one side. Airway examination is not possible. How will you proceed?

6. While attempting pre-oxygenation, the patient thrashes around and shouts, not allowing the mask on. How do you respond to this behavior? Attempting to place cricoid pressure also results in a violent response. How will you protect against aspiration? Are any medications indicated? Should they be given intravenously or orally?

7. You induce, get what you think is a good view, and place the ETT in the trachea, but there is no end-tidal CO_2 measurement. What do you do? How do you know you are in the correct place? What is the differential for a "tube in the right place but no CO_2"?

8. After induction, the heart rate hits 160 beats/min, and the blood pressure is 70/50 mm Hg. What are the end-organ implications, and how do you respond? Do you use β-blockers for cardiac protection or β-blockade in the setting of a "physiologic-response tachycardia"?

9. Things settle down after induction, and the heart rate is 130 beats/min. How will you decrease the heart rate and not cause a cardiovascular collapse? What monitors can guide you? How do you respond if the CVP measurement is 3 or 15? What do you do if the pulmonary artery catheter reads 20/5 or 45/33?

10. The patient continues to show instability, with a persistent systolic blood pressure in the 70s. How will you increase the blood pressure? If you use norepinephrine, how will you guide the therapy? The hematocrit level is 31%, but ischemia is evident on the ECG. Will you transfuse? Why or why not? What are the dangers of transfusion?

Postoperative Questions

1. The surgeon finds only ileus, and closes in 35 minutes. Do you extubate? What are extubation criteria? In the setting of ongoing ischemia, do you alter these extubation criteria?

2. The chest radiograph shows a whiteout of both lungs, and pink, frothy fluid is in the ETT. How will you evaluate this pulmonary finding? Will you use CT, or send endotracheal fluid for analysis? What are you looking for? The intensive care unit (ICU) staff members suggest changing the ETT to a larger one so they can suction the fluid more efficiently. Do you do this? How?

3. The patient has developed an air leak around the ETT. She can breathe around it, but her saturation is poor, and she needs positive end-expiratory pressure (PEEP). Her airway is swollen from fluids. How do you evaluate this air leak? What could it be? How will you change the tube? Will you use a tube changer or fiberoptic device? Do you have a tracheostomy kit on standby?

4. The nephrologist is concerned about renal damage during her episode of hypotension. What is a creatinine clearance value? Does this help you?

How? What techniques may help to prevent worsening renal function? Do you use dopamine? Will epinephrine and a higher cardiac output help? Is fluid restriction or fluid administration a good idea? Can insulin help the patient?

5. During a line change, you put a Swan-Ganz introducer into the subclavian artery. Do you pull out or keep it there? Do you apply pressure? You remove the Swan-Ganz line, and a half-hour later, the chest radiograph shows a hemithorax filled with fluid. The patient goes into shock. How do you proceed?

CASE 5: FIXING A BROKEN HEART

Chris Gallagher

A 72-year-old man ("I never went to a doctor in my life.") is admitted with a myocardial infarction (MI). He deteriorates, an intra-aortic balloon pump (IABP) is placed, and he is scheduled for emergent CABG. The cardiologist hears a loud murmur and, by echocardiography, diagnoses a ventricular septal defect (VSD) in the apical segment that will require repair.

Preoperative Questions

1. How does an IABP work? Describe how you time it correctly. What happens if it inflates too soon? Too late? If you turn it off? If it ruptures?
2. How can a 72-year-old man with no earlier history have a VSD? What would be the effect of a long-standing VSD? What is Eisenmenger's syndrome?
3. What special precautions will you take regarding lines as you set up this room? How do you prevent air bubbles? Paradoxical embolus? How can this occur if pressure is higher on the arterial side?
4. What additional laboratory studies do you need before going to the OR? Are blood typing and antibody screening sufficient? Will you order blood factors ahead of time? Which ones? Why?
5. What are the hazards of moving a patient with an IABP placed and vasoactive drips running? You see he has dobutamine running in a peripheral line. Do you have any concerns? Will you stop the dobutamine? Why or why not? What if you see the line is infiltrated? Is there any special treatment for the arm?

Intraoperative Questions

1. You have three, 20-gauge, peripheral intravenous lines in, some with inotropes running. How will you manage the lines for induction? Will you put in additional peripherals? Put in central lines? Which ones? What if the patient groans and complains during placement of a central line?
2. What are your choices of induction agents? Is etomidate a good choice? Is ketamine? Should you use a high-dose narcotic only? Should you use propofol? Which relaxant should you use? What if patient ate 3 hours ago? What are the dangers of succinylcholine if the patient had been lying in bed for 3 days?
3. The surgeon is concerned that bleeding will be a problem. Should you give ε-aminocaproic acid? What is it? How does it work?

4. Cardiac function is poor, and the surgeon suggests you need a Swan-Ganz catheter. Do you agree? How will you place it? If you do place it, and the trace suddenly shows arterial pressure. What could have happened? Now what do you do? Should you withdraw or keep it in place? Should you send a mixed venous blood gas sample for evaluation? What would it show?

5. How will you prepare for separating from cardiopulmonary bypass? The patient's hematocrit is 22%; do you transfuse? Do you wait until you are off bypass? The patient's potassium level is 3.4; should you give him potassium or wait? If the potassium level is 6.8, should you treat or wait? The clamp has been off only 12 minutes, but the surgeon says it is okay to come off. Do you agree or disagree? Why?

6. When the patient comes off bypass, bleeding from the back of the heart is brisk, and the surgeon says to give blood factors. There is a surgical incision in the back of the heart. Which factors will you give and why? Do you have any other suggestions?

7. Each time the surgeon lifts the heart, the IABP has a hard time picking up and following. What is your diagnosis? What can you do to help the situation? Should you trigger off the ECG or the arterial pressure? Should you slow the heart rate or speed up the heart rate?

8. With manipulation, the pacer is having trouble. How does a pacer work? How should you set the pacer? What if it does not pick up? What about this case specifically makes pacing a concern? Describe the conduction system of the heart.

9. At what point do you tell the surgeon to go back on bypass and fix the hole? Should an anesthesiologist make a "surgical recommendation"? Why or why not? What are the dangers of going on bypass a second time? Will the patient have a systemic inflammatory response? What are the dangers of massive transfusion in this setting?

10. The chest is closed, and the surgeon asks for a transesophageal echocardiography (TEE) assessment. What will you be looking for? How will you tell if the VSD is still open? Should you float a Swan-Ganz catheter now? Using the Swan-Ganz catheter, how could you tell if the VSD is still open? If you see a regional wall motion abnormality, what does it signify? How will you manage this? Should you use nitroglycerin or reopen the patient?

CASE 6: CONSCIOUS SEDATION

Chris Gallagher

A 25-year-old, 5-foot 4-inch, 290-pound woman is scheduled for an emergent MRI for possible cauda equina syndrome. When she arrives in the radiology department, she is heavily bejeweled, multiply pierced, and vociferously bemoaning her woes and travails on earth. "I always get conscious sedation for MRI," she states with practiced certainty. With that, she slaps the back of her hand against her forehead and falls back in the gurney with a resounding thump.

Preoperative Questions

1. What further information do you need regarding this patient's history? If she were healthy other than herniated disks and back pain, do you need any

laboratory studies? Do you need a human chorionic gonadotropin determination? What if she says there is no possibility she is pregnant?

2. What is cauda equina syndrome? What history will you elicit? What are the physical findings? Is this an emergency? Is it up to you to decide whether this is an emergency?

3. It is now 3:30 PM, and the patient last ate at 6 AM. Does she have a full stomach? If she went to the emergency room at 8 AM and received Dilaudid and morphine intravenously, does this information change your assessment? Should you give her an antacid, metoclopramide, or anticholinergic therapy?

4. She states she "always gets conscious sedation for her MRI scans." What is conscious sedation? What are the risks of conscious sedation? What are the risks in the setting of MRI? What, specific to MRI, contributes to problems with claustrophobic patients? Can you cancel the case and insist she go to a place with an open MRI?

5. The patient hops off the bed, walks over to the MRI, and lies down on the table without any problems. Does this change anything? If your clinical assessment is that she does not have cauda equina, can you cancel this case? Can you postpone it until she has less of a full stomach?

Intraoperative Questions

1. Describe the special considerations in conducting an anesthetic in an MRI machine. Can she wear jewelry? What dangers are there? What about using a laryngoscope, monitors, or an anesthesia machine?

2. What is your choice of anesthetic and sedation? What methods do you use? Can you use a propofol drip, midazolam and fentanyl, or dexmedetomidine? What are the advantages and disadvantages of each approach?

3. You sedate with propofol, but the patient keeps wiggling around, complaining that her back hurts, and is unable to hold still. The MRI technician says he cannot get a good study. How do you increase sedation? What are the general risks and those specific to MRI?

4. The patient's airway obstructs, and you can no longer see an end-tidal CO_2 trace. What do you do? When you pull her out, you see her airway is obstructed, but by vigorous shaking, you can get her to open her own airway. Should you resedate and send her back in?

5. At what point would you proceed to general anesthesia? What are the risks of general anesthesia compared with sedation? Is one safer than the other? Do you induce on the MRI table or on the gurney? If she has a difficult airway, where is the safest place to intubate her? What if there is a problem with the fiberoptic intubation and MRI?

6. You induce and place a laryngeal mask airway (LMA). When the patient is in the MRI scanner, the end-tidal CO_2 monitor looks funny—partially blocked maybe—and the oxygen saturation level drops from 99% to 83%. What is the differential diagnosis? You pull her out, and you see green fluid in the LMA. What is your next move?

7. On removal of the LMA, you see emesis in the back of her throat. The MRI table does not have a Trendelenburg button. What do you do? If the suction pulls out of the wall, do you go ahead and intubate through the emesis? What is the remedy for aspiration at this point?

8. You intubate, and the oxygen saturation level is 88%. Do you proceed with the rest of the MRI study? What if the diagnosis of cauda equina syndrome

is not yet made? Do you use PEEP? How much? What are the drawbacks and limitations of PEEP?

9. While working on the aspiration, you failed to notice the blood pressure, and now the blood pressure alarm is going off. The patient is on 3% sevoflurane, and you cannot feel a pulse. What do you do? Describe the effects of high inspired potent inhaled agents in the setting of a cardiovascular collapse?

10. Will you extubate at the end of the case? Would you extubate if her oxygen saturation level was 95% on 50% oxygen? A colleague suggests extubating and, if she needs it, giving her continuous positive airway pressure (CPAP) by mask. Is this a good idea? How does mask CPAP work? In what setting is mask CPAP a good idea?

CASE 7: EAR TUBES: WHAT COULD BE EASIER?

Peggy Seidman and Steve Probst
A 20-month-old, 17-kg child with trisomy 21 presents for outpatient bilateral myringotomies for placement of pressure-equalization tubes.

Preoperative Questions

1. What are normal expectations for a child with trisomy 21? What are the cardiac, airway, and gastrointestinal problems? Do you expect parental separation issues? Is line placement different?

2. Go into detail regarding cardiac issues for patients with trisomy 21. What is an endocardial cushion defect? What are the implications of a VSD repair or an atrial septal defect (ASD) repair? Should an intracardiac patch or primary repair be done? Is subacute bacterial endocarditis (SBE) prophylaxis necessary for this case?

3. Is sedation appropriate for this child? If so, which sedative should be used? What if the child were younger? What if the child were older? What if the child did not have trisomy 21? When would it be appropriate for the parents to be present at induction? What if the parents behave inappropriately in the holding area?

4. Is laboratory work necessary? If so, which studies should be ordered? Do you need a chest radiograph, C-spine film, abdominal film, or MRI scan? The child has had corrective heart surgery; do you need a baseline ECG?

5. Discuss the management of the patient's NPO status? Is there any difference for a patient with trisomy 21? Is there any difference if the child is on reflux precautions? Discuss clear liquids versus regular food. If the child's body mass index (BMI) is greater than 35, would that change your NPO management?

Intraoperative Questions

1. Do you perform an intravenous or a mask induction? Why or why not? Which agent would you use and why? What if you have difficulty placing an intravenous line? Do you even need an intravenous line for this case? A colleague suggests you skip it.

2. You do a mask induction with sevoflurane, nitrous oxide, and oxygen, and the child goes into laryngospasm at a 3% sevoflurane end-tidal level. What do you do? Should you increase or decrease the level of sevoflurane?

Should you adjust the nitrous oxide level? Should you awaken the patient or give something intramuscularly?

3. Laryngospasm was not broken with earlier maneuvers (e.g., increasing sevoflurane, turning off the nitrous oxide, maintaining 20 cm H_2O positive pressure). How do you break the laryngospasm? The patient's heart rate is 80 beats/min, and the oxygen saturation level is 35%.

4. Laryngospasm resolves, and the patient is stable. The surgeon is anxious to proceed. How will you manage the rest of the case? Will you use a mask, LMA, ETT, or intravenous line? Should you cancel the case because of airway complications?

5. You choose to intubate. What is your choice of blade and ETT size? You place the 1.5 Wis-Hipple laryngoscope and you see redundant pharyngeal tissue; how do you manage this? A second look with a different blade reveals the same view. Now what do you do?

6. Do you need neuromuscular blockade for intubation? The procedure will require 15 minutes of surgical time according to the surgeon. Can you use suxamethonium? Why or why not? Is rocuronium a better choice? What is the dosage?

7. On 4% sevoflurane, the heart rate drops from 120 to 4 beats/min (yes, 4). You have no intravenous line. What is your treatment plan? Will you use cardiopulmonary resuscitation (CPR), intramuscular atropine, or intramuscular epinephrine? Will you place a line? Will you administer epinephrine or bicarbonate through the ETT? Should you consider intraosseous placement for line access?

8. Several attempts at intravenous access have failed. How many times should you "go peripheral" before you "go central"? Discuss the intraosseous option. What if the child were 10 years old? Where is the best place to establish central access?

9. The surgeon cannot visualize the tympanic membrane, and the case is now of indefinite length. You have been doing the case by mask for 30 minutes. Do you change? Do you place an LMA or ETT?

10. You did the entire case without an intravenous line by using mask ventilation. How do you manage post-emergence delirium? How do you manage pain control? Do you need to give anything for ear tubes? Would you use rectal Tylenol, intramuscular ketorolac, intranasal fentanyl, intramuscular morphine, intramuscular Demerol, or intramuscular ketamine?

CASE 8: UNRELENTING MISERY

Chris Gallagher

A 47-year-old, 50-kg woman has metastatic breast carcinoma. She has a large metastatic lesion in the middle of her femoral shaft and is scheduled for a "prophylactic pinning" because the orthopedic surgeon thinks the bone could snap at any minute. On examination, the patient looks cachectic, drained, and miserable. She has had chemotherapy and radiation therapy, all to no avail. Her bone scan shows lesions everywhere, including her back.

Laboratory test results are remarkable for a hematocrit of 27%, platelet count of 145,000, albumin level just below the lower limits of normal, and normal values for the prothrombin time (PT) and partial thromboplastin time (PTT). The chest radiograph showed disease there, with small effusions on both sides. The ECG showed sinus tachycardia, and her electrolyte levels were all normal.

Intraoperative Questions

1. Should you use invasive monitors? Why or why not? If you decide on an arterial line, would you place it before or after induction? If you decide on a CVP line, would you place it before or after induction? Why?

2. You attempt a left radial arterial line, but you create a hematoma. The patient is groaning and complaining that her entire life consists of needle sticks and nausea from chemotherapy. Do you continue? Do you go to another site? Which site? If you "end up having to go femoral," do you first induce, or do you "topicalize better" and proceed. What are the risks of a femoral arterial line?

3. Just as you are about to induce, a medical student (going into anesthesia) asks whether you consider her to be a "full stomach." Do you perform a rapid-sequence induction (RSI)? What are the risks of RSI compared with modified RSI and with regular induction?

4. You induce with propofol and rocuronium. Just before intubating, you see the blood pressure is 60/40 mm Hg. Do you intubate right away? Do you give her a pressor? If you "release fluids wide open," how much fluid gets in over a minute through a 20-gauge peripheral line? After intubation, the blood pressure is still 60/40 mm Hg. What is your management plan? What is the effect of putting her head down?

5. With incision, the patient moves. Your twitch monitor showed no twitches with train of four and none with tetanus. How does a twitch monitor work? How could the patient move with no muscle twitches? Do you give more relaxant? Does an allergic reaction to the relaxant explain the earlier hypotension?

6. With the patient's poor nutritional status, what problems can you anticipate with your anesthetic? What does a low albumin level mean to us? Is there any effect on the volume of distribution? What is the volume of distribution?

7. As the surgeon drills through the femoral shaft, the end-tidal CO_2 wave suddenly disappears. What could explain this? How can the monitor malfunction? Can it be explained by a kink, pathophysiologic reason, or embolus?

8. You see yellow fluid filling the end-tidal CO_2 sampling line, running all the way back up into the Defend container, and snaking its way up and into the guts of your machine. What effect will this have on your equipment? How did this happen? Explain the possibilities of a fat embolus, regular embolus, and congestive heart failure (CHF). How will you make the diagnosis?

9. The blood pressure drops to 70/45 mm Hg, you lose the saturation waveform, and ST-segment depression occurs. What explains these hemodynamic findings? How will you manage this situation? Explain your choice of hemodynamic support and monitoring.

10. The ETT keeps filling with yellow fluid. Should you use suction? Explain your choice in terms of Starling forces. What if fluid dries and obstructs? She has a 7.0-French ETT in; should you change the tube? If the instability continues, do you cancel the case? What do you tell the surgeon?

Cases from Real Life

Postoperative Questions

1. During transfer to the bed to go to the ICU, the patient goes from a right lateral decubitus position to supine. What physiologic alterations occur with this change? Is there any chance for hemodynamic worsening with this move? Will oxygenation worsen, or will it improve—or can you tell?
2. On arrival to the ICU, the patient arrests. Describe how you proceed through advanced cardiac life support (ACLS) protocol in the setting of the patient's fat embolus. At what point do you open the chest and attempt surgical removal of the embolus from the pulmonary artery?
3. The patient is successfully resuscitated, and TEE is called for. What would you expect to see if an embolus is the correct diagnosis? What would you see if CHF is the diagnosis? What other findings on TEE could help with her management?
4. In the ICU, the patient's blood gas assessment shows a Po_2 level of 55 on 100% oxygen. How can you improve her oxygenation? You institute PEEP, and things get worse. Explain this result. Using TEE, could anything explain this refractory hypoxemia? Can anything related to West's zones 1, 2, or 3 explain this?
5. The husband comes in the ICU and is alarmed at the turn of events. "But she's a no-code!" he yells. She did not want to end up on a ton of tubes and stuff. "Let her go!" How do you respond to this new information? Is she a no-code? What are the ethics of letting her go now?

CASE 9: WHAT WAS THAT POPPING SOUND?

Chris Gallagher

A 38-year-old, previously healthy man presented for clipping of a giant aneurysm in his anterior communicating artery in the Circle of Willis. His laboratory work is fine, results of the physical examination are normal, and his only complaint is blurred vision.

The surgical plan is complex, involving near dismantling of his face to get at this difficult-to-approach lesion. Many hours of dissection are planned, and a tracheostomy is planned as well. The chest radiograph and ECG results are normal. Earlier attempts at "coiling" the lesion failed.

Intraoperative Questions

1. Discuss the risks inherent in placing a tracheostomy, including the possibilities of an airway fire and subcutaneous emphysema. Should you intubate first and then do the tracheostomy, or do the tracheostomy with the patient awake? In what situation would you do the tracheostomy first?
2. Before induction, consider the blurred vision complaint. Is it evidence of increased ICP? What does it mean in the absence of other signs? Are there any risks with "assuming increased ICP" and proceeding "as if he has it for sure"? How do you induce a patient with increased ICP?
3. Which invasive monitors will you use for this long, complicated case? Is there any need for specialized CVP if you are concerned about an air embolus? What are the complications with placing such a CVP line? What constitutes the best placement for a central, internal jugular, external jugular, subclavian, or femoral line?

4. The surgeon performs a fantastically complicated dissection through the face. What are the dangers with dissection around the eye? The heart rate drops to 35 beats/min while pulling on the eye. What is the mechanism, and what is the treatment? How will you paralyze and maintain paralysis to ensure the patient does not buck at the absolute worst time?

5. A bulging brain is a problem as dissection continues. How do you assist the surgeon? Do you use mannitol? What is the mechanism and what are the shortcomings of mannitol? Should you use Lasix? Should you employ hyperventilation? What are the problems with hyperventilation?

6. The surgeon is nearing the base of this monster and asks for "the most hypotension you can possibly give." How do you manage this? Do you use potent inhaled agents? What are the problems with that approach? Do you use narcotics, vasodilators, nicardipine, or pentathol? What are the advantages and disadvantages of each?

7. The blood pressure is 70/50 mm Hg, and there is no ectopy or ST-segment change. The surgeon says, " I need lower pressure, or this guy is going to die." How much lower can you go? What problems do you anticipate? Are there any options at this point other than going lower and lower?

8. A faint "pop" is heard. The blood pressure increases to 280/150 mm Hg, and the heart rate drops into the 30s. What could explain this—syringe swap or infusion of a wrong inotrope? What is the pathophysiologic mechanism? What is your response? What is the best way to control "absolutely out of control hypertension"?

9. The surgeon says, "Oh, damn!" You look over the field, and you see the brain bulging up like a basketball from the skull. The sulci are flattened, and the normal gray of the brain has become fiery red and looks hemorrhagic. What caused this? What options do you have at this point? Should you accept electroencephalographic (EEG) silence or resort to hyperventilation as a desperation maneuver?

10. The organ donation consultant is called. How do you manage the hemodynamics and intracranial issues as preparation is made to transfer the patient to the ICU? What hemodynamic changes can you anticipate in the brain-dead patient?

Postoperative Questions

1. In the ICU, the patient starts putting out 1.5 L of urine each hour. What could be causing this? Is it diabetes insipidus? What is the mechanism? What about mannitol infusion? What is the mechanism of diuresis with mannitol? What is the treatment if the patient has diabetes insipidus?

2. An air leak develops around the cuff, and the patient cannot be ventilated adequately. How can you change the tube? Is the intubating stylet ready? What about fiberoptic access, a tube changer, or direct laryngoscopy? What if the patient is extremely swollen?

3. Plans include harvesting the heart. As you are planning to go back to the OR, the patient becomes hemodynamically unstable. How can you stabilize the patient but not endanger the heart and keep it viable for another organ recipient?

4. During the organ harvest, how do you manage the anesthetic? Do you use muscle relaxants, narcotics, or potent inhaled agents? If the patient is brain dead, do you need to do anything at all? Why or why not?

5. The surgeon asks for heparin as he is about to clamp the aorta and dissect out the heart. You give 3 mL of heparin, thinking it is the 10,000 U/mL concentration of heparin. As the surgeon clamps, you look down and see you gave the 1000 U/mL concentration of heparin, thereby severely underdosing. What do you do?

CASE 10: A GUSHER

Syed Shah

A 35-year-old man with history of intravenous drug abuse, human immunodeficiency virus (HIV) infection, and endocarditis presents for aortic valve replacement. There was no stenosis, but he had moderate aortic insufficiency. His laboratory test results were normal, and the physical examination showed a normal airway. The chest radiograph was normal, as was the CT scan of the chest.

The patient was lined up in the usual way for a cardiac procedure, with a left, radial, 20-gauge arterial line and a right arm, 16-gauge, peripheral intravenous line. Plans were to induce and then place a right intrajugular Cordis and Swan-Ganz catheter. Just before induction, vital signs were all normal.

Intraoperative Questions

1. A colleague suggests you place the Swan-Ganz catheter before induction. Is this necessary? Why or why not? What is the value of pre-induction "numbers" in the setting of cardiac surgery?
2. Would TEE and a CVP line serve just as well to monitor the patient? How about a TEE and a Cordis, a TEE and several big peripheral lines, or a CVP with no TEE? Are there any special considerations for the HIV-positive patient and the use of TEE?
3. Which induction agents should you use? Do you "have to use etomidate" because you are in the heart room? Should you use pentathol, ketamine, or propofol? Describe the pros and cons of each. Does any outcome study show a difference?
4. With laryngoscopy, his heart rate drops into the 30s. What is the mechanism, and is treatment necessary? What should be done in the setting of aortic regurgitation? Should you forge ahead and intubate, or should you treat before you intubate?
5. With sternotomy, the surgeon says "Oh, damn!" What are the implications of such a statement? What are the dangers during sternotomy? What could have gone wrong? Is there any difference when this is a repeat operation?
6. The left arterial line dampens and registers a blood pressure in the 20s and 30s. That is the differential diagnosis for a severely damped arterial line? With retraction, you see bright arterial blood shooting above the level of the screen. What is your management plan at this point?
7. The aorta and left subclavian are torn open by the saw. How do you manage this catastrophe? Address the issues of the anesthetic level, resuscitation, muscle relaxation, rapid transfusion, and dangers of rapid transfusion. When do you get a rapid infuser? Do you use the cardiopulmonary bypass machine to transfuse?
8. You place the patient on femoral-femoral bypass. What is the difference between this approach and conventional bypass? What are the problems

with femoral-femoral bypass? What are the advantages? What if the perfusionists say they cannot get enough flow? How would a blood gas measurement reflect inadequate flow?

9. A blood gas determination shows a pH of 7.03 on bypass. How will you manage this? Will you use bicarbonate or just let adequate perfusion take place? What are the problems with using bicarbonate? How about using tris(hydroxymethyl)aminomethane (THAM)? The blood gas determination also shows a hematocrit of 17%. Should you transfuse? Should you wait until you come off bypass and then transfuse?

10. As you are coming off bypass, a TEE examination shows a perivalvular leak. What is the implication? What if the TEE study shows a small amount of central regurgitation? How would a tissue valve look compared with a prosthetic valve?

Postoperative Questions

1. Concern is raised about the patient's neurologic status. How do you evaluate this in the immediate postoperative period? Would you use muscle relaxants, narcotics, or sedatives? Do you go to CT right away? Would bispectral (BIS) index monitoring be helpful? Would an EEG study help? What is the timing for each of these methods?

2. The patient's lactic acid level is progressively increasing. What could be causing this? Something in the gut or leg? What if the patient has an IABP? What if the amylase level rises? Does this indicate pancreatitis? What is the treatment? What is abdominal compartment syndrome, and how do you treat it?

3. Bleeding is noticed in the chest tubes. How much bleeding is acceptable? When would you need to re-explore? The surgeon says to give more fresh-frozen plasma (FFP). Do you agree? Why or why not? How would you diagnose tamponade?

4. Two days later, the blood pressure is 70/60 mm Hg, the heart rate is 130 beats/min, and the cardiac output is 8 L/m. What is your diagnosis? Is something other than sepsis possible? What is the treatment? The surgeon is horrified when he sees what you are doing. Explain the rationale for the use of any vasoactive drugs.

5. The neurologic workup shows no brain activity after 1 week. What are the criteria for brain death? Do you need blood flow studies? Is a clinical examination alone sufficient? Do you need a CT or EEG study? Do you try carbon dioxide and see if that stimulates breathing?

CASE 11: GUMMING UP THE PULMONARY WORKS

Shaji Poovathor

A 66-year-old woman, who is 5 feet 5.5 inches tall and weighs 108 kg, is admitted in the ICU for treatment of documented pulmonary embolism and deep venous thrombosis of her right lower extremity. She has a history significant for hepatitis C, arthritis, bladder cancer, asthma, and diabetes. Her current medications include dexamethasone (replacing her home prednisone dose, which she was on for the past 2 years), sliding-scale insulin, Atrovent and albuterol nebulizer on an as-needed basis, and heparin drip running at 800 units/hr, being titrated per protocol. She is on a nasal cannula at 2 L/min.

Her oxygen saturation ranges from 95% to 97%. She is awake, alert, and oriented. Her vital signs are a heart rate of 98 beats/min, blood pressure of 165-180/90-105 mm Hg, temperature of 37.7°C, and respiratory rate of 28 to 35 breaths/min. Her airway examination result is Mallampati class 2, with a full range of neck motion, and she has no upper or lower teeth. You get a call from the general surgeon that she now has an "acute abdomen" with air under the diaphragm. She goes into the OR with an indwelling right-side, triple-lumen catheter. The heparin drip is off. Stress-dose steroid medication is administered.

Intraoperative Questions

1. What monitors do you want to use in this patient and why?
2. Do you want an arterial line before or after induction? Why or why not?
3. How would you induce this patient? What is your induction agent of choice? Why?
4. On induction, the patient desaturates to 88%. What is your response?
5. The blood pressure is 90/40 mm Hg. Her oxygen saturation level is 77%, and the saturation level is slowly declining. What are your first reflex thoughts and actions?
6. What are you going to do with the ventilatory settings? Would you use PEEP? If so, how much PEEP?
7. The surgeon opens the peritoneum and finds bile spillage throughout. After a while, as he retracts the first part of duodenum to look for any possible perforation, the heart rate drops to 40 from 89 beats/min. What is your first response?
8. One hour into the procedure, the peak airway pressure rises to 44 from 31 cm H_2O. What is the differential diagnosis, and what is your response?
9. Would you extubate this patient in the OR? Why or why not?

Postoperative Questions

1. You decide to keep the patient intubated. What type of ventilatory mode would you prefer in this patient? Why?
2. The surgical ICU resident tells you that the heparin drip needs to be restarted. What is your response?
3. As you are about to leave the ICU, the nurse calls you and shouts, "Her oxygen saturation is 95%." What is your response to the nurse?
4. You take care of the situation in the previous question, and then you go down to the OR to set up for another case. The same nurse calls and tells you, "The patient's saturation is now 85%." What is your response, other than exclaiming *damn* again?
5. What is the difference between low-molecular-weight heparin (LMWH) and unfractionated heparin?

CASE 12: TRAUMATIC DISORDER DURING PREGNANCY

Ellen Steinberg and Jian Lin

A 32-year-old, gravida 3, para 2 woman who was at about 35 weeks' estimated gestational age is brought to the shock-trauma department immediately after a motor vehicle accident. She has obvious extensive orthopedic injuries and other undetermined injuries and had to be extricated from her car. You arrive in the emergency room (ER) as part of the trauma team.

Preoperative Questions

1. What are the initial steps for evaluating a pregnant trauma patient?
2. How should the patient be positioned during the evaluation?
3. What, if any, radiologic procedures should be performed on this patient? Why or why not? Would your choice of radiologic evaluation be affected if the pregnancy were at 8 weeks' estimated gestational age? What about 17 weeks' estimated gestational age?

Intraoperative Questions

The patient has had two prior cesarean sections. Her blood pressure is 100/60 mm Hg, and her pulse is 110 beats/min. She weighs 300 pounds. She is responsive and breathing spontaneously, feels a bit short of breath, and is complaining of severe pain. The fetal heart rate is 60 beats/min. The obstetrician wants to do an immediate cesarean section in the shock-trauma department!

1. How will you proceed?
2. What are the anesthetic considerations in this situation?
3. What are the indications for an emergency cesarean section in the shock-trauma department?
4. What is the CPR protocol for pregnant women? What is the optimal time from the start of cardiac arrest to delivery of the fetus in terms of maternal-fetal morbidity and mortality? Is CPR effective in the pregnant patient?
5. What problems would you anticipate intraoperatively in this patient?

CASE 13: THORACO WHACKO

Roy Soto and Robert Trainer

The chief of surgery asks you to come to the vascular clinic to evaluate a thin, elderly patient who is a potential candidate for surgery. The patient is an 80-year-old, 50-kg man with a large thoracoabdominal aneurysm. The surgical plan is endovascular repair of the aneurysm under local anesthesia in about a month, but the patient first requires a debranching procedure, in which the celiac, mesenteric, and renal arteries are detached from the aneurysm wall and reattached elsewhere. This is done to ensure good blood flow after the endovascular procedure; otherwise, the endovascular graft would occlude all of these vessels. The patient uses no medications other than inhalers and has been using home oxygen therapy for 3 months after a bout of pneumonia. He uses the oxygen "only when I sleep," and he has fair exercise tolerance, claiming that he can climb a flight of stairs without a problem. Preoperative dobutamine echocardiography reveals an EF of 55% and no reversible ischemia. The procedure will require 3 hours, and the surgeon asks you several questions.

Preoperative Questions

1. Can you do this procedure under spinal or epidural anesthesia only?
2. Would it matter if the surgeon makes a horizontal chevron incision or a typical midline incision?
3. Will you be able to extubate this patient?

You decide that the patient is "good to go," and tell him and the surgeon as much in the clinic. You choose a combined epidural and general anesthesia technique. Chart review reveals that the patient was taking oral steroids for about a month, but that he stopped 3 months ago.

Intraoperative Questions

1. What is your detailed plan for monitoring, induction, maintenance, emergence, and perioperative pain management?
2. What is your plan for fluid management?
3. Should he have been given a course of perioperative steroids? If so, why and how much of what kind? Back up your answer with evidence-based literature.

CASE 14: LITTLE CASE WITH A BIG CONCERN

Roy Soto and Robert Trainer

A 95-year-old man is brought to the OR for cystoscopy and transurethral resection of a bladder tumor (TURBT). You have seen his name on the add-on schedule for days, and you have prayed that he not come to your room, but alas, there is no avoiding it. He is all yours now! He lives alone and has a nurse who visits him daily. He was doing well and managing to get around his apartment with a walker until he developed painless hematuria. He was admitted and treated for a urinary tract infection (UTI). He developed urosepsis, developed CHF, and had a significant MI. His medical history is significant for hypertension, critical aortic stenosis, a few MIs (including the week before the proposed operation), and CHF, which is "fairly well controlled" with Lasix as needed. The cheerful cardiology note mentions an EF of 25% and states that he is "at high risk for a perioperative event even with a low-risk procedure."

He comes to the preoperative area slightly confused but looking reasonably well. His blood pressure is 95/50 mm Hg, and his heart rate is 70 beats/min. He has slight rales identified on the bilateral lung examination, but he seems to be in no respiratory distress while lying flat on the gurney.

1. What are the anesthetic goals of managing a patient with critical aortic stenosis?
2. What are the anesthetic goals of managing an elderly patient with CHF?
3. What are the anesthetic goals of managing a patient with a recent MI?
4. What is your detailed anesthetic plan, including monitoring, induction and regional technique, airway management, maintenance, pain control, and fluid replacement?

CASE 15: HEARTBREAK HOTEL

Zvi Jacob and Robert Trainer

A 3-year-, 2-month-old girl with dilated cardiomyopathy initially presented when she was 7 months old. She had a history of ventricular dysrhythmias identified on Holter monitoring. She recently was found to have many dental caries. Current medications include digoxin (60 μg every 12 hours), carvedilol (4 mg every 12 hours), enalapril (2.5 mg every 12 hours), and aspirin (40.5 mg once daily). Pertinent physical findings include height (37 inches) in the 40th percentile and weight (28 pounds) in the 20th percentile. Her respiratory rate was slightly elevated at 30 breaths/min. Otherwise, the child was resting comfortably. Her skin was pink, and pulses were strong and symmetric in all extremities. Lungs were clear to auscultation bilaterally (CTAB), and pulse oximetry showed her oxygenation was 99%. Cardiac examination revealed a point of maximal impulse displaced to the left, mid-lower costal area, with a grade 3/6 blowing holosystolic murmur best heard at the left, lower sternal border and with a 2/4 mid-diastolic rumble at the apex.

An echocardiogram performed immediately preoperatively showed dilated cardiomyopathy. The left ventricle was severely hypokinetic, with a regional wall motion abnormality (RWMA), especially in the septal area. The left atrium was severely dilated, and severe mitral regurgitation was seen. Other pertinent laboratory test results include a B-type natriuretic peptide level within normal limits, chem-8 test results within normal limits, hematocrit of 32.5, and ECG results showing a sinus rhythm with left atrial and left ventricular enlargement at 96 beats/min.

The plan was discussed with the parents and the oral surgeon to avoid epinephrine in local anesthetics and to include ampicillin for subacute bacterial endocarditis (SBE) prophylaxis.

1. What is the incidence of pediatric cardiomyopathy?
2. What are your concerns about this patient?
3. How would you monitor this patient?
4. Would you use a volatile anesthetic in a patient with already depressed myocardial function?
5. As the case proceeds, the patient's blood pressure and heart rate begin to drop. What agent would you use to rescue this patient?

CASE 16: SOME CHOLECYSTECTOMIES ARE MORE INVOLVED THAN OTHERS

Robert Katz and Timothy Ueng

A 38-year-old woman with a history of hypercholesterolemia, who had an anterior wall MI 2 years earlier, is scheduled for a cholecystectomy. At the time of her MI, she also had a cerebrovascular accident, with resultant bilateral leg weakness. CT of her head shows an old frontal lobe infarction. Her EF is 30%. She is pregnant, at term, and will need a cesarean section. Laboratory test results, miracle of miracles, are normal.

Preoperative Questions

1. What are the American College of Cardiology/American Heart Association (ACC/AHA) recommendations regarding preoperative cardiac evaluation in this patient?
2. Should β-blockade be instituted in the preoperative period? If so, how far in advance of surgery should it be done?
3. What additional cardiac stress does term pregnancy incur?
4. What other physiologic changes of pregnancy increase perioperative risk in this patient?
5. What anesthetic options would you present to this patient? Which will you recommend?

Intraoperative Questions

1. What perioperative monitoring do you recommend?
2. Would you put in a pulmonary artery catheter? Why or why not?
3. Would you do a spinal for this case? Why or why not?
4. If you choose general anesthesia, what induction agents will you use?
5. If you choose general anesthesia, what maintenance agents will you use?
6. What anesthetic technique or techniques will you choose? Describe the pros and cons.
7. If you choose an epidural, what agent or agents will you use? Would you use a local anesthetic containing epinephrine?
8. The infant is delivered with Apgar scores of 9 and 9. Five minutes later, the patient suffers a cardiac arrest. What is your differential diagnosis?
9. What clinical signs, symptoms, or monitor readings would support the various diagnoses in your differential?
10. The patient is intubated. CPR is begun. The cardiac rhythm returns to sinus, and the patient regains consciousness. Would you continue with the cholecystectomy? Why or why not?

CASE 17: FROM RUSSIA WITH LOVE

Igor Izrailtyan

A 64-year-old Russian Cossack in the ICU is recovering from right pneum onectomy. He is now septic and scheduled for an exploratory thoracotomy to drain suspected purulent material. His laboratory test results are consistent with sepsis, with a high white cell count, tachycardia, and low blood pressure (90/60 mm Hg). He is not intubated but is in respiratory distress.

Preoperative Questions

1. What are the implications of sepsis in this patient? What are all the hemodynamic parameters you may see? What will an echocardiogram show?
2. Because the patient is septic, will you delay this case? Will you recommend they drain under local anesthesia in the ICU? Is it your place to tell a surgeon what procedure to do?
3. The preoperative potassium level is 7.5, but the patient has no history of renal disease. What will you do? Will you proceed or wait for a repeat procedure? How does hemolysis affect your laboratory test results?
4. Define respiratory distress in the ICU. Would you intubate before moving the patient to the OR? Do you need an ABG determination? If the ABG evaluation shows a P_{O_2} of 61 mm Hg, do you need to intubate? What if the value is 51 mm Hg? Should you wait for the controlled conditions of the OR?
5. Is a thoracic epidural a good idea? Why or why not? The surgeon says it will help with splinting, and the family wants him to be comfortable. What is your response?

Intraoperative Questions

1. What monitors will you place? Defend which side you will put the central line on. Explain the dangers of left-sided central lines. The resident says he never puts in subclavian lines. Is this a good patient to practice on?

2. What is the best way to isolate the remaining lung? Do you need to worry about isolating the lung because there is only one? What are the dangers of bronchial blockers in patients after recent surgery?

3. This patient is 6 feet 5 inches tall and weighs 120 kg. Are there any special concerns given the weight and the height? How do you determine how deep to place the ETT?

4. You notice a leak on the ventilatory circuit. What are the potential sources of leaks in the system? What devices are built into the system to detect leaks or detect line crossovers?

5. As you are trying to bag ventilate the patient, the leak suddenly becomes catastrophically large, and you cannot move any air. What do you do? Can the surgeon help you?

6. Is there any advantage to a double-lumen tube in this case? How would it work in the post-pneumonectomy setting? Should it be right or left sided?

7. While attempting to place a different ETT, you notice (how did you miss this?) that the patient has an old tracheostomy site. Can using the tracheostomy site help? How?

8. The saturation drops to 65%, and the patient develops multifocal ectopy. Do you treat with lidocaine or amiodarone? Do you not treat with anything and keep working on the saturation alone?

9. At the end of the case, would you extubate this patient? Would you keep a single-lumen tube in? How about a bronchial blocker or a double-lumen tube? What are the problems of sending the patient to the ICU with a double-lumen ETT?

10. The ICU staff members say they are unfamiliar with the double-lumen ETT. What in-service training will you offer them? What are other options? Should you change the tube the next day or in a few days? What are the problems with sedation with a tube sitting on the carina?

CASE 18: TO LIVE FOREVER, NEVER SEE A DOCTOR

Frank Stellacio

An 82-year-old man has studiously avoided contact with doctors and thereby lived a full and happy life. Alas and alack, Old Man Time catcheth us all, and last year, this fine specimen got short of breath, suffered a mild cerebrovascular accident on the right side. During workup, they found coronary artery disease and aortic stenosis (they always find something they can bill for). So, one AVR and a three-vessel CABG later, he is back on the road. Current medications include Plavix, but he has been off it for 10 days. The patient is also hypertensive but well controlled with atenolol. Now he is scheduled for a suprapubic prostatectomy under an epidural because the surgeon does not want us to do this with the patient asleep. The PT, PTT, and INR are normal. His hematocrit is 29%, but all other laboratory test results are normal. His EF is 60%, so the cardiac cutters did not do him too wrong.

Intraoperative Questions

1. The patient is on Plavix, but the coagulation study results are normal. What are the implications of Plavix therapy? What does the Society of Regional Anesthesia say about it? Are these guidelines or standard of practice? What is the difference?

2. An epidural is placed without problems. Which local anesthetic would you use? Why? Is there any advantage of one over another? Would you include narcotics or epinephrine? Why or why not?

3. The patient complains of shortness of breath. How will you tell the difference between a high block resulting from CHF and aspiration? Do you need to stop the case and get a chest radiograph? Do you need to intubate? Why or why not?

4. You give 2 L of fluid. What do you expect his hematocrit to be now? The patient is hypertensive. How does that change your interpretation of the hematocrit? When should you transfuse?

5. Midazolam (4 mg) is given early in the case. What are the implications of this amount in an 82-year-old man? What are the differences in pharmacology in the geriatric and younger populations? What about the volume of distribution?

6. The case goes well, but the suction shows 2500 mL of reddish fluid. How will you determine the blood loss in this case? What is the difference if the red fluid is "clear enough to be able to read a newspaper through it" versus dark red? The surgeon says, "There is urine mixed in." Does that change your thinking? According to our friend the surgeon, the patient is "pissing like a horse." He does not specify whether a Palomino or an Arabian.

7. You transfuse 2 units of blood while the patient is awake, and the surgeon assures you. "That is enough." How will you determine whether this really is enough? The patient is on atenolol; are there any problems associated with that?

8. You place the Foley catheter at the end of the case, and the Foley is bloody. The surgeon assures you, "It will clear." How do you interpret this? How would you determine whether there is a significant amount of blood in the abdomen? How much blood can you "hide" in the abdomen? Where else can significant amounts of blood hide?

9. In the PACU, the patient is initially stable, but the ECG shows that the patient goes from a normal rate and that the complex widens. How do you evaluate this? How could heavy bleeding cause what looks like a hyperkalemic response?

10. Do you redose the epidural at the end of the case? What if you are concerned with ongoing bleeding? What is the effect of sympathectomy? What is the effect in the setting of β-blockade?

Postoperative Questions

1. Now the Foley catheter has frank blood pouring out. You are transfusing 4 units of blood. At what point do you place invasive monitors? He had none before. Do you place a triple-lumen or a Cordis line?

2. Do you start plasma component therapy? Do you use platelets, FFP, cryoprecipitate, or Amicar?

3. The wide complex continues. Is it related to the blood? How much potassium do you get from a bag of blood or from a bag of old blood? Should you request "young blood" for this young-at-heart guy?

4. The platelets arrive and are type A positive, but the patient is A negative. Can you transfuse this bag of platelets? What are the rules of engagement regarding FFP, platelets, and cryoprecipitate and blood type?

5. His blood pressure drops as you are transfusing. There are signs of ischemia, and he is complaining of chest pain. Do you start a phenylephrine drip to increase perfusion? Even if the blood pressure goes up, have you actually increased perfusion? What is the difference between perfusion and pressure?

CASE 19: HIP CHECK

Chris Gallagher

A 74-year-old woman, who has been wheelchair bound for years, presents for open reduction and internal fixation (ORIF) of a right hip fracture. Truth to tell, she is not sure how long it has been fractured! It has been "hurting for a while," but because she moves around so little, it might have been broken for some times. Her medical history is most remarkable for her debilitated state. She has arthritis, no exercise tolerance (she is unable to do much for herself), and carries the mushy diagnosis of multi-infarct dementia. Medications include digoxin (no one at the skilled nursing facility knows why; presumably, she has "something wrong with her heart") and metoprolol (same reasoning). Since admission, she has been put on subcutaneous heparin. Laboratory test results are remarkable for a sodium level of 128 mEq/L, potassium level of 3.2 mEq/L, and hematocrit of 27%. The ECG shows sinus tachycardia and an old inferior infarct.

Preoperative Questions

1. What is multi-infarct dementia? Compare it with other causes of dementia? What are the implications for anesthesia and for obtaining consent?
2. The patient is debilitated and does no activity. Do you need further evaluation of her cardiac status before proceeding? Because she has a hip fracture that cannot wait too long, is it worth pursuing this further? What is the risk of waiting longer?
3. Discuss the implications of the following in her history: arthritis, low sodium level, and low potassium level. Should you move to correct the electrolyte abnormalities before proceeding? Why or why not?
4. Her ECG shows tachycardia. What are the possible reasons? What are the problems with tachycardia? She is on metoprolol; how can she be tachycardic? Does she need more β-blockade? What are the dangers of this approach?
5. A check radiograph shows atelectasis and possible pneumonia, and the radiologist will not commit. What are the implications of atelectasis? What are the implications of pneumonia? Should you proceed with surgery? If you delay, what about the pulmonary embolism risk?

Intraoperative Questions

1. Do you use any invasive monitors? A colleague suggests you "keep a finger on her pulse and use etomidate" rather than subject her to an awake placement of an arterial line. Is this approach as good? Is there any evidence to show an arterial line is needed?
2. Her wrists are curled up, cutting off access to her radial arteries. Where to now? Should you use a brachial site? What are the risks? Should you use an axillary site? What are the risks? Should you use a femoral site? What if you try femoral access but go too deep and get intestinal "juice" in the needle?

3. You cannot get a good airway examination, but she looks "arthritis scary." She will not cooperate with an awake intubation—no way, no how. How do you secure the airway? Should you try a breathe down, asleep fiberoptic, or awake fiberoptic approach with some curious concatenation of sedatives?

4. You successfully intubate but have a hard time hearing her breath sounds. How will you make sure you do not have a right main stem intubation? Should you look at the markings on the ETT? Use a fiberoptic assessment? It is too much of a hassle?

5. You have a triple-lumen subclavian line in on the right. The distal port does not aspirate but the proximal two do. Do you transfuse through this line? Is there any troubleshooting you can do? What could be wrong? What could be "really bad" wrong?

6. The surgeon is unpleasantly surprised, telling you that her whole pelvic girdle is as fragile as tissue paper and falls apart with manipulation. How will this affect your management? Are there special risks? Is there need for more access? What do you do in the middle of the case?

7. Ventricular ectopy occurs. How do you tell "serious" ectopy from "harmless" ectopy? What is the mechanism of ventricular ectopy? How will you tell it from a reentrant rhythm? What diagnostic maneuvers do you employ? The potassium level is 2.8 mEq/L; is this the cause? Why or why not? What is the treatment?

8. "Oh, damn. I forgot about doing a regional to keep her from getting deep venous thrombosis or a pulmonary embolism!" you say to yourself. The case is finishing. Do you put in a regional for postoperative pain relief and to decrease clot risk? Would such a maneuver help now? What is the thinking behind regional anesthesia to decrease pulmonary embolisms?

9. The case finishes, and the patient is on her side, fully awake and alert. Can you extubate her on the side? Why or why not? Is it safer than on her back? Could you extubate someone prone at the end of the case? How do you ventilate in such a case?

10. Just as you move the patient supine and are loosening the tape on her ETT, her face becomes completely gray, her blood pressure drops, the end-tidal CO_2 gets cut in half, and she goes into ventricular tachycardia. Why caused this reaction? What is the treatment, including the ACLS protocol?

CASE 20: BITING OFF MORE THAN YOU CAN CHEW

Chris Gallagher

A 280-pound, mentally impaired, 38-year-old man needs extensive dental work under general anesthesia. He is institutionalized, prone to panic attacks, but soothed by Barney tunes (you could not make this stuff up). He takes Dilantin for a seizure disorder. Laboratory test results were unobtainable, because drawing blood would have taken an act of Congress. He is in the holding area, and surprise, surprise, he has no intravenous line. He will not cooperate in any way with an airway examination. A caregiver from the institution has a CD of *Barney's Greatest Hits*.

Intraoperative Questions

1. How do you do an airway examination when you cannot do an airway examination? What do you look for, without spooking the patient, that will tip you off one way or another?

2. How do you obtain intravenous access in this patient? What are the intramuscular options? Should you play the Barney CD? Do Barney karaoke? Breathe down? How do you breathe down a 280-pound, uncooperative patient? Which agent should you use if you do this? Why?

3. You breathe him down but still cannot find anything peripheral. How do you get access? Are there any special tricks for placing a peripheral line?

4. You have the patient breathing spontaneously and need to use a fiberoptic scope to place the ETT. The surgeon prefers the nasal route but understands you have issues. What do you do? Should you use oral or nasal intubation? Should you do one and then switch?

5. While placing the nasal tube, the patient gets light, and green liquid is seen in the posterior pharynx. What is your management plan? Should you turn the patient to his side? Should you soldier on and get the tube in? Should you then use suction, steroids, or antibiotics? Is there any case in which you would use antibiotics?

6. You have intubated the patient and suctioned out some green liquid. Do you proceed with this case or cancel? What are the risks of canceling or proceeding? If you cancel, do you keep the patient intubated? Why or why not?

7. You proceed, and the oxygen saturation drifts from 98% down to 91%. The surgeon says there is another hour of work. How will you manage this low saturation level? Is it time to cancel? If you choose PEEP, what are the problems with PEEP? What is the best method of ventilation? What would make you get an "ICU ventilator"?

8. The patient bucks violently (the sevoflurane ran to empty, and you did not notice it) and sits bolt upright, knocking over all equipment and one person. How will you get the situation under control? How do you determine whether the patient is still intubated? If he has been extubated, then what?

9. To get things under control, you give 150 mg of propofol. Thirty seconds later, the BIS goes to 5. What does this mean, and what are your concerns? What is the BIS? Why does propofol have that effect? How soon should it "return to normal"? What do you do if it is still low (in the teens) 30 minutes later?

10. Do you extubate at the end of this case? The surgeon says the patient will be a wild child and that it may be best to get the tube out. Do you agree?

Postoperative Questions

1. True to form, the patient is a wild child and goes nuts in the PACU. How will you sedate him? How will you know this is just "him" and not an intracranial event?

2. The mother goes ape when she finds out he is on a ventilator. How do you explain to her the events of the aspiration and the treatment plan? If she asks whether you did something wrong, what do you say?

3. The plan is to keep him intubated overnight. Does he need an arterial line? What if this is just for "airway protection"? What other methods besides arterial blood gases can you use to keep track of his ventilatory status overnight?

4. In the morning, the patient's ABG determination shows a Po_2 of 65 mm Hg on 50% oxygen and 5 cm H_2O of PEEP. Can you extubate? What else goes into the decision? How does the aspiration influence you?

5. The ICU nurses say that they can halve the dose of propofol if they keep playing the Barney CD. What are your options? Should you pipe Barney over the entire hospital intercom system? Should you offer headphones to the ICU staff so they do not go nuts? Should you put on a Barney suit and sing live? Why or why not?

CASE 21: HOW FAR CAN YOU GO?

Roy Soto and Matthew Tito

A 70-year-old man presents for urgent, right-sided carotid endarterectomy (CEA) after frequent episodes of transient ischemic attacks. He has a history of hypertension and heavy tobacco use. His blood pressure is 180/105 mm Hg, heart rate is 48 beats/min, and respiratory rate is 12 breaths/min. His medications include metoprolol and LMWH. His preoperative hematocrit is 29%.

Preoperative Questions

1. Would you treat this patient's blood pressure before surgery? Why or why not?
2. What is your target for this patient's intraoperative blood pressure? What blood pressure do you use as a baseline when calculating intraoperative blood pressure goals? For this particular surgery, is a higher or lower blood pressure preferable? Why?
3. Does this patient require a preoperative transfusion? Why or why not? Would you have blood available for this patient? Would you type and cross-match or type and screen for antibodies? How many units will you use? What hematocrit do you want to maintain in this patient and why?
4. Does this patient need a cardiac workup before going to surgery? Why or why not? What specific information would you want? How would this information change your anesthetic management?

Intraoperative Questions

1. The surgeon requests regional anesthesia for this patient. How do you respond? Does the LMWH alter your plan in any way? How do LMWH and heparin work?
2. Suppose you are doing general anesthesia for this case because the patient refuses to stay awake during the procedure. How do you induce him? Why do you use etomidate, not propofol? Can you use propofol? Will you keep the patient paralyzed throughout the procedure? Would you give an opiate as well? If so, how much and why?
3. How do you monitor this patient? When do you place your arterial line and why? Is there any difference if the case is done under general or regional anesthesia? Do you use EEG monitoring? What is a stump pressure? Why do surgeons place a shunt during some CEAs?
4. Intraoperatively, the patient remains hypertensive, with a mean arterial pressure above 100 mm Hg. How do you manage his blood pressure?
5. Your treatment results in a drop in pressure to 70/40 mm Hg. How do you manage this? Does his bradycardia alter your treatment plan? Why or why not?
6. The patient develops ST depression and T-wave inversion during this episode of hypotension. How do you respond? If the ECG changes reverse

themselves when the pressure is raised, and the surgery has not yet started, do you cancel the case and wake the patient? Why or why not?

CASE 22: ROAD WARRIOR

Roy Soto

A 60-year-old man involved in a motor vehicle accident is scheduled to undergo intramedullary rodding of an open, right femur fracture. The patient has multiple abrasions on his face, chest, and legs. A cervical collar is in place. His blood pressure is 105/60 mm Hg, heart rate is 96 beats/min, and hematocrit is 31%. Left-sided rib fractures are seen on the chest radiograph, and nonspecific ST changes with premature ventricular contractions are observed on the ECG.

Preoperative Questions

1. What criteria are used to evaluate the cervical spine? What information would you want to obtain from C-spine films? How useful is a lateral C-spine film?
2. How would you diagnose myocardial contusion? What are the physical findings? What are the ECG and echocardiographic findings? How about getting creatine phosphokinase (CPK) and troponin levels?
3. Would you order a type and screen or a type and cross of blood products? What is the difference? Would type-specific blood be adequate? What is trauma blood? What are the implications of administering trauma blood before switching to type and cross blood?

Intraoperative Questions

1. Is an arterial line indicated? Why or why not? How would you assess volume status? Should central venous pressures be measured? Pulmonary artery pressures?
2. How will you manage the airway? Does anesthetic management include C-spine considerations? If awake intubation is chosen, how would you anesthetize the airway? What induction agent and muscle relaxant would you select? What agents will you use for maintenance? Would you use a BIS monitor?
3. Ten minutes after intubation, peak airway pressure increase to 45 cm H_2O. How do you respond? What is the differential diagnosis? How do you diagnose and treat tension pneumothorax?
4. Two hours into the operation, the patient's blood pressure is 80/40 mm Hg and heart rate is 120 beats/min. How do you respond? The estimated blood loss is 1 to 2 L. After transfusing 3 units of packed red blood cells, the patient continues to bleed. The surgeon requests FFP. How would you proceed? Would you consider obtaining a thromboelastogram (TEG)? What information can you obtain from a TEG? What other tests can you do to assess coagulation?
5. During closure, tachydysrhythmia ensues as the heart rate increases from 105 to 150 beats/min. Rhythm appears to be a narrow complex. How would you respond? What are the causes? Suppose the blood pressure is 70/40 mm Hg; how would you respond? If the blood pressure is 120/80 mm Hg, what pharmacologic agents would you consider? A medical student suggests adenosine. What is your response?

CASE 23: TREATING LEUKEMIA AT HOME

Frank Stellacio and Igor Pikus

A 4-year-old old boy with leukemia was treated at home by parents who opposed chemotherapy for religious reasons. They instead treated the child with homeopathic herbal therapy. Their hand is forced by circumstances, and the child is now scheduled for a line placement. His platelet count is 50,000, and the hematocrit is 21%. The child is listless, and the parents are hovering and praying.

Intraoperative Questions

1. Why is the child listless? What is the differential diagnosis? Do you need a diagnosis before you can induce?
2. Comment on the platelet count and its implications. Explain the implications of the hematocrit. Do you need to transfuse right away in the OR?
3. You need an intravenous line, but you are doing this operation to get an intravenous line. How do you handle this dilemma? What if you cannot get peripheral placement? Is there any technology to help get a peripheral line? Will ultrasound help?
4. You need to place a central line. How do you place a central line in a child? Is it any different from placement in an adult? What are the special problems with a central line in a child? What are the problems with placement of intrajugular, subclavian, and femoral lines?
5. How will you induce? Is a sick kid with leukemia considered to be a "full stomach"? You breathe him down, and he vomits while in phase 2. What do you do?
6. The surgeon places the line and tries to flush it. Just after he flushes it, the technician notices that concentrated heparin was given by mistake and that the patient just got 10,000 units of heparin. What can you anticipate will happen in this patient with a low platelet count and hematocrit? Will you reverse? Is "waiting it out" an option?
7. As you get ready to extubate, you notice bright red blood in the mouth. Will you extubate? The patient is bucking, and the surgeon says, "Come on, get the damn thing out!

Postoperative Questions

1. You are called emergently to the ICU to intubate this patient that night. Do you use suxamethonium in this emergent situation? Why or why not?
2. You arrive, and the patient is covered in blood. The ICU staff attempted extubation several times to no effect. What problems do you anticipate, and how will you handle the problems? You look in and see only blood. What are the options?
3. What are the options regarding a surgical airway? Are they different for a child? Can you place an LMA and perform a tracheostomy later?
4. You intubate, but the face is covered in blood. How do you secure the ETT? Do you use tape or string? Do you sew? How? What are the dangers of accidental extubation, and how you will prevent it?
5. How do you sedate this 4-year-old child? What are the long-term problems with infusion of propofol or etomidate? Does the child need stress-dose steroids? Does he need an infusion of platelets?

CASE 24: HARD TO SWALLOW

Zvi Jacob

A 28-month-old, male toddler is referred to the ER in your institution for management of a suspected foreign body in his airway. At home, the mother attempted removal of the object from the right nares. During these attempts, he suffered minimal nose bleeding, which quickly resolved. After no success, the mother sought further treatment in the ER. Several unsuccessful attempts to remove the object were made by the ER resident.

The medical history indicates the boy has always enjoyed good health. He last ate 5 hours earlier. On evaluation, he has a respiratory rate of 35 breaths/min and an oxygen saturation level of 97% on blow-by oxygen. He is using accessory muscles of respiration to a moderate degree. On auscultation, the toddler has somewhat diminished breath sounds over the right lung and has mild expiratory wheezing. Chest radiography is pending.

Preoperative Questions

1. What type of history is typical for a foreign body in the airway?
2. Who are at risk for foreign body aspiration? What is the natural history of most choking episodes?
3. Does the absence of symptoms in the ER or absence of radiographic abnormalities exclude an airway foreign body?
4. What are the most common objects aspirated?
5. What types of foreign bodies are most dangerous to the lung tissue? Which ones are the most lethal?
6. What interventions can be tried before arrival in the OR if the patient is rapidly deteriorating?
7. When should the case be done? Are there any risks associated with waiting or with not waiting?
8. How would you treat the patient's current symptoms?

Intraoperative Questions

1. Should this patient be premedicated? Explain.
2. What technique would you use for induction of anesthesia? Discuss RSI and inhalation induction.
3. How would you manage a complete airway obstruction during induction?
4. How would your anesthetic management and the risks change between an acute and a chronic foreign body presentation?
5. Describe the options for removal of airway foreign body (e.g., rigid bronchoscopy, bronchotomy).
6. Are you going to intubate after the foreign body removal?
7. What are the expected postoperative complications after the foreign body removal? What would you prepare?

CASE 25: DONUT INTERRUPTED

Peggy Seidman and Chris Page

You are sitting and having a donut and coffee in the preoperative testing center when you hear a disturbing sound, a baby crying. No good can come of this. The resident comes to present the story. A former 28-week preemie, now 5 months old and 7 kg, is scheduled for treatment of benign intracranial hypertension as an outpatient. He has albuterol treatments daily, takes prednisone, and has the *cutest* little nasal cannula on. "WHOOOOAAA," you say.

Preoperative Questions

1. What are the criteria for outpatient surgery in children, infants, and former preemies? How old is this baby in terms of postgestational age?
2. What information about the neonatal intensive care unit (NICU) course is critical? What about airway management and length of intubation?
3. What is the significance of airway and breathing issues, home oxygen delivery, current home monitoring, and the child's medications?
4. What would be a normal weight and vital statistics for a child with this history? What preoperative laboratory test results do you want, if any?
5. What are the NPO guidelines for this patient? Is outpatient surgery a good choice? The surgeon wants to do his easy cases first and this one last. Is this a good decision?
6. How long does it take for you tell the mother *no way* for day surgery and book the child as the first case of the day in the main OR?

Intraoperative Questions

1. Can mom come to the OR? Does this child need midazolam? What is 1/8 L of O_2?
2. Should you use straight regional anesthesia? Where and when will you get intravenous access? Can you use spinal, caudal, or caudal with or with out a catheter? Which local anesthetic will you use? Will you add epinephrine, clonidine, or a narcotic? When was the last time you did one of these? What the heck is a sugar nipple?
3. Can you use mask induction? What induction agent will you use? What is the risk of mask induction in a patient this age? What are the advantages of sevoflurane in this age group and with this lung pathology?
4. Can you use intravenous induction? What access will you use? When and where will you induce? Will you even be able to get an intravenous line in this infant? What are the hourly fluid needs for this child and this operation? Which fluid will you use?
5. For airway management, will you use an LMA, ETT, or mask? The surgeon expects to be 35 minutes at the most.
6. For postoperative pain control, will you use a narcotic or caudal block? What would you use for a single-shot caudal block? What is an ilioinguinal block, and is it better or worse than other methods? What other medications would help with postoperative pain?
7. You decide to intubate so as not to lose the airway during your block and the operation. What size tube should you start with? What is a leak test, and how do you do it? Do you use a cuffed or uncuffed tube? Does the history of a 3-week intubation in the NICU worry you?
8. What are the extubation criteria for this infant? Is a deep extubation advisable? What are the risks and benefits of a deep extubation?
9. Give this baby a latte! What are the data regarding intraoperative caffeine in preemies having general anesthesia? What the heck does caffeine do? What is the right dose? What is the right caffeine? How much caffeine is in a cup of coffee or a shot of espresso?

Postoperative Questions

1. What monitors should be used in the PACU and for how long? Should this child be monitored over night? If so, which monitors should you use? Should the patient be transferred to the pediatric intensive care unit (PICU)?
2. The infant is screaming in the PACU, and the nurse wants to give fentanyl. What do you want? Does all screaming indicate pain? What are the advantages of nursing and sugar for soothing infants? What are the advantages of a parent in this situation?
3. The infant is breast-fed and will not take sugar water from a bottle. Mom wants to feed in the PACU. Now what?

CASE 26: HELLP, I NEED SOMEBODY

Joy Schabel and Chris Martin

A 22-year-old, very edematous, primigravida, nullipara patient presents to labor and delivery for an immediate cesarean section because of HELLP syndrome. She is receiving intravenous magnesium sulfate. The patient last ate a sandwich 4 hours earlier. The fetal heart rate is 100 to 110 beats/min, with poor beat-to-beat variability. There are frequent late decelerations. The mother's blood pressure is 160/95 mm Hg, heart rate is 100 beats/min, respiratory rate is 20 breaths/min, and temperature is 98.6°F. The airway examination reveals she has a Mallampati score of 3 and a swollen tongue. She has a platelet count of 71,000, aspartate aminotransferase (AST) level of 210 IU/L, and alanine aminotransferase (ALT) level of 225 IU/L. Her PT and PTT values are not available.

Preoperative Questions

1. What is HELLP?
2. Is the fetal heart rate normal?
3. What are late decelerations? What is their significance?
4. What is the number 1 determinant of fetal well-being?
5. Should the case be delayed until the patient is NPO for 8 hours? Why or why not?
6. Is there any information from the history and physical examination that you need to obtain before proceeding with the cesarean section?
7. What is your anesthetic plan and why?
8. Suppose you had chosen to perform a spinal anesthetic. Describe your preload fluid management.
9. Would you treat the patient's blood pressure preoperatively, and if yes, how?
10. What monitoring would you use for this patient and why?

Intraoperative Questions

1. A spinal anesthetic is performed. Brisk bleeding occurs at the spinal insertion site after the needle is withdrawn. What would you do?
2. Three minutes after the spinal anesthetic is placed, the blood pressure drops to 70/40 mm Hg. What do you do?
3. There is no improvement in the blood pressure after several boluses of ephedrine, phenylephrine, and fluid. What do you do?

4. As the obstetricians are closing the uterus, the patient suddenly complains of chest pain. Her respiratory rate is 24 breaths/min. Pulse oximetry shows a level of 95%, but it was 99% earlier. There is a 2-mm ST depression in leads II and V_5. What is your differential diagnosis and the most likely diagnosis? How do you respond?

5. After 50 minutes, the obstetricians are still operating and the patient complains of incisional pain. What do you do?

Postoperative Questions

1. After 1 hour in the recovery room, the patient has had no urine output. Urine output was only 50 mL intraoperatively. What do you do?
2. The urine output does not improve after fluid boluses. What is your differential diagnosis? How do you respond?
3. You place a Swan-Ganz catheter, and the pulmonary capillary wedge pressure (PCWP) is 48 mm Hg. What do you do?
4. The patient becomes very lethargic and weak. What is the differential diagnosis, and how do you respond?
5. List the systemic magnesium levels at which a patient will lose the deep tendon reflex, have respiratory arrest, and have cardiac arrest.

CASE 27: OBSTETRICS AND A BAD AIRWAY

Jay Bhangoo and Misako Sakamaki

A 32-year-old, gravida 2, para 2 woman had a cesarean section 18 hours earlier. The cesarean section was uneventful, with 1200 mL of estimated blood loss and 200 mL of urine output. The patient is 4 feet 7 inches tall and weighs 95 kg. She has some vaginal bleeding and received 2 units of packed red blood cells, producing a hematocrit of 25%. She was NPO before the cesarean section. The patient is coming back to the OR for dilation and curettage (D&C). Her medical history is positive for asthma and hypertension, for which she takes albuterol as needed and Lopressor, respectively.

Preoperative Questions

1. What other laboratory studies or history would you like?
2. How would you premedicate this patient?
3. Would you do regional or general anesthesia for this case?
4. If you choose regional, would you do a spinal or an epidural? The patient did have a labor epidural, which was used for the cesarean section.
5. Is this patient considered NPO?

Intraoperative Questions

1. You chose to do a spinal. What local anesthetic are you planning to use? What are the downfalls of using lidocaine?
2. You decided to do spinal anesthesia. It worked beautifully, but the surgeon cannot control the bleeding with a simple D&C. The surgeon must open the belly and possibly do a hysterectomy. Do you continue the spinal or convert to a general anesthesia?
3. You decided to continue with the spinal. The surgery is taking more than 3 hours, and the patient is starting to feel the pain. What is your next move?

4. You have to put the patient to sleep. How do you do it?
5. You did an RSI with propofol and suxamethonium intubation. You cannot intubate. You could barely ventilate with two people. What is your next step?
6. While you are attempting to intubate the patient, she is bucking. The surgeon wants you to paralyze her right away. What do you tell the surgeon?
7. The surgeon tells you that the patient is oozing. He wants you to give FFP. What is your response?

CASE 28: ON CALL IN LABOR AND DELIVERY

Ursula Landman and Jeffrey Pan

You have just taken over cases in the labor and delivery department on a Friday evening, and the obstetric anesthesiologist tells you as she is leaving, "There is a 30-year-old, 450-pound, primigravida, nullipara woman in room 4 who is being induced with no epidural, and there is still no intravenous line. Her blood pressure is 120/70 mm Hg, pulse is 70 beats/min, and respiratory rate is 15 breaths/min. The fetal heart rate is in the 140s. No medical or surgical history is available. The patient has been taking prenatal vitamins, and she has no known drug allergies. There were many attempts at delivery during the afternoon, without success. The obstetric anesthesiologist said that the patient wants general anesthesia if she is to have a cesarean section, but the obstetrician says that he does not need anesthesia. The obstetric anesthesiologist has left.

1. Do you establish a mutually agreed on plan for anesthesia with the obstetrician and the patient?
2. If so, how do you proceed? The obstetrician is waiting and wants to start the pitocin.
3. There is an incomplete preoperative chart written by the day team. What do you do to evaluate the situation?
4. Epidurals are usually done with a 17-gauge, 3.5-inch Tuohy-Schliff needle. Would you want an alternative?
5. Would you want any additional equipment in the vicinity? If so, what items?
6. After the patient is in labor for about 15 hours, the obstetrician plans to do a cesarean section because of failure to progress. There is still no epidural. What do you do?
7. You have been attempting an epidural for about 2 hours without success? What do you do?
8. After 2.5 hours and many attempts, cerebrospinal fluid flows out of the Tuohy. Do you place a spinal anesthetic or try for an epidural still?
9. The obstetrician is getting very impatient; it is the wee hours of the morning now, and he would like to get started. What do you do?
10. The fetal heart rate should be checked how often?
11. What are the two components of the fetal heart rate monitor?
12. Is it better to have a Doppler transducer or a fetal scalp electrode?
13. What is the normal baseline fetal heart rate?
14. What is the difference between an early and a late deceleration?
15. Describe the management for fetal distress.
16. The obstetrician begins to worry about neonatal apnea. Can you state the difference between primary and secondary apnea?
17. Define Apgar score.

CASE 29: WINDOW TO MY SOUL

Chris Gallagher and Anshul Airen

A 52-year-old man, after an aortic valve replacement (AVR) 3 weeks ago, presented for a follow-up visit. He complained of shortness of breath and an inability to sleep lying flat at night, which surprised the cardiac surgeon because this man had a good EF preoperatively, and his valve replacement went swimmingly. His medications (metoprolol, Coumadin) are in order, and his laboratory test results are in order. He is compliant with the Coumadin and has an INR in the therapeutic range. The chest radiograph shows a widened mediastinum, and echocardiography shows a fluid, loculated pattern around the heart. He is scheduled for creation of a pericardial window.

Preoperative Questions

1. What is a therapeutic range for an INR? Why do heart valve patients have to take anticoagulants? What happens if they do not take their anticoagulants? What if they take medications that interfere with their anticoagulants or potentiate them?
2. What are the potential sources of pericardial effusion? What other conditions manifest like this? What are the physiologic effects of a rapid fluid buildup or a slow fluid buildup? What other physical signs will you look for?
3. The transthoracic echocardiogram (TTE) shows a pericardial effusion. What "windows" does TTE have? Compare it with TEE? Do you need TEE before you begin? Why or why not? What will TEE add?
4. This man had a heart operation 3 weeks earlier. Can you anticipate any problems related to his recent surgery? What will you look for in the anesthetic record? What will you do if you cannot find the old anesthetic record?

Intraoperative Questions

1. The man talks in complete sentences and can lay flat. Do you need an arterial line before induction? Why? Are there other options for beat-to-beat blood pressure measurement? What are the advantages and disadvantages of each?
2. You have a 20-gauge intravenous line in that runs pretty well. Do you need more volume access before induction? Can you wait and "put in a 16" after induction? How about a central line? Which kind will you use? The surgeon says, "This will be real quick." Will his statement affect your actions?
3. Can you do this case under local anesthesia with sedation? How? In what cases would you prefer to do this under local anesthetic? What physical findings tip you to "really bad tamponade physiology" compared with "this is no big deal"?
4. You go with sedation, but as the surgeon progresses, he "drifts left" and causes a pneumothorax (you can see the lung). What physiologic changes can you anticipate? Because this is "open to air," will the patient be any worse off? Compare a tension and a nontension pneumothorax.
5. How will you induce in this "not so bad" pericardial window patient? How would this differ from the patient who is in "a bad way"? Would you use ketamine, etomidate, or propofol?
6. You induce without an arterial line and are surprised that the cuff is taking so long to cycle. How does a blood pressure cuff work? How long will it take

to let you know there is no pressure or a pressure of 300 mm Hg? Is there any other way to "get the pressure faster"?

7. The cuff gives you a pressure of 74/40 mm Hg, but the heart rate is still 53 beats/min. How will you treat this? Will you use splash and slash and get in right away? Will you use Neo-Synephrine, ephedrine, or epinephrine?

8. You give Neo-Synephrine, and the heart rate falls to 29 beats/min. What is your response to this? What is the reason for the drop? What is the interaction with β-blockers?

9. While the surgeon is digging his finger under the sternum, you see unifocal ectopy. What is the reason for this? Do you need a blood gas determination? If a test showed a potassium level of 3.4 mEq/L and you have only peripheral lines, should you replete the potassium? How? How fast? Should you give antiarrhythmic therapy in the meantime?

10. The surgeon says he needs to do a small left thoracotomy to get at the effusion. How do you respond? Do you add more lines? What are your postoperative ventilation plans now? What if the surgeon asks for lung isolation?

CASE 30: A MASSIVE PROBLEM THAT SNUCK UP ON US

Rishi Adsumelli and Igor Pikus

A 50-year-old woman is scheduled for endoscopic laparotomy for suspected ovarian carcinoma. She presented to the ER last night with breathlessness and orthopnea. Examination shows that she has ascites. Her medical history was significant for myasthenia gravis with thymoma, for which she underwent thymectomy 8 years earlier and fully recovered. She is not on any medications. A chest radiograph revealed a widened upper mediastinum and bilateral pleural effusion. The gynecologic oncologist says that the type and screen, hematocrit and hemoglobin, and serum chemistry profile (including β-human chorionic gonadotropin) results are ready, and he wants to operate as soon as possible.

Preoperative Questions

1. What is the differential diagnosis for widening of the anterior mediastinum?
2. How do you proceed?
3. The CT scan shows compression of the tracheobronchial tree in the region of the carina. There is possibly a 40% compression. What else will you do?
4. How about pressure-volume loops?
5. What else can be done to rule out dynamic obstruction?
6. Echocardiography shows some external compression of the right atrium, but there is no significant obstruction to the filling and flow, and the patient has normal systolic function. Bronchoscopy shows no dynamic obstruction or distortion of the lumen. Do you want any additional consultations?
7. What do you do about bilateral pleural effusion?

Intraoperative Questions

1. How would you proceed with the anesthesia?
2. Which things will you keep in the room?

3. How do you position this patient for induction?
4. Considering the massive ascites, do you want to do an RSI?
5. Would you use muscle relaxants?
6. After induction, you place the patient in the supine position, and you notice that the pulse oximeter is showing a value of 92% and the end-tidal value dropped to 25. What do you do?

CASE 31: NOTHING TRIVIAL IN THE OUTPATIENT CENTER

Andrea K. Voutas

A 42-year-old woman presents to the ambulatory surgery center for a laparoscopic ovarian cystectomy. Her medical history is significant for morbid obesity (BMI of 45), asthma controlled with inhalers with rare wheezing, and a two pack per day smoking habit. She denies any abdominal pain, nausea, or vomiting. She has no allergies and is NPO. Oxygen saturation levels are between 95% and 96% on room air.

The patient denies a history of hypertension, chest pains, or palpitations, and she has fair exercise tolerance. She carries groceries into the house and can climb a flight of stairs without shortness of breath. She has not had any emergency room visits for pulmonary symptoms, nor has she been treated with systemic steroids. She does have sputum production in the morning but denied any recent upper respiratory infections. Her only medications are the inhalers (PRN), and she has no allergies. On further questioning, it is revealed (by her husband who is seated beside her) that she snores excessively at night, waking him up. He also reports that she turns often and sometimes vocalizes. She denies daytime sleepiness. You ask if she has had a sleep study. Although she has not, you make a presumptive diagnosis of obstructive sleep apnea.

Preoperative Questions

1. What are the anesthetic concerns for this patient?
2. What other information would you like in the patient's history?
3. Define obstructive sleep apnea and obstructive sleep hypopnea.
4. Discuss the pathophysiology of obstructive sleep apnea.
5. Discuss the systemic effects of obstructive sleep apnea.
6. Discuss the parameters measured in a sleep study and how the severity of obstructive sleep apnea is graded.
7. How is the perioperative risk of obstructive sleep apnea determined?
8. What is this patient's perioperative risk of obstructive sleep apnea?
9. What are you going to pay particular attention to during your physical examination?
10. On examination, her blood pressure is 140/90 mm Hg, her heart rate is 88 beats/min, and her airway has a Mallampati score of 1 to 2. Her cardiac examination reveals regular heart rate and rhythm without any murmurs, gallops, or rubs. Examination of her lungs reveals decreased breath sounds bilaterally, but they are clear. What laboratory data and tests would you want?
11. Is this case appropriate for an ambulatory surgery center? If this patient were scheduled to have a laparoscopic cholecystectomy instead, would this center be appropriate?
12. Would you consider any premedications for her?

Intraoperative Questions

1. The patient is induced in a rapid-sequence fashion, intubated by direct laryngoscopy without incident, and maintained on a combination of a propofol infusion and sevoflurane. What are your concerns intraoperatively?
2. The case proceeds relatively uneventfully, except for a constant debate between you and the surgeon about how much Trendelenburg positioning the patient can tolerate. Her lungs remain clear, with occasional rhonchi. Her oxygen saturation levels are 95% to 96% on 50% FIO$_2$ throughout. How will you extubate this patient?
3. The patient is awake and extubated. You start to disconnect the monitors, leaving the pulse oximeter on while you turn to jot down a few last notes on your anesthesia record. You suddenly hear those terrifying low tones of the pulse oximeter, look up, and find the patient has dozed off and the saturation level is 79%. You spring into action and stimulate the patient. The oxygen saturation rises to between 93% and 94%. You proceed to transfer the patient to the PACU. How long should you monitor the patient in the PACU?
4. How will you manage postoperative pain?

CASE 32: THE BIG HIT

Bharathi Scott and Chris Collado

A 58-year-old man is scheduled for CABG on pump. He has the usual history of unstable angina, diabetes, and hypertension. The cardiac catheterization report shows triple-vessel disease with a normal left ventricular EF. You are thrilled that finally you have a routine CABG this week. No big deal—been there and done that. Just as you are walking down to the floor to see the patient, the friendly cardiologist says, "The patient's platelet count has dropped, and we are waiting for the antibody test. I think the patient has heparin-induced thrombocytopenia. We stopped heparin yesterday and started him on argatroban."

1. What is HIT? Explain the differences between type 1 and type 2 HIT.
2. How is HIT diagnosed?
3. What are the preoperative considerations from an anesthesiologist's point of view?
4. What are your options regarding anticoagulants?
5. What is the mechanism of action of the alternative agents?
6. What is the dosing regimen?
7. What are the advantages and disadvantages of the available alternative drugs?
8. How will you monitor the level of anticoagulation?
9. How will you reverse the anticoagulation?
10. When the cell saver technician wonders what he should use for anticoagulation, what will you tell him?

CASE 33: HOME IS WHERE THE OXYGEN IS

Carlos Mijares and Wei Song

A 50-year-old woman with metastatic ovarian cancer is scheduled for exploratory laparotomy. She has a 40 pack-year smoking history. She cannot walk more than 30 steps without having to stop because of shortness of breath. She requires nasal cannula oxygen for sleep at night. She also has significant ascites. A room-air ABG assessment shows a pH of 7.35, P_{O_2} of 55 mm Hg, and P_{CO_2} of 46 mm Hg. Her blood pressure is 121/56 mm Hg, heart rate is 112 beats/min, and hematocrit is 28%.

Preoperative Questions

1. What is the life span for a patient with ovarian cancer? What would you tell the patient about the operation preoperatively?
2. Do you need any further workup on this patient? What tests would you order?
3. Does the patient need any workup for cardiac function? Does the patient need cardiac catheterization?
4. Does the patient need any pulmonary function tests? If so, what tests do you order?
5. Would you drain the ascites before surgery? Why or why not?
6. Do you think the patient needs oxygen 24 hours each day? How much oxygen would you give the patient: 2 L/min, 4 L/min, or 6 L/min? Why?
7. How do you interpret the ABG results?
8. Would you transfuse the patient preoperatively? Why or why not?
9. Would you premedicate this patient?

Intraoperative Questions

1. What monitors do you choose for this patient? Would you put arterial line and central line in this patient? What about using a Swan-Ganz catheter?
2. You decide to place an arterial line before induction, but the patient is very anxious. Would you give sedation?
3. How would you induce this patient? What agents would you use? Would you use ketamine? What muscle relaxant would you choose? What is the Hoffman reaction?
4. What factors can affect the Hoffman reaction?
5. What agent would you use for anesthesia maintenance? What are your concerns?
6. After opening the abdomen, the patient's blood pressure suddenly drops. What is your differential diagnosis?
7. During surgery, peak airway pressure suddenly increases. What is your differential diagnosis? Can capnography allow early detection of an endobronchial intubation?
8. How do you diagnose pneumothorax? Would you place a chest tube?
9. What intravenous fluid would you use: crystalloid or colloid?
10. The patient's SpO_2 slowly drops into the low 90s. What would you do? How does PEEP work?

12

Grab Bags

CASE 1: EAR TUBES

Chris Gallagher and Robert Chavez
A woman is scheduled for one ear tube, and the surgeon is fast. You induce with 100 mg of propofol, turn her head, and as the surgeon is placing the tube, a massive amount of emesis, fully formed food, pours out of her mouth. You have only a mask on her. How do you manage this situation?

CASE 2: RADIATION THERAPY FOR A MENTALLY RETARDED MAN

Chris Gallagher and Robert Chavez
A 50-year-old, severely retarded man needs 18 radiation treatments for esophageal cancer. He has a port you can access for giving intravenous fluids. How will you manage his sedation so he can hold still during the few minutes the radiation beam needs to be focused on his esophagus?

CASE 3: KNIFE IN THE BACK

Chris Gallagher and Robert Chavez
An 18-year-old man is stabbed in the middle of his back, and the knife is still sticking out. The knife wound has produced Brown-Séquard syndrome. How will you secure the airway given the knife sticking out of his back, and how will you maintain the anesthetic?

CASE 4: FEVER IN THE INTENSIVE CARE UNIT

Zvi Jacob
On day 5 after an exploratory laparotomy, the patient's temperature is 39.2° C, heart rate is 102 beats/min, blood pressure is 74/50 mm Hg, SpO_2 is 94%, and FIO_2 is 0.6. What is your differential diagnosis? How would you proceed? Discuss sepsis management in the intensive care unit (ICU).

CASE 5: SMOKING CESSATION

Zvi Jacob
A 45-year-old woman who is a heavy smoker presents for an elective operation. What are your recommendations regarding smoking cessation? Discuss smoking and its complications during the perioperative period.

CASE 6: TACHYCARDIA AFTER KNEE ARTHROSCOPY

Zvi Jacob

A 40-year-old man is admitted to the postanesthesia care unit (PACU) after knee arthroscopy. His heart rate suddenly increases from 83 to 155 beats/min. How would you proceed? If he has supraventricular tachyarrhythmia (SVT), please explain your management plan.

CASE 7: BONE PAIN AND SARCOMA

Zvi Jacob

A 20-year-old woman has severe bone pain caused by metastatic Ewing sarcoma. How would you treat her? Describe the different treatment options.

CASE 8: INTRAVENOUS FLUIDS

Zvi Jacob

Discuss the intravenous fluid solutions (e.g., crystalloids, colloids) used in the operating room (OR).

CASE 9: SEDATION IN A HALO

Chris Gallagher

A 65-year-old man with Parkinson's disease is in a halo for a stereotactic brain procedure to relieve his symptoms. Describe how you will conduct sedation given the airway limitations.

CASE 10: SWAN-GANZ CATHETER

Chris Gallagher

You are starting hearts at a new hospital and are surprised that everyone gets a Swan-Ganz catheter. Explain whether they should or should not and why? What are the options in the ICU if no Swan-Ganz catheter is available?

CASE 11: POSTOPERATIVE RIGIDITY

Chris Gallagher

A 25-year-old man who underwent testicular torsion repair develops rigidity and tachypnea in the PACU 30 minutes after emergence. How will you further evaluate and treat this situation?

CASE 12: PERIPHERALLY INSERTED CENTRAL CATHETER AND DESATURATION

Chris Gallagher

A 20-year-old intravenous drug abuser has a peripherally inserted central catheter (PICC) in for long-term antibiotic therapy. He is in your ICU, and his saturation keeps dropping every time his visitors come in and for about 30 minutes afterward. What is going on?

CASE 13: AORTIC VALVE REPLACEMENT IN A PREGNANT PATIENT

Chris Gallagher

A pregnant woman requires emergent aortic valve replacement because of a stuck valve. She is at 20 weeks' gestation, and you cannot wean her from bypass. It looks like only norepinephrine can save her, but a colleague reminds you that norepinephrine is contraindicated in pregnancy. What are the options? Which do you pick?

CASE 14: SUBCUTANEOUS EMPHYSEMA

Chris Gallagher

A 62-year-old man with esophageal cancer needs an esophagectomy. While placing the double-lumen endotracheal tube (ETT), some difficulty is encountered. After placement, subcutaneous emphysema occurs, and the ventilator alarms. What may have occurred, and how do you manage this?

CASE 15: PATIENT IN THE TRIPOD POSITION

Chris Gallagher

A 45-year-old woman comes into the emergency room (ER) and assumes the tripod position while keeping her chin forward, drooling, and exhibiting a high fever. She has a psychiatric history. What is the differential diagnosis, and how do you manage this situation?

CASE 16: ATTENTION DEFICIT DISORDER AND ELECTROPHYSIOLOGIC STUDY

Chris Gallagher

A 26-year-old man with attention deficit disorder (ADD), Asperger's syndrome, and developmental delay is scheduled for an electrophysiologic study. The mother is at the bedside. The cardiologist tells you he can do this under sedation but is concerned because of the young man's diagnoses. How will you evaluate and manage this situation?

CASE 17: FIRE ALARMS

Chris Gallagher

You are in the middle of an appendectomy and the fire alarm goes off. "We have been told to evacuate, no kidding, because the hospital is on fire," the coordinator tells you. What do you do?

CASE 18: ETOMIDATE FOR SEDATION

Chris Gallagher

Few or no carotid endarterectomies are being done at your hospital because almost everything is getting stented. The interventional radiologists ask for some guidance on sedating patients for this procedure, specifically asking about giving etomidate for sedation. What do you tell them?

CASE 19: EPIDURAL PLANNED BUT THE PROTHROMBIN TIME IS HIGH

Chris Gallagher

A patient has excruciating pain from bony metastases to the spine and needs a pain service consult. Systemic medications can no longer control the pain. A high thoracic epidural is planned, but the patient's prothrombin time is high because of liver involvement. How do you advise? Do you place the epidural? Do you use more systemic medications or different ones?

CASE 20: MEDIASTINAL MASS

Chris Gallagher

A patient with an anterior mediastinal mass is scheduled for radiation therapy. She is having this done because the lesion is so big they do not dare operate on her, but she cannot lie flat for the radiation therapy. You are asked to help sedate her. What is your input?

CASE 21: ANKLE PAIN

Brian Durkin

A 50-year-old woman complains of burning pain in her left lower extremity. She twisted her left ankle 6 weeks earlier, and her pain has never improved. Her blood pressure is 115/49 mm Hg, pulse is 70 beats/min, respiratory rate is 16 breaths/min, weight is 65 kg, and height is 5 feet 6 inches. What is your plan? Does she need magnetic resonance imaging (MRI)? Do you know what the problem is? What medicine would you prescribe? What tests would you order?

CASE 22: BLOOD PATCH IN A JEHOVAH'S WITNESS

Brian Durkin

You are asked by your obstetrician-gynecologist colleagues to place an epidural blood patch in a 34-year-old woman who delivered a healthy baby by cesarean section under spinal anesthesia 3 days earlier and now complains of a persistent headache. She is 5 feet 1 inch tall, weighs 90 kg, and is a Jehovah's Witness. What is your plan?

CASE 23: PATIENT CANNOT MOVE LEGS

Brian Durkin

You are called to evaluate a patient in the PACU who has undergone a right total hip arthroplasty under epidural anesthesia. The case was completed 1 hour earlier, and the patient complains that he cannot move his legs. What is your plan? Would you order an MRI scan? Would you call a neurologist?

CASE 24: PAIN CONTROL IN THE POSTANESTHESIA CARE UNIT

Brian Durkin

You are called by the nurse to the PACU to evaluate a patient who complains of continuing pain in his leg. The nurse tells you that she has given the patient 300 µg of fentanyl in the last 20 minutes and that "it has not touched him." What is your plan? Would you give more fentanyl? Would you give morphine? Would you give hydromorphone? What is the equivalent dose of 5 mg of morphine if you have only fentanyl to give? How about hydromorphone?

CASE 25: NEPHRECTOMY AND HEPARIN

Brian Durkin
You have taken a donor nephrectomy patient to the OR and placed a thoracic epidural before induction of general anesthesia. The surgeon tells you he is administering subcutaneous heparin (5000 units) before the incision. What do you tell her? What if the case called for intravenous heparin at a dose of 7000 units? What about 20,000 units? What if the surgeon wanted you to place a nasogastric tube and squeeze down clopidogrel (75 mg), followed by tinzaparin?

CASE 26: CELIAC PLEXUS BLOCK

Brian Durkin
You are asked to provide anesthesia to a patient who has stage IV esophageal cancer and is going to have a computed tomography (CT)–guided neurolytic block of the celiac plexus. He has intractable pain and is unable to assume the prone position. Medicine at home includes methadone and ondansetron. What is your anesthetic plan? What structures are at risk from this procedure? What postoperative concerns do you have?

CASE 27: EPIDURAL STEROIDS

Brian Durkin
You are asked by your obstetrician-gynecologist colleagues for a favor. They want you to place an epidural steroid injection in a 32-year-old woman who is 27 weeks' pregnant. They have already called a spine surgeon, who has refused to operate on her herniated L5-S1 intervertebral disk. She is in excruciating pain; she requires intravenous hydromorphone by patient-controlled analgesia; and her visual analog scale (VAS) pain score is 9/10. What are your concerns? What is your plan? Why not operate? Can this operation be done under local anesthesia? What nonmedication therapies can be offered?

CASE 28: LASER FOR POLYPS

Roy Soto
A 7-year-old boy presents for laser treatment for laryngeal polyps. What complications are you concerned about? How do you prevent an airway fire?

CASE 29: OPEN REDUCTION AND INTERNAL FIXATION OF A WRIST

Roy Soto
After a fall, a 17-year-old, healthy boy presents for wrist open reduction and internal fixation (ORIF). Do you do regional anesthesia? What kind of regional

anesthesia do you perform? The surgeon is quick and tells you he will finish in an hour. Can you do the block by giving one single injection?

CASE 30: MASSETER SPASM

Roy Soto

A 19-year-old, healthy man with a history of masseter muscle spasm (MMS) is admitted on the floor the night before a laminectomy. You are seeing him, and no old medical records are available. Do you obtain a baseline creatine phosphokinase (CPK) level? If the CPK is normal, what do you do next? The old medical records arrive. He had two operations after the episode of MMS. Suxamethonium was used for both operations without any problems. What do you think?

CASE 31: PREECLAMPSIA

Roy Soto

A 20-year-old parturient with severe preeclampsia is scheduled for a cesarean section. She is taking magnesium. What are the signs of magnesium toxicity? How would you monitor her magnesium therapy? How would you manage her blood pressure (180/110 mm Hg) in the OR? If the patient undergoes a general anesthetic, what muscle relaxant would you choose?

CASE 32: PANCREATECTOMY

Roy Soto

A 60-year-old man is scheduled for pancreatic resection. Where would you insert an epidural catheter? What local anesthetic or opioids would you infuse? What infusion rate would you use? What strategies would you employ to minimize respiratory depression? How would you treat hypotension resulting from an epidural?

CASE 33: CEREBRAL ANEURYSM

Roy Soto

A 48-year-old woman is scheduled for clipping of a giant middle cerebral artery aneurysm. How would you manage the blood pressure at the moment of clipping? Would you hyperventilate or hypoventilate the patient? What strategies would you use for cerebral protection and for hypothermia? Would you use etomidate or a barbiturate?

CASE 34: VIDEO-ASSISTED THORACOSCOPIC SURGERY

Igor Izrailtyan

A 27-year-old man is scheduled for video-assisted thoracoscopic surgery (VATS) to address recurrent pneumothorax. The double-lumen endotracheal tube (ETT) is in the correct position, but the lung keeps coming up. The peak inspiratory pressure is 22 cm H_2O on volume control ventilation. What would you do?

CASE 35: ASTHMA

Frank Stellacio

A 31-year-old man with severe asthma (you name it, he is on it, and that means steroids, too) is scheduled for emergency appendectomy. He is wheezing and says he has been faring badly lately. Poor life management has resulted in undertreatment (money earmarked for asthma inhalers has instead gone for fine wines with screw-off caps sold with paper bags wrapped around them to increase the ambience). How do you induce?

CASE 36: ASTHMA AND APPENDECTOMY

Frank Stellacio

Talk about déjà vu! You do an emergency appendectomy in a severe asthmatic, and after intubation, you cannot move any air at all. What do you do?

CASE 37: TRIGGER POINTS

Chris Gallagher

Trigger point injection is harmless, right? What are the complications associated with this harmless procedure?

CASE 38: HEAD INJURY

Chris Gallagher

For severe traumatic brain injury, what are the current recommendations regarding hyperventilation, steroids, and anticonvulsants?

CASE 39: UNSTABLE NECK

Chris Gallagher

A patient with neck pain after a motor vehicle accident (MVA) requires intubation, but there are no x-ray films yet. How do you intubate this patient? Is manual in-line stabilization a proven benefit? Do stabilization maneuvers make visualization more difficult?

CASE 40: PULMONARY ARTERY CATHETER KNOT

Chris Gallagher

The chest radiograph shows a pulmonary artery catheter has knotted. How will you remove this catheter?

CASE 41: AIRWAY FIRE

Chris Gallagher

During placement of a tracheostomy, the endotracheal tube (ETT) bursts into flames. What steps do you take?

CASE 42: STEROIDS IN A MUSCULAR MAN

Chris Gallagher

A heavily muscled man comes in to your outpatient center for knee arthroscopy. You ask about steroid use, and he admits to it. Does this change your management plan? What if he took ephedra, Garlique, or St. John's wort?

CASE 43: LEFT BUNDLE BRANCH BLOCK

Chris Gallagher

A 67-year-old man with vasculopathy is scheduled for a femoral-popliteal operation. You are concerned about ischemia, and he has a left bundle branch block. How will you detect myocardial ischemia in this patient?

CASE 44: CARBON MONOXIDE

Chris Gallagher

On a Monday morning, your first case, a man with an abdominal aortic aneurysm (AAA), has an astounding finding on his blood gas determination: a high carbon monoxide concentration. How did this happen, what do you do, and how do you prevent this in the future?

CASE 45: AIRWAY IN A PREECLAMPTIC PATIENT

Chris Gallagher

Everything else has failed, and you have to go with a general anesthetic for a severely preeclamptic patient. What special precautions do you take regarding her airway? What is your concern about intracranial hemorrhage?

CASE 46: MONOAMINE OXIDASE INHIBITORS

Chris Gallagher

A depressed patient on monoamine oxidase (MAO) inhibitors presents for an emergent operation for testicular torsion. Describe an "MAO-safe" anesthetic. What are the concerns about using MAO inhibitors?

CASE 47: TRACHEOSTOMY AND LUNG ISOLATION

Chris Gallagher

A 70-year-old woman with a tracheostomy requires lung isolation for a left upper lobectomy. How will you achieve lung isolation in a patient with a tracheostomy?

CASE 48: PARENTAL PRESENCE

Chris Gallagher

A mother wants to be in the room during induction for her 4-year-old son. The child gets oral midazolam, and his mother is freaking out because he is "acting so funny." What do you tell her? Should she come back to the room now, or should you keep her out?

CASE 49: HYPOTHERMIA FOR HEAD INJURY

Chris Gallagher

A head-injured patient is normothermic. A colleague suggests instituting mild hypothermia to improve this patient's outcome. Is it a good idea? How will you do it? How will you ensure the core "goal temperature" is reached? What are the risks?

CASE 50: CARBON DIOXIDE INSUFFLATION IN VIDEO-ASSISTED THORACOSCOPIC SURGERY

Chris Gallagher

During a video-assisted thoracoscopic surgery (VATS) procedure, the surgeon insufflates CO_2 to facilitate visualization. The pressure is only 10 cm H_2O but the blood pressure drops into the 80s. What is happening, and what should you do?

CASE 51: CONSTRUCTION IN THE OBSTETRICS DEPARTMENT

Ellen Steinberg

You have three obstetric rooms, and construction is occurring at the hospital. There is a scheduled elective section for placenta previa. Something weird has happened with the suction in two of the three rooms. Suction works only in the third room. Do you "go back" or not? Why or why not?

CASE 52: FLOW VOLUME AND ANTERIOR MEDIASTINAL MASSES

Chris Gallagher

A 52-year-old patient with an anterior mediastinal mass has no symptoms whatsoever and has normal flow-volume loops. Do you need to take any special precautions with induction? What if the patient is symptomatic? Is there any difference if the patient is a 6-year-old child? How is the physiology different?

CASE 53: APROTININ (Note: this is for historical purposes only as aprotinin has recently been pulled from the market.)

Chris Gallagher

A 64-year-old man is scheduled for repeat, repeat coronary artery bypass grafting (CABG), and there is great concern about bleeding. The patient has renal insufficiency with a creatinine level of 2.6 mg/dL. The surgeon suggests you use aprotinin. Do you have any concerns regarding renal function or regarding the grafts already there?

CASE 54: BOTOX

Chris Gallagher

A 7-year-old child with cerebral palsy is scheduled to have a Botox injection in his hamstrings to decrease spasticity and help with pain control.

How will you conduct the anesthetic? Do you have any concerns regarding the Botox?

CASE 55: TRANSJUGULAR INTRAHEPATIC PORTOSYSTEMIC SHUNT PROCEDURE

Chris Gallagher

What concerns do you have during a transjugular intrahepatic portosystemic shunt (TIPS) placement? Do you give fresh-frozen plasma (FFP) ahead of time "just in case"?

CASE 56: VAGINAL BIRTH AFTER CESAREAN SECTION

Chris Gallagher

A woman is adamant about proceeding with labor despite a previous cesarean section. How do you advise her, and what plans do you make? In the face of a well-functioning epidural, how will you detect *the* complication?

CASE 57: MULTI-ACCESS CATHETER INSERTION GONE BAD

Chris Gallagher

Insertion of a multi-access catheter (MAC) for dialysis goes awry, with the line hitting the subclavian artery, producing a large loss of blood and necessitating big fluid resuscitation, all in an achondroplastic dwarf who is now in respiratory distress with a laryngeal mask airway (LMA). How do you manage this situation, which lands in your lap when you walk by the PACU?

CASE 58: DELIRIUM IN AN ELDERLY PATIENT

Chris Gallagher

Your surgicenter sees a lot of elderly patients and a lot of postoperative delirium. What is this condition? Design a protocol to minimize this complication.

CASE 59: NERVE BLOCK AND COUGHING

Chris Gallagher

While performing an infraclavicular block on a slender, 25-year-old athlete, the patient suddenly coughs, increases his respiratory rate, and says he cannot get his breath. What is your diagnosis and management plan?

CASE 60: HEADACHE

Chris Gallagher

A 22-year-old, postpartum patient calls you from home complaining of blurred vision and headache. She had an epidural 2 days earlier. What is your response?

What is the differential diagnosis? What more sinister things could it be, and how can you tell?

CASE 61: CEREBROSPINAL FLUID DRAINAGE

Chris Gallagher

You are performing anesthesia for clipping of a cerebral aneurysm. Part of your plan is cerebrospinal fluid (CSF) drainage. What are the benefits of CSF drainage? What are the risks? You look down and realize you left the stopcock turned the wrong way, and you have drained 100 mL of CSF. What now?

CASE 62: PHEOCHROMOCYTOMA

Chris Gallagher

An indigent patient with a pheochromocytoma is scheduled for elective resection of the tumor. No insurance company will touch him, so he has not gotten any preoperative care. His blood pressure is 170/90 mm Hg. Do you proceed? Why or why not? If you do not proceed, how will you optimize this patient's status?

CASE 63: CERVICAL EPIDURAL

Chris Gallagher

You are providing sedation at a pain clinic for a 50-year-old, morbidly obese, demanding patient. The procedure planned is a cervical epidural, requiring sedation in the prone position. How will you provide sedation?

CASE 64: PAIN RELIEF AFTER KNEE SURGERY

Chris Gallagher

A patient will be sent home after an anterior cruciate ligament repair. Pain relief is being provided by a continuous peripheral catheter infusing a local anesthetic. What do you advise the patient? What are the risks of such a maneuver?

CASE 65: EQUIPMENT CHECK

Chris Gallagher

What does the negative-pressure leak test look for in your machine check? What are the risks to the patient if you skip this test and a problem occurs?

CASE 66: EQUIPMENT CHECK

Chris Gallagher

An elderly gentleman arrives in the OR with a pacemaker in his left upper chest. Your colleague tells you to "keep a magnet handy, just in case." What is your colleague telling you? Is that advice valid? What is the function of a magnet in such a setting?

CASE 67: CONSENT

Chris Gallagher

Do you need a separate consent for anesthesia procedures? Why or why not? What if a well-informed patient asks that you create one for him ad hoc? Will you? Why or why not?

CASE 68: GASTROSCHISIS

Chris Gallagher

During a gastroschisis repair, the surgeon asks you for guidance on "when to stop pushing stuff in." How will you do this? What are the circulatory effects of this repair? What are the respiratory effects?

CASE 69: PYLORIC STENOSIS

Chris Gallagher

A 4-week-old infant undergoes repair of pyloric stenosis. How will you manage pain control in this baby? Will you use narcotics or acetaminophen? What are the risks of each? If you use a local anesthetic, which one and how much?

CASE 70: COCAINE USER

Chris Gallagher

A 30-year-old cocaine abuser requires sedation in the ICU after a close encounter of the 9-mm kind purees his liver. Is long-term propofol a good solution? Compare it with dexmedetomidine. Are fentanyl and midazolam as good or better? Give your reasons for each answer?

CASE 71: SEIZURE DISORDER

Chris Gallagher

A 10-year-old child with a long history of a seizure disorder, who is on four different anticonvulsants and still suffering breakthrough seizures, is scheduled to have an appendectomy. Are there any special considerations for the anesthetic choice? What is the effect of anticonvulsants on narcotic metabolism? What is the effect of neuromuscular blocking agents?

CASE 72: CRANIAL MAPPING

Chris Gallagher

A neurosurgeon needs an awake and cooperative patient for a cranial mapping procedure. This patient has claustrophobia but says, "I will try, but I may freak out, Doc." Design a sedative analgesic for this case.

CASE 73: DIASTOLIC DYSFUNCTION

Chris Gallagher

A 75-year-old man comes to you for a hernia repair. An ambitious cardiologist figured "something must be wrong with this guy" and did a transthoracic echocardiogram on him. He comes to you with a diagnosis of moderate diastolic dysfunction. What does this mean, and how will this diagnosis alter your anesthetic? Should you cancel until the diastolic dysfunction is treated? How would you treat it?

CASE 74: SLEEP APNEA

Chris Gallagher

Describe the postoperative complications and concerns in the ambulatory patient with sleep apnea. How do you decide whether the patient can go home or needs overnight observation?

CASE 75: RENAL FAILURE

Roy Soto

A 44-year-old patient with renal failure is scheduled for an arteriovenous (AV) graft. He also has coronary artery disease and had a stent placed 2 weeks earlier. Do you proceed with the AV graft or wait an additional 4 weeks? What are the risks of waiting? What are the risks of not getting the AV graft?

CASE 76: NERVE GAS

Chris Gallagher

Word comes to you that terrorists have used a nerve gas bomb nearby. What is the mechanism of action of these agents, and what should you be prepared to treat?

CASE 77: CENTRAL LINE STERILITY

Chris Gallagher

You are placing a central line and had a hell of a time doing it. You finally get the wire in, and it then brushes your ungowned forearm. How do you manage this? What is the relative risk of infection compared with sticking again? Is there any way to make the next stick less problematic?

CASE 78: KIDNEY PROTECTION DURING ABDOMINAL AORTIC ANEURYSM

Chris Gallagher

During cross-clamping in an AAA procedure, the surgeon asks that you start renal-dose dopamine and give "a lot of mannitol." Do you agree with this management plan? What is your strategy for protecting the kidneys?

CASE 79: MYASTHENIA GRAVIS

Roy Soto

A 59-year-old man with a history of myasthenia gravis presents for direct laryngoscopy under general anesthesia to enable laser therapy for vocal cord polyps. Pyridostigmine (750 mg/day) controls his symptoms. Would you consider succinylcholine for this case? Why or why not? How would you dose it if you did? A colleague suggests a succinylcholine drip. What is your response? How would you determine adequate return of neuromuscular function for extubation?

CASE 80: UREMIA AND PLATELET FUNCTION

Roy Soto

A 44-year-old woman with end-stage renal disease requiring dialysis requests an epidural for labor analgesia. Does uremia affect your choice of anesthetic technique? Why or why not? How does uremia affect coagulation? What tests can be performed to assess platelet function?

CASE 81: MANDIBLE FRACTURE

Roy Soto

A 19-year-old man presents for repair of bilateral mandibular fractures. He is thin and is otherwise healthy, but he cannot open his mouth more than 2 cm because of the pain. What is your plan for airway management? Would your plan change if the patient were obese? Why or why not? At the conclusion of surgery, the patient's teeth are wired closed. What is your plan for extubation? Assume the patient has respiratory distress in the recovery room. How would you prepare for reintubation?

CASE 82: PREGNANT NURSE

Roy Soto

An OR nurse tells you she has just found out that she is pregnant and asks you if she should avoid working in the OR. What is your response? Would your response be different if she were in her third trimester? Why or why not? She also asks about the risks of working in the recovery room. What is your response?

CASE 83: GENERAL ANESTHESIA IN A PREGNANT PATIENT

Roy Soto

A patient who is 20 weeks' pregnant comes to the OR for laparoscopic chole-cystectomy. She asks you what the anesthetic risks are for her fetus. What is your response? Would you recommend fetal heart rate and contraction monitoring? Would your decision be different if she were 37 weeks' pregnant? Why or why not?

CASE 84: KID WITH A BAD AIRWAY

Peggy Seidman

An 8-month-old infant has a large cystic hygroma shown by the CT scan to compress trachea and right upper bronchus with collapse of the right upper lung. The surgeon insists on an MRI/MRA scan to discern the vascular supply before excision. Should sedation be done in the MRI scanner? Is sedation of an 8-month-old infant ever a reality? Is an LMA acceptable for airway management during general anesthesia?

CASE 85: EPIDURAL AND COMPLEX REGIONAL PAIN SYNDROME

Joy Schabel

A 33-year-old parturient is requesting an epidural for labor analgesia. Her history is significant for complex regional pain syndrome (CRPS) in the left upper extremity. She sees a chronic pain specialist and had a spinal cord stimulator placed at C7-8 to help manage her chronic pain. What is CRPS, and how does a spinal cord stimulator decrease a patient's pain from CRPS? Would you place an epidural for labor analgesia in this patient? Why or why not? What if the stimulator was placed at L1-2?

CASE 86: PREMATURE INFANT AND PATENT DUCTUS ARTERIOSUS

Robert Katz

A 3-day-old, premature infant (29 weeks' gestational age) comes to the OR for repair of a patent ductus arteriosus. The infant is lethargic in the holding area. What is your differential diagnosis?

CASE 87: PERICARDIAL WINDOW

Chris Gallagher

A 65-year-old patient scheduled for a pericardial window comes to you sitting bolt upright and is short of breath. As you seek a pulse, you feel an irregular tapping, but when you look at the electrocardiogram (ECG), you do not see atrial fibrillation? What could account for this disconnect between what you feel and what you see?

CASE 88: TRANSESOPHAGEAL ECHOCARDIOGRAPHY PROBE PLACEMENT

Chris Gallagher

A cardiologist is having a hard time placing a transesophageal echocardiography (TEE) probe. How can you help him in an awake patient or in an intubated patient? Is there any concern if this is a patient with a thoracic gunshot?

CASE 89: BURNS

Chris Gallagher

After a routine AAA procedure in which all went well (thank God for small favors), you make a disturbing discovery as you take down the drapes. The patient appears to have burns wherever the Betadine pooled. What could account for this, and how will you prevent it from happening again?

CASE 90: CORNEAL ABRASIONS

Chris Gallagher

The ICU nurses tell you that several patients have been complaining of eye pain and have been found to have corneal abrasions. You review the records, and all seems in order. Describe a mechanism for how corneal abrasions can occur in the ICU when their eyes were appropriately covered in the OR?

CASE 91: OBESE PREGNANT PATIENT

Rishi Adsumelli

A 32-year-old parturient with a history of two previous cesarean sections presents in labor at 11 PM (when else?) the night before her scheduled cesarean section. She weighs 480 pounds and stopped off for a chimichanga (vegetable— she is watching her weight) 1 hour before. The obstetrician says, "Guess what? We cannot monitor this baby at all! Ay caramba!" (he also likes Mexican food, so we have a kind of Latin theme here). We need to do the section immediately. It is your move, amigo. What do you do to get ready? What are the concerns of the obstetrician and anesthesiologist? What happens if you cannot pick up a heart beat? What is the risk of a uterine rupture? What are the anesthetic options? What problems do you expect with an epidural or with spinal anesthesia? Discuss continuous spinal anesthesia.

CASE 92: WHIPPLE IN A DIABETIC PATIENT

Rishi Adsumelli

A 45-year-old man was admitted to the hospital with a complaint about abdominal pain. The patient had a history of diabetes and pancreatic cancer, and he has undergone chemotherapy, radiation therapy, and a Whipple procedure. The attending oncologist consults you for a pain management strategy for this patient. How would you evaluate this patient's pain? What are the potential causes of this presentation?

On physical examination, you find decreased sensation in the hands and feet. What diagnoses are you leaning toward? A CT scan of the patient's abdomen shows recurrence of the tumor in the liver and the retroperitoneal area. How would you treat this patient? What is the myth about pain treatment in cancer patients?

13

Answers to Stem Questions

CASE 1: YOU CRACK ME UP

Intraoperative Questions

1. Besides the usual monitors recommended by the American Society of Anesthesiologists (ASA), what additional monitors would you place?

An arterial line is placed after induction. You do not need the beat-to-beat pressure monitoring on induction, and the patient is somewhat less than cooperative. Why make both your lives miserable if you do not have to? You definitely want it after induction, because this is no "routine bronch" with jagged glass in his trachea. If things go kablooey, I would rather have an arterial line than not.

There was no need for a central venous pressure (CVP) line because I could get good peripheral access, and this was not a volume case. If something bizarre happened, and the surgeon needed to open the chest, I would put one in. When *they* are in the chest, *we* should be in the chest. This may be overkill, but when something goes wrong in a chest case, that is not the time to start getting central access.

2. Does induction for a fiberoptic bronchoscopy differ from induction for a rigid bronchoscopy? If so, how? How are the goals different?

Yes, for fiberoptic bronchoscopy, life is relatively routine for us: induce, intubate, secure the airway, and then go through the endotracheal tube (ETT). Not a ton of stimulation.

For rigid bronchoscopy, it is a different situation. We have to surrender the airway, ventilation is not superb (there is no cuff sealing the airway), and the stimulation is in a continuous state of "laryngoscopy plus direct tracheal stimulation." Muscle relaxation has to be good enough to intubate at all times. Rigid bronchoscopy is a pain, pure and simple.

3. Does placement of the ETT pose a potential threat to the placement of the foreign body? What if the foreign body were a peanut?

Yes, the ETT can push the foreign body farther down the trachea, making it hard to fish out. However, if a foreign body is right in the trachea, it can cause complete occlusion, and pushing the foreign body farther down may at least allow you to ventilate one lung. These cases of a foreign body in the trachea are always touch and go. Talk over the game plan with the surgeon ahead of time, and get a feel for exactly what is where. If it is a peanut, you can even hit it and break it into smaller pieces (God Almighty, what a pain!). Sometimes, a judicious mix of techniques may help, such as alternating between ventilating with an ETT, surrendering to the bronchoscope, and going forward one step at a time. Flexibility and ingenuity are the keys.

4. You induce and attempt to mask ventilate, but the heavy beard and mustache impede effective gas exchange. How do you modify your technique?

Wake up the patient, and dry shave him with a flat razor—that is what you do! After your oral board examiners regain consciousness, you modify your response to the following. Put a large Steri-Drape over the face, poke a hole in the mouth area, and you have a better seal. At first, it looks like you are smothering the patient, but people will get over that when they see how well you are ventilating. Alternatively, you can push on and intubate right away. With big beards, suxamethonium is a good idea so you can get "in there" right away. If the mustache alone is impeding your view (assume you did not do the Steri-Drape trick), put a piece of tape on the mustache, smashing it flat so you can see to intubate.

5. You attempt to place an 8.0-French ETT, but as sometimes happens, you cannot get a big tube in, and you are able to place a 7.0-French ETT. The surgeon says, "I cannot do this through a 7.0!" How do you help the surgeon out?

With the smaller tube in, make sure you effectively ventilate, get the saturation level up, ensure the vital signs are okay, and get your anesthetic going. Do not let the surgeon rush you. Then exchange the ETT over a tube changer, keeping in mind that you do not want to push the foreign body farther down the trachea. Like the Wicked Witch of the West said, "These things must be done delicately, delicately." When doing the exchange, grease the living bejeebers out of the larger tube and try wiggling it back and forth as you advance it. If you cannot achieve this, tell the surgeon about your dilemma and suggest he use a smaller scope. He will get mad at you and curse you to your seventh generation going forward and backward, but what can you do?

6. Fiberoptic bronchoscopy fails. How do you conduct your anesthetic to allow for rigid bronchoscopy?

You have established that you can intubate, and you now must make sure the patient is well anesthetized (look at the BIS monitor and be ready to give a bolus of propofol). Prepare for suboptimal ventilation (which you always get with a rigid bronchoscope) by making sure you are on 100% oxygen, tilting the patient's head up to give more functional residual capacity (FRC), and making sure you have complete neuromuscular relaxation. Suction the mouth out, and then hand over the airway to the surgeon. And tell him to hurry up!

7. The surgeon has a hard time getting a big rigid bronchoscope into the trachea, and the patient desaturates to the mid-80s. He is still attempting to get the scope in. What do you do?

Push him aside, reintubate, and get the saturation level up. He will need a smaller bronchoscope. Do not let the surgeon flounder while the patient expires.

8. With the rigid bronchoscope in, the surgeon attempts to grasp the glass stem of the crack pipe, but it keeps "crumbling" every time he grabs it. What can you do to help?

Tilt the patient's head down, and hit him on his feet. Do not laugh. This may work the crack pipe "downhill" a little and let the surgeon get a better stab at it. Even if you have never seen this sort of thing before, keep thinking. You can also try to put the fiberoptic scope through the rigid scope, go through the crack pipe, and snag it from within. This is what we ended up doing.

9. The determination for a blood gas sample sent for evaluation in the middle of this epic struggle shows a pH of 7.23, PO_2 of 65 mm Hg, and PCO_2 of 69 mm Hg. What is your interpretation, and how do you intend to improve the patient's status?

This situation is clearly poor ventilation. Do everything you can to improve ventilation, including stopping the case temporarily, establishing a better airway, reintubating, and ventilating back to less life-threatening numbers.

10. After several attempts, the surgeon says, "Maybe we should wake him up and cancel this?" Are there any other alternatives?

This is where you must have the voice of the consultant. In effect, the lungs cannot handle it, but you cannot leave a guy with a hunk of glass in his trachea. You need to consider getting a machine to do what the lungs are doing by putting him on cardiopulmonary bypass (CPB). Go on bypass, provide oxygenation that way, open the chest, cut open the trachea, and fish out the foreign body. This may seem radical, but it is one way to solve the problem. When all the easy routes are gone, you must go with the difficult route.

Postoperative Questions

1. On the way to the postanesthesia care unit (PACU) the Foley catheter falls under a gurney wheel and snaps off. The end of it is not on the floor, but you cannot see anything on examining the patient. What do you do?

The balloon may have kept a portion of the Foley in the bladder, and you now have a foreign body in the genitourinary tract and possible urethral damage. Call the urology department for an emergency consultation. Document everything that happened, and explain what happened to the patient. Far-fetched as this may sound, it does happen, usually when a catheter laboratory disaster or a level 1 trauma comes rolling in for immediate repair. Things fall off the bed in the chaos, and kaboom!

2. The glass stem is out, but the patient continues to cough violently. Is there anything else on the differential diagnosis for severe coughing? Is there anything you can do to alleviate this patient's distress?

Something is awry in the chest, so go for the basics first: physical examination (decreased breath sounds can mean a pneumothorax, which can produce a cough) and a chest radiograph looking for pneumothorax or another foreign body you missed (perhaps you knocked a tooth out during the case, and it got into the tracheobronchial tree). Coughing can result from fluid overload. After you have ruled out all the baddies, a diagnosis of exclusion is irritation to the trachea from the scratching of the glass and the bronchoscope. Symptomatic treatment with narcotics or lidocaine may help (always watching for respiratory depression).

3. A persistent sinus tachycardia of 120 beats/min gets the PACU nurse's attention. How do you evaluate this? Is it a concern in a 44-year-old patient?

Yes, tachycardia is always a concern. All 44-year-old patients can have ischemia (this man is not a poster child for health awareness, after all). Evaluate tachycardia by rounding up the usual suspects (e.g., pain, hypoxemia, hypercarbia), and get a 12-lead electrocardiogram (ECG) (tachycardia causes ischemia, and ischemia can cause tachycardia). After you have ruled out anything treatable (e.g., anemia is unlikely because this was not a blood loss case, but you do not lose anything by ruling out the easy ones), treat the tachycardia by judicious use of β-blockade (i.e., esmolol drip or metoprolol), aiming at getting the heart rate down to 80 beats/min. Dig around in the patient's records, and see what his usual heart rate is (maybe it is always this high). Unfortunately, this man probably has no old records to go by.

How It Actually Happened

I was in the middle of another thoracic case when the computed tomography (CT) fellow came in, threw up the chest radiograph, and said, "You have to see this to believe it."

The universal sentiment of the room was this: How the hell do you suck that big piece of glass into your trachea in the first place? And after you do that, how the hell do you not go to the hospital for 2 days?

Those amazing humans! This patient was not the world's easiest intubation (remember, this book is about real live cases, not just stuff we dreamed up). Masking was tough. We had to put in a smaller tube, switch to a bigger tube, and then we all groaned when we had to go to rigid bronchoscopy. We knew the surgeon would have a hard time getting that damned bronchoscope in (what is bronchoscopy but the ultimate in laryngoscopy?). Sure enough, the surgeon could not get a big rigid scope in and had to go with a smaller rigid scope. At that point, we were doing the same sort of ventilating that you do with a rigid bronchoscope (i.e., no balloon to inflate, lots of air leaking, and a crummy gas, just as in the previous questions).

After several attempts at grabbing the pipe, with pieces of glass crumbling off (it was sickening to hear that glass crunch). We almost despaired. The surgeon said, "Maybe we should wake him up and cancel this." I said, "No way! He cannot go around with that thing in his lung!" Everyone and their second cousin piled into the room and all manner of suggestions flew around:

- Use a femoral-femoral bypass, cut open the trachea, and pull it out.
- Put a flexible scope through the middle of it and pull it out.
- Put him head down and pound on his feet to get it to "jiggle" up the trachea (we tried that and shook him and did all kinds of stuff, but it would not budge).

The "fiberoptic scope through the middle" approach appealed to us, but the stem was long, and we were scared that it would break apart during the tight turn through the oropharynx, leaving all kinds of broken glass in his posterior pharynx. Then we had an "aha" moment and got it (cover up the stuff below for a little bit, and think it through before you read on).

We did a tracheostomy, shortening the distance to the crack pipe stem, and taking the turn in the hypopharynx out of the equation. After the tracheostomy, we could ventilate better (the ST segments finally came down). We then slipped the flexible fiberoptic scope through the middle of the crack pipe stem, "J'd" it to hook it, and pulled it out through the tracheostomy site. The whole room cheered.

While in the hospital, the guy kept coughing, with small bits of broken off glass occasionally flying out of his tracheostomy. He eventually stopped coughing up glass, his tracheostomy site healed over, and he is back on the streets again, ready for more thrills.

CASE 2: EXCEDRIN HEADACHE

Preoperative Questions

1. What would be your neurologic examination of this patient?

Because this is an urgent procedure, the purpose of this examination is to rapidly document the baseline neurologic status of the child. The examination should include the Glasgow Coma Scale (GCS), which is composed of three parameters: eye response, verbal response, and motor response. Clinical evidence of high intracranial pressure (ICP) should be sought (i.e., vomiting, papilledema, confusion, behavioral changes, and Cushing's triad of bradycardia, systolic hypertension [with widened pulse pressure], and a change in respiratory pattern).

2. What would be the anesthetic relevance?

This information can help evaluate whether any of the cranial nerves are affected or if there is a problem with spinal fluid flow. High ICP elevates the risk for vomiting and aspiration during induction of anesthesia.

3. How will you assess elevated ICP?

During the preoperative evaluation, consider the symptoms elicited in the medical history and the physical examination (e.g., vomiting, increasing level of confusion, headaches, Cushing's triad). Imaging studies showing a mass effect on the brain may help confirm the diagnosis.

4. Is magnetic resonance imaging (MRI) necessary? Is other imaging needed?

Brain imaging studies are necessary for the surgical team to plan the correct procedure. No other imaging studies are needed at this point.

5. What laboratory studies will be helpful?

Helpful tests include preoperative levels of electrolytes (e.g., potassium, sodium), blood urea nitrogen and creatinine levels, a complete blood cell count, and type and cross for two units of packed red blood cells (PRBCs).

6. How will your findings affect your plan for premedication?

There is no need for preoperative sedation in a child who is already lethargic and confused.

7. How will you assess the patient's volume status?

In this case, preoperative intravascular fluid depletion is expected. Findings such as confusion, dry mucosal tissues, hypotension, and low urine output support it. Intravascular fluid treatment should be reviewed before induction, and good intravenous access should be achieved (i.e., two large-bore intravenous catheters).

8. What type of fluid will you use for this case?

Any kind of crystalloid solution is appropriate for this case.

9. Will you add dextrose-containing solutions? Explain why or why not.

No. Dextrose-containing solutions should be avoided because of the risk of causing brain edema in the presence of an injured blood-brain barrier.

10. What monitors will you use? When a CVP monitor is indicated, how will you place it?

Standard ASA monitors, including the ECG and those for blood pressure, heart rate, CO_2, and temperature, are required. Intra-arterial blood pressure monitoring, precordial Doppler, and a central venous line should be placed. The CVP line is placed immediately after induction, and its position should be verified by an intraoperative chest radiograph.

11. Will you include a precordial Doppler monitor?

Yes, it should be included, because it will help in the detection of an air embolism.

12. What blood products should be available?

Two units of PRBCs should be available in the OR.

Intraoperative Questions

1. Describe your anesthetic plan for induction, maintenance, and emergence.

After initial optimization of the intravascular volume, the patient should be brought into the OR, monitors placed, and the patient preoxygenated. Intravenous induction uses a modified rapid-sequence induction (RSI) with propofol, rocuronium, lidocaine, and fentanyl boluses. Anesthetic maintenance should include a combination of sevoflurane, propofol, and fentanyl infusions and intermittent rocuronium boluses for muscle relaxation.

2. Please explain your anesthetic goals for this case. Are they different from those for adult patient management?

The anesthetic goals are to avoid further brain injury and ischemia, avoid elevating the ICP, and maintain hemodynamic stability.

3. What are the risks during induction?

The risks during induction include vomiting, aspiration, and wide changes in hemodynamic status, hypoxia, and an increase in ICP.

4. Discuss ways of controlling ICP during anesthesia.

There are several ways to control ICP:

- Reducing cerebral blood flow by hyperventilation and constricting cerebral blood vessels or by causing deliberate hypotension. Hyperventilation used to be done widely, but the concern for cerebral ischemia makes us recommend attaining eucarbia now.
- Increasing cerebrospinal fluid (CSF) removal, which can be achieved by placing a CSF drain
- Minimizing the brain mass by elevating the head and optimizing venous return or by using diuretics
- Reducing the cerebral metabolic rate by inducing mild hypothermia and using general anesthesia and adjuvants such as barbiturates

5. During intracranial dissection, the patient suddenly becomes hypotensive and tachycardic. What is the differential diagnosis? If there is venous air embolism (VAE), what are the potential risks?

The differential diagnosis includes bleeding, arrhythmia or cardiac ischemia, pulmonary embolism, and venous air embolism. Intraoperative VAE can range in severity from being asymptomatic to causing severe injury or death. Factors that determine the morbidity of an episode of VAE include the rate and volume of air entrained and the status of the patient at the time of the embolism.

The lethal dose of intravascular air in humans is unknown, but accidental injections of between 100 and 300 mL have been fatal. The mechanism of death from massive air embolus is circulatory obstruction and cardiovascular collapse resulting from air trapped in the right ventricular outflow tract. VAE that does not cause immediate death can cause paradoxical embolization by acutely increasing right atrial pressure, resulting in right-to-left shunt through a patent foramen ovale. Pulmonary microvascular occlusion also can occur; the air can produce increasing obstruction to blood flow, undergo resorption, or result in increased dead space. Bronchoconstriction may result from release of endothelial mediators, complement production, and cytokine release. Morbidity and mortality from air embolism are directly related to the size of the embolus and the rate of entry. Doses of air greater than 50 mL (1 mL/kg) cause hypotension and dysrhythmias, and 300 mL of air entrained rapidly can be lethal. Bronchoconstriction results in increased airway pressure and wheezing. Other manifestations of air embolism include hypoxemia, hypercapnia, and decreased end-tidal CO_2 (because of increased functional dead space). Hypotension, cardiac dysrhythmias, and cardiovascular collapse occur as air entrainment continues.

6. What methods are used to make the diagnosis? Which is the most sensitive?

The most important method is to closely monitor the patient and have a high index of suspicion. Transesophageal echocardiography (TEE) is the most sensitive monitoring technique for VAE, and it is able to detect 0.02 mL/kg of air administered by a bolus intravenous injection. Doppler ultrasound is a fairly sensitive monitoring technique. A Doppler ultrasound probe can detect 0.25 mL of air.

The pulmonary artery catheter is the next most sensitive monitor. Air entering the pulmonary circulation causes mechanical obstruction and reflex vasoconstriction due to pulmonary hypoxemia, resulting in increased pulmonary artery pressure. Mass spectrometry for end-tidal nitrogen is as sensitive as the pulmonary artery catheter. End-tidal CO_2 is a standard intraoperative monitor that is used in almost every surgical procedure, but it is not specific for air embolism. The least sensitive monitor is the precordial or esophageal stethoscope. A "millwheel murmur" indicates a massive air embolism. When a millwheel murmur is heard, cardiovascular collapse is imminent.

7. What is your management plan for VAE?

The primary goals are to prevent further air entry, reduce the volume of the entrained air, and support the cardiovascular system while air is resorbed. The surgeon should be informed as soon VAE is suspected. The surgeon should flood the surgical field with irrigating solution, control open blood vessels, and apply bone wax to exposed bones. The FIO_2 should be increased to 1.0. If N_2O is used, it should be discontinued when an air embolism occurs. If a CVP catheter has been placed in the right atrium, air can be aspirated through the catheter.

The optimal site for the tip of the catheter is at the junction of the superior vena cava (SVC) and the right atrium. If significant amounts of air have entered the circulation, the jugular veins can be manually occluded. This prevents additional air from being entrained while the surgeon obtains hemostasis. If surgical conditions permit positioning the patient in the left lateral decubitus position, it can help to keep air in the right atrium from entering the ventricle. The blood pressure should be supported by administering fluids and inotropic drugs such as epinephrine. If possible, the operative site should be positioned below the level of the heart; this increases venous pressure at the operative site and reduces air entrainment.

8. Will you extubate this patient?

At the conclusion of the case, assuming the patient is hemodynamically stable and after performing a positive-pressure leak test, the patient may be extubated in the operating room (OR) if certain extubation criteria are met: adequate tidal volume, awake and following commands, and full reversal of muscle relaxation. Emergence should be smooth, with minimal coughing and bucking.

CASE 3: CT AND A BAG OF CHIPS

Preoperative Questions

1. How can you honorably get the hell out of doing this case without dumping it on some unsuspecting colleague and incurring his or her eternal wrath?

Uh, you cannot. Next question, your honor.

2. What possible horrors accompany the smirking surgeon's comment, "They had a time of it last year"?

He is no doubt making reference to the challenges associated with the morbidly obese, including poor pulmonary function and poor cardiac function. You will have problems with the airway, ventilation, and hemodynamics. Intubation may be difficult, and if intubation fails, mask ventilation will also be difficult, set against a background of quick desaturation, in the very person (i.e., poor heart and prone to arrhythmias as evidenced by the automatic implantable cardioverter defibrillator [AICD]) you do not want to desaturate. Oh, what a tangled web we weave.

Ventilating a 330-pound man is difficult enough, but you are now inside a CT scanner, you cannot tilt the patient's head up (to scrape up a little FRC help), and he is prone, with his abdominal contents pushing up his diaphragm, making ventilation difficult. A hemodynamic remedy is tricky. Too little fluid, and the pressure will go down; too much fluid, and you will overload his lungs.

3. How will you determine the degree of the patient's pulmonary compromise?

You can do a million-dollar pulmonary function test (PFT) workup, but your best interrogation is obtaining a history: "Can you lie flat? How much can you do?" Conduct a physical examination looking for the usual bad things, such as a fast respiratory rate, weak accessory muscles, puffing (i.e., evidence of auto–positive end-expiratory pressure (auto-PEEP) at room-air saturation. At a glance, you can tell the pulmonary cripple. These patients do not come to cryoablation unless they are in horrible shape in the first place; everyone with a shred of alveolus comes to the OR to have this excised.

4. Cryoablation will be done, but no cautery will be used. How do you manage the AICD? Is this different from "a regular case"?

You always have to be ready to open, heaven forbid, in case bleeding is encountered. Do the usual things you do for an AICD. Have the programmer people turn it off, place Zoll pads to be able to defibrillate, and have them turn the AICD on when you are done with the case. This fits under the rubric, "If you bring an umbrella, it will not rain."

5. How do you explain the risks of general anesthesia in these circumstances to this patient?

Honesty tinged with compassion is the best policy. Tell the patient you will do everything to make sure his breathing and heart are taken care of during the case, but realistically, he is at high risk for complications. Explain that any complication that comes up will be treated as quickly as possible and that you will call in consults to help. The biggest potential problem is being on a ventilator postoperatively. I also would explain awake intubation, because this is my method of choice for securing the airway.

6. The surgeon and interventional radiologist concur that this is the only way to get the tumor. Do you need any further workup or laboratory studies? The patient has had a chest radiograph, ECG, and hematocrit determination.

Make sure there is no coagulopathy; know the platelet count, prothrombin time (PT), and partial thromboplastin time (PTT). This is not idle fishing (get every test known to man); you must make sure this fellow does not bleed because opening up this guy would present a host of problems.

7. The patient's rhythm is entirely paced. Discuss how this affects your assessment of the patient and the plan for your anesthetic. Does a magnet have any place here?

Entirely paced means that you do not turn off the pacer part of the AICD! During interrogation of the AICD, ask the tech person, "Is there anything, anything at all, underneath that paced rhythm?" It is reassuring to know that there is some native "bail out" mechanism in the heart. (The best place to look all this stuff up is Marc Rozner's annual talk on pacers in the ASA refresher courses. Rozner is so damned smart my head aches when I talk to him, and he is funny as hell and has a great irreverence for all things and all people. Buttonhole him at the next ASA meeting, and see for yourself what I am talking about.) This is one of the few times during the oral exam that I would quote a reference and say, "Rozner says do not put a magnet on the AICD because you cannot be sure what it will do." I do not see anyone hassling you for questioning Rozner on pacers. It would be like questioning Buddha on enlightenment.

Intraoperative Questions

1. Physical examination shows a large tongue, thick neck, and an inability to lie down flat for any length of time. How will you secure the airway, keeping in mind you are "off site"?

The prime rule of off-site work is to equip it like it is not an off-site area. This man is a bad airway case, so I would roll all the necessary equipment (e.g., fiberoptic scope, topicalization supplies) into the off-site area and perform an awake intubation. No short cuts are allowed because we are "not where we usually are." Even if this eats up a lot of time, I would do it because this guy will desaturate like crazy if you attempt intubation, fail, and try to mask ventilate.

2. As you are topicalizing and sedating for an awake intubation, the surgeon says, "They did not do this last year when they operated on him." Does this change your management plan? What do you say to the surgeon?

When this happens, I tell the surgeon, "Maybe last time it was a better anesthesiologist." If I am convinced someone will be hard to intubate, I perform an awake intubation, regardless of the patient's history. The earlier person may have had difficulty and not recorded or admitted it. The patient's airway may have worsened (e.g., gained weight, more arthritis, tumor invasion) since the last time. Caution says to do the right thing, so do the right thing.

3. How do you manage sedation for this patient? How do you manage if a baseline arterial blood gas (ABG) determination puts the patient in the 60/60 club?

You are skating on thin ice here because supplementary oxygen may deprive him of his hypoxemic drive to breathe and he is sensitive to respiratory depression. The most important part of the sedation will be the detailed explanation at the beginning. The more he is "on my side," the better. For sedation, I would use dexmedetomidine with a small dose of midazolam, avoiding narcotics altogether. I would be meticulous in the topicalization process, stopping if he is poorly topicalized and re-topicalizing rather than shoving ahead by adding heavier sedation. If this takes a while, it takes a while.

4. Do you need additional monitors other than the ASA standards?

Use an arterial line. Anticipate respiratory trouble after the procedure (they are making a hole in his already feeble lung). A cuff will take forever to cycle on his big arm. With an ejection fraction (EF) of 30% and prone position, you will need beat-to-beat blood pressure capability.

5. You intubate successfully and move the patient to the prone position. Inspiratory pressures go up, and you are delivering only about 200 mL of tidal volume. What do you do?

This, amigo, is what we call a *problema grande*. He needs to be in this position to do the case, and you are sort of stuck. Make sure nothing preventable is wrong (e.g., right main stem intubation). It will be hard to tell by breath sounds (i.e., poor lungs and his size), so look with the fiberoptic scope. Try to adjust the ventilator—anything to keep him at least "in the ballpark" stable. Use frequent small breaths or whatever it takes. If that does not work, get an intensive care unit (ICU) ventilator (they are better than ours), and try to adjust that. Given what they need to do, I would even live with suboptimal ventilation as long as the saturation level stays above 88% (after all, that is his baseline), because this procedure is the guy's only shot at a cure.

6. After several ventilator adjustments, the end-tidal CO_2 level persistently remains at 75. Do you adjust the ventilator again? How? Do you cancel the case? What are the risks of a high CO_2 level?

Hypercarbia is a problem, but again, this procedure is this guy's only shot at curing his cancer, so if he is not showing signs of end-organ intolerance (i.e., ectopy) and this is really the best that can be done, I would tell the interventional radiologist my concern and live with the high CO_2 level while encouraging swiftness on the part of my colleagues. I would call in an ICU specialist to double check my vent settings and see if he or she can come up with anything better. Short-term high CO_2 with no other option along with "this is the only chance for a cure" is a risk I would take.

7. Oxygen saturation drops to 89% when the patient is fully inside the CT scanner. What do you do?

I would fix everything I could fix (e.g., tube position, suction, β-agent if patient is bronchospastic, addition of PEEP), but I would otherwise live with this situation because this is probably as good as you are going to get in this patient in this position. Assuming a risk for a shot at a cure when the other options are to cancel case or open up and operate is worth it. As in "regular thoracostomies," you can live with a saturation level in the 80s for a while to facilitate the resection, and I would do the same here.

8. How do you maintain anesthesia? Do you need muscle relaxants? If so, which muscle relaxants do you use?

Use 100% oxygen, sevoflurane, vecuronium, or other muscle relaxants. You do not *need* the relaxation to do the procedure, but movement at the wrong time could move the cryo probe and damage nearby vessels or the heart! Just as you would maintain muscle relaxation in a retinal case, in which movement can be a disaster, you maintain relaxation in this case to prevent a disaster.

9. At the end of the case, describe how you will ascertain this patient's readiness for extubation. Do you take any special precautions regarding the hypoxemic drive to breathe? Do you give any special considerations to the preoperative baseline CO_2 level?

Get the patient in a good position: out of the CT scanner, supine, and on a bed where you can sit him all the way up. Then go through the usual criteria: complete neuromuscular relaxation reversal, good inspiratory pressures, good saturation, and an ability to control secretions and follow commands. Then address any special considerations; because he had a high baseline CO_2 level, you can accept a high level at end of the case (i.e., back to baseline). The hypoxemic drive to breathe question is a killer because you want as much oxygen on him as possible (as you do at the end of any procedure in case the patient obstructs, gets overnarcotized, or has residual weakness), but you do not want to give him a high oxygen level because it undermines his drive to breathe. I would keep him intubated, get him to the PACU or ICU, and have him evaluated carefully over an hour or so, seeing how he does on continuous positive airway pressure (CPAP) with progressively lower FIO_2 values until you can see how he will react. Ideally, you will be able to extubate him when he is on 30%.

10. Immediately on extubation, the patient breathes 40 times per minute, says he is short of breath, and keeps insisting you let him hang his feet down. What is your diagnosis? What is the treatment? Do you let him hang his feet down?

Let him hang his feet down! This shortness of breath is most likely volume overload; poor lungs and a poor heart means he is easy to overload. Let him pool his fluid in his legs (it is like instant Lasix) to decrease his central filling pressures. The patient has probably done this maneuver before and knows it works. After that, place a Foley catheter, get a chest radiograph, and give furosemide to shed excess intravascular fluid and aid his breathing.

How It Actually Happened

I did everything short of pulling the fire alarm and emptying out the hospital to get out of doing this case, because it had "you will have a bad day" written all over it. It did.

God looks out for drunks and fools, so I must have been drinking that day, because the patient came down with a working intravenous line. Thank you, Lord, and yes, I will have another drink.

Airway land looked bad, with a tongue so big I think Mallampati has to come up with a class 5 view next time around. Ignoring all blandishments of "they did not do him awake last time," I damned well did him awake this time. For my money, difficult is difficult. Maybe last time, someone much more talented than I am intubated him with ease, but I was not about to take that chance. We were off-site, too, so if I screwed up the intubation and he shifted into facultative anaerobe mode, he would be dead seven ways from Sunday by the time anyone got there to help me.

Sedation was light as possible because his baseline blood gas determination showed we were dancing on the knife edge in terms of O_2 and a CO_2. Luckily, he was stoic, and the topicalization worked. We took our time, knowing a rush job would lead to a botched intubation attempt and bleeding.

Going prone was epic, and fitting 330 pounds on that skinny CT table was no easy feat. I wanted to tie him down with battleship chains, but they do not allow those in the CT scanner, so we used tons of tape and every Velcro strap available in three counties.

Ventilation was an industrial effort, with high P_{CO_2} persisting throughout the case. We tried every different setting a ventilator can have, wiggling and re-adjusting until we finally got the CO_2 to a level just a little above his baseline. We considered a unit ventilator, but by then, the case was done.

We stuck to caution the way white sticks to rice and kept the man intubated postoperatively, taking him to the PACU intubated. There, we placed him on CPAP and observed him for 30 minutes, determining when the time was right. We had him sitting bolt upright to help increase FRC and decrease his work of breathing. Were we not clever little medicos, heading off trouble before it starts?

Not so fast, slick. After extubation, he did fine for about 7 nanoseconds (a long-term success in my book), and then he started panting fast, puffing, and was unable to say a sentence. His saturation level dropped into the upper 80s. Damn!

A Foley catheter, Lasix, and breathing treatments at least moved him out of "reintubation-ville." The chest radiograph showed pulmonary edema. We moved him to the unit upstairs, where he continued to improve overnight. Just before we sent him up, he insisted that we let him swing his legs over the bed and hang them down. I will be batter-fried and served on a stick at the county fair, but that guy got better the second he hung those feet down. He must have deposited a liter of fluid in each of those legs, uncongested his lungs, and fixed himself right up.

The best part happened the next day. I went to the unit, saw the nametag on his door, and found no one in there. "He has been transferred to the floor, or he has been transferred somewhere more celestial," methinks.

Then I *heard* him. I walked around the corner, and there he was, sitting up in bed and reaching into a large bag of Salt & Vinegar Kettle Baked Potato Chips—good for the waistline and fluid status! "Hey, Doc!" he shouted.

"We switched rooms this morning," the ward clerk explained, "but did not change the name plates yet."

Crunch, crunch, crunch. "Want some?" he asked as he held the bag forward. He was sitting and dangling his feet down, probably titrating *dangle* to *salt load* with the finesse of a Cirque de Soleil juggler. "Heard you had some trouble yesterday. Hope I wasn't too much trouble," he said with big smile on his face. "Nothin' you can't handle, right?"

"Think I will take a few chips, now that you offer."

CASE 4: SOMETHING IS DISAGREEING WITH MY STOMACH

Intraoperative Questions

1. Invasive monitors are part of your plan, but the patient's mental status presents challenges. Which invasive monitors will you use, and how will you get them in, given these circumstances?

Can you get an arterial line in a mentally impaired patient? Yes, but it would be a struggle, and someone with tachycardia, positive troponin levels, and instability does not need to undergo a long struggle to place a line. Realizing that "induction is the big baddie," I would immediately have the blood pressure cuff on, and I would have the surgeon keep a finger on the femoral artery, ready to stick it as soon as her eyelids flutter with the start of induction and to tell me if the pulse disappears. I would induce with a reduced dose of an agent known for its stability (e.g., etomidate), aware of the fact that nothing guarantees stability if the patient is on the nth degree of sympathetic support.

2. Describe the hemodynamic response to sepsis and how this plays against a background of evolving myocardial infarction (MI)?

Sepsis does everything bad for the patient with evolving MI or tachycardia (e.g., shortening diastole, increasing work load), and at the same time, the perfusion pressure drops from systemic vasodilation. Bad news all around!

3. Bleeding may be a concern. Should you use ε-aminocaproic acid? What is it, and how does it work?

ε-Aminocaproic acid binds to plasminogen and plasmin. Binding prevents conversion of plasminogen to plasmin and prevents plasmin from degrading to fibrinogen and fibrin. All this chicanery results in decreased fibrinolysis. Decreased formation of the degradation products of fibrinogen and fibrin decreases platelet function. Patients are less likely to develop "medical bleeding," a coagulopathy. There is some evidence that blood loss and use of bank blood is decreased with the use of ε-aminocaproic acid, and it does not have much of a down side, so I would use it.

4. This patient has a full stomach and an intra-abdominal abscess. How will you induce? Which induction agent will you use? Which muscle relaxant will you use? What are the potential complications associated with muscle relaxants?

You have an aspiration risk plus a hyperkalemic risk (i.e., intra-abdominal abscess) from succinylcholine. I would induce with etomidate (for the hemodynamic reasons given earlier) and rocuronium in a modified RSI. The risk with long-acting relaxants is a failed intubation, and you do not have the option of waking the patient in 5 minutes and going to plan B.

5. The patient has buckteeth, and she holds her head off to one side. Airway examination is not possible. How will you proceed?

You are stuck, because you may be looking at a bad airway in a patient who will not cooperate with an awake intubation, and you do not have a lot of time. Hell, this could be a board question!

Look over the neck as best you can, find an old intubation note if possible, get friends around to help you out, have a fiberoptic scope and an intubating stylet around (or whatever else you are good at—light wand, Shikani), and proceed. You will not be able to adequately sedate and topicalize her, so you will have to induce and take your best shot. Tell the surgeon and have a tracheostomy kit handy.

6. While attempting pre-oxygenation, the patient thrashes around and shouts, not allowing the mask on. How do you respond to this behavior? Attempting to place cricoid pressure also results in a violent response. How will you protect against aspiration? Are any medications indicated? Should they be given intravenously or orally?

Do not make her more mad; just keep the mask near her. You can try the trick that works for claustrophobic people: put the end of the circuit in her mouth like a straw rather than the mask on her face.

Cricoid pressure should not be placed or even used! What heresy! Cricoid pressure does not occlude the esophagus, has never been shown to prevent aspiration risk, makes it harder to mask, and makes it harder to intubate. No one ever is taught how hard to push (did you get taught with a strain gauge in your residency?). Moreover, it does not matter how hard you push, because it pushes the esophagus off to the side.

No medications have been shown to decrease aspiration risk, so I would skip the whole litany of antacids, propulsives, and the rest. If there is no proof for it, I do not use it.

7. You induce, get what you think is a good view, and place the ETT in the trachea, but there is no end-tidal CO_2 measurement. What do you do? How do you know you are in the correct place? What is the differential for a "tube in the right place but no CO_2"?

Use alternative methods to see if you are in the right place: mist in the ETT, breath sounds, no gurgling over the stomach, and compliance. If really pressed, put a fiberoptic scope down the damn thing and look for rings.

If the tube is in the right place and no CO_2 is coming out, you are not measuring it (i.e., machine malfunction); the patient is producing CO_2, but it is not getting to you (i.e., obstructed ETT); CO_2 is not being delivered to the lungs (i.e., massive pulmonary embolus or complete cardiovascular collapse), or the patient has not produced CO_2 for a long time (e.g., if you correctly intubated King Tut's mummy, you would not get any CO_2, because he has not made any for a few thousand years).

8. After induction, the heart rate hits 160 beats/min, and the blood pressure is 70/50 mm Hg. What are the end-organ implications, and how do you respond? Do you use β-blockers for cardiac protection or β-blockade in the setting of a "physiologic-response tachycardia"?

Sepsis and hypovolemia (in effect, sepsis is hypovolemia) account for these vital signs. To make life even worse, an allergic reaction (such as to the rocuronium) would give a similar hemodynamic picture. The end-organ result is low perfusion and high demand on the heart, and this hypotension can starve other organs (e.g., kidneys, gut) of needed perfusion. The patient will go into shock, preserving flow to a few key organs (e.g., brain, heart) while sacrificing others.

β-Blockade will most likely kill this patient, because this is a physiologic response to keep alive. You need to provide fluids and vasopressor support.

9. Things settle down after induction, and the heart rate is 130 beats/min. How will you decrease the heart rate and not cause a cardiovascular collapse? What monitors can guide you? How do you respond if the CVP measurement is 3 or 15? What do you do if the pulmonary artery catheter reads 20/5 or 45/33?

The best way to get the heart rate down is to "fix anything that you can fix" (e.g., acidosis, light anesthesia, hypovolemia, anemia), and after the patient is stable, you can start a cautious amount of β-blockade to try to get that heart rate down a little. If the CVP value is 3, the patient is hypovolemic. If it is 15, the patient is most likely "full," and you should work on vasopressor support. Similarly, the low pulmonary artery catheter reading goes along with hypovolemia, and the higher one corresponds to full; use inotropes, not more volume.

Overriding all these attempts to read the numbers and make the diagnosis is a better monitor that can take the guesswork out of it, the TEE. Rather than divining what is happening through numbers, take a look!

10. The patient continues to show instability, with a persistent systolic blood pressure in the 70s. How will you increase the blood pressure? If you use norepinephrine, how will you guide the therapy? The hematocrit level is 31%, but ischemia is evident on the ECG. Will you transfuse? Why or why not? What are the dangers of transfusion?

Use norepinephrine, and if there is no response, use a vasopressin infusion. Therapy is always guided by the same mantra: Start at a reasonable dose, then dial up, and make sure a response occurs. If there is no response, do not forget simple things, such as an infusion that is not getting in or not hooked up or a pump that is not working.

At 31%, we are above the magic number ("keep the hematocrit above 30"), which has some basis in fact; hematocrit levels lower than 24% and higher than 34% are best in the cardiac setting. I would not transfuse more, risking a mismatch (e.g., clerical error) and transfusion-related acute lung injury for no benefit.

After optimizing the hematocrit to improve things on the ECG, I would work on other aspects of the myocardial oxygen supply and demand teeter-totter, such as increasing the perfusion pressure or decreasing demand.

Postoperative Questions

1. The surgeon finds only ileus, and closes in 35 minutes. Do you extubate? What are extubation criteria? In the setting of ongoing ischemia, do you alter these extubation criteria?

No. Extubation criteria (e.g., negative inspiratory force, adequate oxygenation, ability to protect the airway) are always overshadowed by whether the patient is stable enough to handle a respiratory stress in addition to everything else. With recent ischemia, inotropic support, possible acute respiratory distress syndrome (ARDS) (sepsis and a hypotensive episode could certainly send the patient in that direction), the last thing she needs is an extubation and a hypoxemic event.

2. The chest radiograph shows a whiteout of both lungs, and pink, frothy fluid is in the ETT. How will you evaluate this pulmonary finding? Will you use CT, or send endotracheal fluid for analysis? What are you looking for? The ICU staff members suggest changing the ETT to a larger one so they can suction the fluid more efficiently. Do you do this? How?

There is no need for CT; this is ARDS, given her history. Treatment is supportive, with PEEP titrated to adequate blood pressure (do not make the PEEP too high!) and adequate oxygenation (do not make the PEEP too low!). You could send the fluid for analysis to make sure something else was not superimposed, such as aspiration, but that would be a low-yield study. Do not change the tube unless you need it for adequate oxygenation. In her current unstable state, a botched tube exchange could finish her off. This fluid is not something you want to keep suctioning out (unless it inspissates and blocks the ETT). Every time you suction the fluid out, you create conditions for more fluid sucking into the lungs.

3. The patient has developed an air leak around the ETT. She can breathe around it, but her saturation is poor, and she needs PEEP. Her airway is swollen from fluids. How do you evaluate this air leak? What could it be? How will you change the tube? Will you use a tube changer or fiberoptic device? Do you have a tracheostomy kit on standby?

Your hand is forced. Get help. Do this with extra people and gizmos around (e.g., fiberoptic scope, tube changer). Place the patient on 100% oxygen before you attempt anything. With the patient paralyzed (use your best shot; you do not want her biting down and fighting you), look in and see if the cuff herniated above the cords. If it has, suction the mouth, deflate the cuff, and advance the tube. If the cuff has broken, change over a tube changer, watching all the while with a laryngoscope. Have the tracheostomy kit nearby, just in case.

4. The nephrologist is concerned about renal damage during her episode of hypotension. What is a creatinine clearance value? Does this help you? How? What techniques may help to prevent worsening renal function? Do you use dopamine? Will epinephrine and a higher cardiac output help? Is fluid restriction or fluid administration a good idea? Can insulin help the patient?

The creatinine clearance rate gives you a better idea of the degree of kidney compromise. This will not change the kidneys or magically bring them back to life, but it does give you a good picture of where you are and something you can follow. For example, if the creatinine clearance is very low (e.g., 10% of normal), you may start dialysis right away.

Do not use dopamine? It has been proved useless.

What about higher cardiac output? Give epinephrine or another inotropic infusion if the patient needs it for hemodynamic reasons. Unfortunately, the kidneys will not spring back to life if only we can get the cardiac output above X.

By all means, administer fluids, guided by CVP, common sense (e.g., blood pressure, acid-base status, urine output), and TEE. Do not starve the kidneys for fluid.

Administer insulin. Ideally, the glucose level was under good control *before* the big hypotensive hit, because high glucose levels have been shown to worsen renal insults. You cannot go back in time, so pay close attention to glucose levels now, and keep them under control.

5. During a line change, you put a Swan-Ganz introducer into the subclavian artery. Do you pull out or keep it there? Do you apply pressure? You remove the Swan-Ganz line, and a half-hour later, the chest radiograph shows a hemithorax filled with fluid. The patient goes into shock. How do you proceed?

The subclavian is not compressible, and if you pull out, the patient may exsanguinate. Keep it in, call the surgeon, and go to the OR. Pull it out there with the surgeon ready to open the chest on a moment's notice. Even with the chest open, this is a hard hole to fix.

If you pull out and get in trouble, go with big fluid resuscitation from below (femoral), and open as soon as possible. Use the femoral approach because as the surgeon is struggling up high, he or she may be clamping vessels like mad and cut off fluid resuscitation from above.

How It Actually Happened

A desperate search for a crack in the floor into which I could disappear proved fruitless, and the case went my way. As happens, the patient arrived with the "usual lines from the medical ICU"—a 24-gauge line in her left index finger (I swear it!) and a 22-gauge line in her left antecubital fossa that ran when we held her arm flat. Dobutamine was supposedly running into it, but who knows? Her mental impairment was severe, but being creatures of habit, we kept shouting, "Hold still! Do not move your arm!" A lot of good that did.

She was a poster child for sepsis, with a flushed look, sweaty face, a heart rate banging away to beat the band, and faint pulses. Her abdomen was swollen, giving that "this is a *real* full stomach" feeling. Her airway was difficult to examine, but you could definitely make out buckteeth. The immediacy of things said we had to go back and just go for it. To delay was death.

Crucial in the considerations was her tachycardia, which we all recognized as the worst possible thing for someone with impaired coronaries and an evolving MI, but we knew any of the "usual suspects" that decreased the heart rate were not readily available:

- Should we use a β-blocker? She was pounding away as a compensatory measure for sepsis, so blocking her could have killed her.
- Should we fix the pain? This much distention was going to get fixed only by surgical repair. We did not have the luxury of giving narcotics until she was comfortable or placing a regional with narcotic or local anesthetic.
- Should we fix the fluids and hematocrit? We were so "lineless," and getting lines would require general anesthesia, so we were again painted into a corner.

I corralled extra hands and promised them all a hefty holiday fowl of their choosing, and we went back to the room. The plan was to secure that airway (more on that later), place lines, send samples for laboratory tests, fix everything we could fix, and try as soon as possible to "physiologically" get the heart rate down.

As we rolled, we debated about using suxamethonium. Did she have intra-abdominal abscess leading to fatal hyperkalemia? Possibly; it has been reported. God help us if we cannot get that airway in this full-stomach, cardiac-compromised nightmare. We swallowed hard and went with suxamethonium.

There was no fatal hyperkalemia. You could argue otherwise, but remember, this is the red meat edition of *Board Stiff*, and we tell it like it happened.

The airway was not the greatest, but an intubating bougie saved our bacon. The rest of the case was "seek and destroy badness." The hematocrit was 25%, and we transfused it up to 32%. CVP (no surprise) was low. Big-time fluid resuscitation, mostly with blood, was needed.

For renal protection, the smart money was on fluid resuscitation, staying away from things that have no proven benefit (renal dopamine has gone the way of the eight track cassette), staying away from things that actively hurt the patient (furosemide worsens the hypovolemia), and using just about the only thing that has any proven merit: good glucose control. Ideally, you control the glucose level before the insult occurs; we were in mid-insult by the time we got her.

Once in the unit, the desire to suction away that nasty pulmonary edema fluid was quickly put to rest. Sucking out pulmonary edema fluid just promotes more pulmonary edema fluid! You are contributing to the problem.

It is time for true confessions. The subclavian artery stick did not occur with this patient, but rather occurred with another one. I added it in here to flesh out the postoperative questions. We opted for the surgeon to be around when we pulled it, and ultimately, the surgical staff had to go in and repair it. Bad luck, that.

CASE 5: FIXING A BROKEN HEART

Preoperative Questions

1. How does an intra-aortic balloon pump (IABP) work? Describe how you time it correctly. What happens if it inflates too soon? Too late? If you turn it off? If it ruptures?

The IABP is your friend; it is the only way to get more from the heart without beating it with inotropes. It has problems, and it causes complications, but those are mainly in the leg (Captain Ahab and Long John Silver did fine with one leg, although to my knowledge, neither benefited from an IABP).

The balloon, placed by means of the femoral artery and extending up to the takeoff of the subclavian artery, inflates during diastole and deflates during systole. Perfect timing places the inflation in the dicrotic notch. It has twin benefits:

- Inflation during diastole increases diastolic perfusion, aiding coronary perfusion (recall that coronary perfusion occurs during diastole).
- Deflation during systole provides a kind of suction effect, helping propel forward flow.

What happens if the timing is not correct? If it inflates too late, you lose all the benefit of diastolic augmentation. If it inflates too soon, it is hard to expel blood from the heart with a sky-high resistance.

If you turn it off, a clot can form on this large intravascular object. The balloon inflates with helium (this thin gas allows the quick inflation and deflation).

If it ruptures, you get a helium embolus in the arterial circulation. Fortunately, this absorbs into the bloodstream quickly and does not tend to kill you. However, you now have a useless IABP and need to replace it.

2. How can a 72-year-old man with no earlier history have a ventricular septal defect (VSD)? What would be the effect of a long-standing VSD? What is Eisenmenger's syndrome?

If this man has had a VSD since birth, he would long ago have developed complications. The constant flow from the high-pressure side (left ventricle) to the low-pressure side (right ventricle) would have overwhelmed the right side, leading to Eisenmenger's syndrome (i.e., left and right sides have equal pressures). This condition has a high mortality rate and is essentially inoperable, except for heart transplantation. This VSD is a result of an MI. A portion of the septum died, necrosed, and turned into a hole.

3. What special precautions will you take regarding lines as you set up this room? How do you prevent air bubbles? Paradoxical embolus? How can this occur if pressure is higher on the arterial side?

Careful with bubbles! Go over all the intravenous lines with a fine-tooth comb, and make sure you do not inject any air. Although the higher pressure on the arterial side should prevent a bubble going from right to left (i.e., from the low-pressure side to the high-pressure side), there is no guarantee. If a bubble does go across (i.e., paradoxical embolus), it can go anywhere it wants in the arterial system, including the brain (stroke), kidney or gut (infarction), or an end artery in an extremity (infarction). That is a high price to pay for being careless with bubbles.

4. What additional laboratory studies do you need before going to the OR? Are blood typing and antibody screening sufficient? Will you order blood factors ahead of time? Which ones? Why?

You want to make sure the kidneys are okay. Order tests for creatinine and potassium. The starting hematocrit is important, because if it is low, you may need to put blood in the pump. Obtain a preoperative ECG to have for postoperative comparison and a chest radiograph (we are doing a chest procedure). If you have time, a type and cross is preferable to a type and screen, although in a pinch, you could use the blood type and screen. I would order platelets ahead of time, because the IABP chews up platelets, and this is sure to be a long pump run because of coronary artery bypass grafting (CABG) and a tough septal defect to repair.

5. What are the hazards of moving a patient with an IABP in and vasoactive drips running? You see he has dobutamine running in a peripheral line. Do you have any concerns? Will you stop the dobutamine? Why or why not? What if you see the line is infiltrated? Is there any special treatment for the arm?

The main problem is the possibility of pulling out some life-saving component. If you pull out the IABP, you lose its good aspects and gain a significant bad aspect—a big hole in the femoral artery spilling blood all over your tennis shoes. Peripheral lines are bad places for inotropic drips, because infiltration could lead to skin sloughing (treatment is warm soaks, arm elevation, and a surgery consult if skin or muscle death occurs). Switch that dobutamine to a central line as soon as possible.

As a general rule, every intravenous or other line that comes from a medical area, such as the ICU, floor, or catheter laboratory, is infiltrated and useless until proved otherwise. Never trust them, get rid of them, and replace them.

Intraoperative Questions

1. You have three, peripheral, 20-gauge intravenous lines in, some with inotropes running. How will you manage the lines for induction? Will you put in additional peripherals? Put in central lines? Which ones? What if the patient groans and complains during placement of a central line?

Peripheral lines from medical areas are worthless. Because this is going to be a Big Kahuna operation, place a Cordis. With some sedation and a sufficient local, you should be able to put this in without making the patient suffer too much. If, however, the patient is truly uncooperative, put in a decent peripheral line, induce, secure the airway, and then put in a central line.

2. What are your choices of induction agents? Is etomidate a good choice? Is ketamine? Should you use a high-dose narcotic only? Should you use propofol? Which relaxant should you use? What if patient ate 3 hours ago? What are the dangers of succinylcholine if the patient had been lying in bed for 3 days?

Etomidate is a good choice because this patient is unstable, and etomidate, given judiciously, can provide stability at induction. Ketamine can increase heart rate too much. A high-dose narcotic can also provide stability, but using reduced doses of any other agent (i.e., propofol or thiopental) would work just as well. Etomidate is not a magic or unique bullet, but it is what I would use.

If the patient ate recently, I would use succinylcholine as part of an RSI. During the RSI, I would *not* use cricoid pressure, because cricoid pressure does not occlude the esophagus (merely pushes it to the side), cricoid pressure makes it hard to ventilate (in case you miss on your intubation), and it makes it harder to intubate. As long as we are ragging on cricoid pressure, it is worth noting that cricoid pressure is based on a Preliminary Communication paper written by a Dr. Sellick in 1961. He had 26 patients in the study (if you want to call it a study) and was extremely vague about the exact technique used (some patients with full stomachs had an inhalation induction). No one is taught how much pressure to apply (were you?), and no study has shown any kind of an outcome benefit. So to hell with cricoid pressure!

If the patient had been immobile, there is a danger of hyperkalemia with the use of succinylcholine. I would do a modified RSI with rocuronium.

3. The surgeon is concerned that bleeding will be a problem. Should you give ε-aminocaproic acid? What is it? How does it work?

ε-aminocaproic acid (Amicar) prevents fibrinolysis, and there is some evidence for its efficacy so I would use it.

4. Cardiac function is poor, and the surgeon suggests you need a Swan-Ganz catheter? Do you agree? How will you place it? If you do place it, and the trace suddenly shows arterial pressure, what could have happened? Now what do you do? Should you withdraw or keep it in place? Should you send a mixed venous blood gas sample for evaluation? What would it show?

It is a bad idea to put a Swan-Ganz catheter in a patient with a hole connecting left and right. The Swan-Ganz catheter on the right may worm its way into the left side. If you do this and see arterial pressure, you have crossed to the other side. Pull the thing back and throw it out. If you did send a mixed venous gas, what you would get is a non-mixed arterial gas.

5. How will you prepare for separating from cardiopulmonary bypass? The patient's hematocrit is 22%; do you transfuse? Do you wait until you are off bypass? The patient's potassium level is 3.4; should you give him potassium or wait? If the potassium level is 6.8, should you treat or wait? The clamp has been off only 12 minutes, but the surgeon says it is okay to come off. Do you agree or disagree? Why?

Follow the ABC approach to separating from bypass:

Airway: Turn on the ventilator, and make sure the lungs go up and come down again.

Bureaucracy: Make sure everything "medical" about the heart is optimal, including the potassium level, hematocrit, temperature, acid-base level, and time since the clamp was off (at least 20 minutes).

Circulatory: Focus on rhythm, rate, and contractility.

Before you get to the big epinephrine drip wide open—OOH, AAH—make sure everything else is taken care of. Then you may not need all the epinephrine.

If the hematocrit is 22%, transfuse now. The blood will get a little beat up, but I want that hematocrit above 24% (evidence exists that levels below 24% are bad) before I attempt to come off. The first shot is the best shot, so have everything just so before the big jump.

If the potassium level is 3.4, give 20 mEq before coming off. The patient gets a lot of mannitol from the pump, and the potassium level will likely drop lower, leading to ectopy. Get the potassium level above 4 before starting.

If the potassium level is 6.8 and the rhythm is good and urine output is brisk, hold off on treating, because the level will come down. If the patient requires pacing, treat with glucose and insulin, but not in an attempt to drive it way down just to get the potassium level below 6; an overshoot could get the potassium level too low, and you will have rhythm troubles.

When the surgeon says come off 12 minutes after unclamping, you should light a cigarette, and tell him or her that you will come off when the cigarette is done (about 8 minutes later if you take slow, infrequent drags). The idea is that you want to give the heart 20 minutes of perfusion and rest to wash out the evil humors of bypass. This is part of the optimizing process before coming off bypass.

6. When the patient comes off bypass, bleeding from the back of the heart is brisk, and the surgeon says to give blood factors. There is a surgical incision in the back of the heart. Which factors will you give and why? Do you have any other suggestions?

To hell with the factors; an incision in the back of the heart that is bleeding needs a stitch, not a factor. This is a formula for disaster, with more and more bleeding, more "hiking the heart to take a look back there," and plunging blood pressure every time the surgeon lifts. In the meantime, the surgeon continues to say, "It is still bleeding. Give more factors." This is where you need to take charge and say, "I'm heparinzing. We need to recannulate, go on bypass, stop this heart, and fix that hole in the backside. Period."

7. Each time the surgeon lifts the heart, the IABP has a hard time picking up and following. What is your diagnosis? What can you do to help the situation? Should you trigger off the ECG or the arterial pressure? Should you slow the heart rate or speed up the heart rate?

There is nothing worse than a surgeon who hesitates to do surgery. The IABP can trigger an automatic mode (not linked to anything and a good idea only when on bypass and you want it to wiggle every now and then) or, more commonly, can trigger off the ECG or the arterial pressure trace. When the surgeon lifts the heart, the ECG complex may get so small (the electrical vector changes as the heart moves) that the IABP cannot recognize it. The blood pressure may drop so low that the IABP does not see it either. You should jump across the drapes, throttle the surgeon, and have him or her read the answer I gave earlier to question 6.

8. With manipulation, the pacer is having trouble. How does a pacer work? How should you set the pacer? What if it does not pick up? What about this case specifically makes pacing a concern? Describe the conduction system of the heart.

A pacer, set in the inhibit mode, will not fire when it sees the heart has already fired a complex. Setting the pacer in the inhibited mode is a good idea, because it then fires only when needed. If the pacer does not pick up, the wire may be in a scarred area, and you may need to turn up the amperage, or the surgeon may need to replace the wire to a more favorable spot. With the surgeon lifting up the heart, the pacer will have a hard time reading anything, because the vector of a complex varies wildly as the heart moves around. The surgeon touching the heart can trigger a complex, and lifting the heart may short out the pacing wires as the wires touch a retractor or something else. What a mess!

The conduction system of the heart starts at the sinoatrial (SA) node, travels down to the atrioventricular (AV) node, and then punches through and runs down the septum (the very septum that had a hole in it, is now repaired, and may have a "chopped up wiring system") to the apex. It then comes around and back up as the complex conducts. Pacing is crucial here because operative mischief is square in the middle of the conduction path.

9. At what point do you tell the surgeon to go back on bypass and fix the hole? Should an anesthesiologist make a "surgical recommendation"? Why or why not? What are the dangers of going on bypass a second time? Will the patient have a systemic inflammatory response? What are the dangers of massive transfusion in this setting?

Now. Go back on now. The anesthesiologist should make a surgical recommendation when the patient needs it. That is why we have to know our job and their jobs as well, and a good anesthesiologist does. No shrinking violets, please.

Going on bypass a second time is a pain in the ass, and it will cause more systemic inflammatory responses and more coagulopathy problems. You may be in there quite a while dealing with bleeding, but it is better than letting the patient bleed to death through a surgical hole.

10. The chest is closed, and the surgeon asks for a TEE assessment. What will you be looking for? How will you tell if the VSD is still open? Should you float a Swan-Ganz catheter now? Using the Swan-Ganz catheter, how could

you tell if the VSD is still open? If you see a regional wall motion abnormality, what does it signify? How will you manage this? Should you use nitroglycerin or reopen the patient?

Make sure the VSD is closed. Do a color study, and see if there is any flow across the old VSD site. Floating a Swan-Ganz catheter now will not add any useful information. If you see a new regional wall motion abnormality, it may indicate ischemia (perhaps a graft kinked, clotted, or dissected). Rather than try any medical means of reopening the vessel, reopen the chest itself, and take a look. A fresh graft is susceptible to all sorts of problems, and it is better to open now and fix it now than to let the patient go on to an infarction.

How It Actually Happened

If you have not yet worked out the questions yourself, do not read this section! I am happy to share with you all the thrills and chills of the case, but you are not reading this book as you would an Agatha Christie murder mystery. You are reading this book to test yourself, so go back, and tackle all the questions first. I will not be there to take the test for you, so do your work.

This poor guy came down with the balloon pump thumping, and he had that "what the hell happened?" look on his face. He had lived his entire life vice free and was fit for a 72-year-old man (looked 55). Just a few hours before, he was living the good life, and now here he was, hanging by a thread with a brand new hole in his heart.

More's the pity, but we were not there to weep or keen. Into the room lickety split, because we knew an MI bad enough to kill the septum—so bad a hole went through it—was nothing to mess with. We scoured the lines for air bubbles, admonished ourselves for not doing so routinely, and set about untangling lines. The dobutamine in the peripheral line was vexatious, but we lucked out and found he had a venous catheter in his groin and hooked up the dobutamine to that.

Because he was stable on what he is taking now, we decided not to change it. We did not place a Swan-Ganz catheter because we did not want to push it through the VSD. If you are a creature of habit and always put in Swan-Ganz catheters, it is easy in a VSD case to do what you always do. That is why you must stop and think about what you are doing!

He had poor cardiac function, so we induced with etomidate and suxamethonium. He was not a true full stomach, but with all the pain he had and the balloon pump, I was not sure he had emptied his stomach too well. Sure enough, there was a big VSD, and the surgeon had to cut out a big hunk of the septum and a hunk of the posterior wall. The conduction system was ripped to shreds, and he became pacer dependent.

The real hook in this case was a dog-ear area on the closure of the posterior wall. Coming off was not too terrible (a lifetime of good living served this man well), but bleeding in the back would not stop. Extensive "lifts and looks" threw off the pacer, which threw off the balloon pump, and everything went downhill. I was just about to say, "We could play this game all day. Just re-heparinize, re-cannulate, go back on, fix the hole, and let's get out of here!" Thank God, the surgeon came to the same conclusion at the same time. It is better to go back on, fix the damn thing, and come off again than to engage in endless, dangerous lifts and looks.

After the hole was fixed, the bleeding stopped (surprise, surprise), and we did not have to give any more factors. Even the largest platelet cannot plug a hole in the aorta. We lived to fight another day. And so did the patient!

CASE 6: CONSCIOUS SEDATION

Preoperative Questions

1. What further information do you need regarding this patient's history? If she were healthy other than herniated disks and back pain, do you need any laboratory studies? Do you need a human chorionic gonadotropin determination? What if she says there is no possibility she is pregnant?

You want to know whether this is really an emergency. She seems to be moving around pretty well for someone with an acute neurologic condition. If go you must (if this is real, time is limited), you will need the quick, anesthesia-oriented history that we need on all our patients:

- Personal or family history of problems with anesthesia
- Quick rundown on a review of systems, looking for heart and lung trouble in particular

The only laboratory test needed is a urinary level of human chorionic gonadotropin (hCG). Even if she protests to high heaven that this would be the Immaculate Conception Part II, you still need to know.

2. What is cauda equina syndrome? What history will you elicit? What are the physical findings? Is this an emergency? Is it up to you to decide whether this is an emergency?

Cauda equina syndrome is paraplegia and diffuse injury to the cauda equina roots. It can be caused by direct needle trauma, ischemia, neurotoxic drugs, bacteria, or an epidural hematoma (which is the one thing you could operate on and fix). The history should focus on paresthesias and weakness. If someone says, "This is what it may be," and you say, "She is faking," but she does end up having something, you may feel stupid and be penniless for the foreseeable future. So no matter your suspicions, it is not really for you to claim it is not an emergency and deny the MRI.

3. It is now 3:30 PM, and the patient last ate at 6 AM. Does she have a full stomach? If she went to the emergency room (ER) at 8 AM and received Dilaudid and morphine intravenously, does this information change your assessment? Should you give her an antacid, metoclopramide, or anticholinergic therapy?

After severe pain starts, all bets are off on gastric emptying. Normal function of the gastrointestinal tract requires parasympathetic input primarily. When the patient is in pain, the sympathetic system predominates. Add narcotics, which slow gastric emptying, and you have no idea whether the patient has emptied her stomach. No outcome study has shown that any of the antiaspiration drug regimens have done anything to reduce aspiration risk, so I would give none of the suggested drugs.

4. She states she "always gets conscious sedation for her MRI scans." What is conscious sedation? What are the risks of conscious sedation? What are the risks in the setting of MRI? What, specific to MRI, contributes to problems with claustrophobic patients? Can you cancel the case and insist she go to a place with an open MRI?

Conscious sedation means the patient is able to respond to commands. It does not mean a "room air general" and having to chop off her foot to get her attention or scream bloody murder to get the respiratory rate up to 2 breaths/min.

The risk of conscious sedation is that you will overdo it and cause respiratory depression. The MRI causes claustrophobia; it is loud, the patient is far away and hard to get to, and movement throws off the finicky scanner. Your best bet is to give "unconscious sedation" (intubated, general anesthesia) rather than risk this. If time is really of the essence, you do not have time to refer her to an open MRI place.

5. The patient hops off the bed, walks over to the MRI, and lies down on the table without any problems, does this change anything? If your clinical assessment is that she does not have cauda equina, can you cancel this case? Can you postpone it until she has less of a full stomach?

This looks more and more ridiculous, but as I explained in the answer for question 2, it is not our call to make. Common sense would say a quick conversation with the evaluating physician is a good idea. There is no use waiting a few more hours; they said it was an emergency, so you have to go.

Intraoperative Questions

1. Describe the special considerations in conducting an anesthetic in an MRI machine. Can she wear jewelry? What dangers are there? What about using a laryngoscope, monitors, or an anesthesia machine?

Primum non nocere (first do no harm) is the byword for physicians. In the MRI scanner, it is *primum getum ridum allum metallum*. Get all the rings and piercings out. You should have an MRI-friendly setup, with an anesthesia machine, monitors, and blades—all nonmetal. Do not get near the machine with the metal cart! Remove your own watches, wallets, ninja swords, Medals of Honor, and anything else that may mess with the monster magnets in the MRI beast.

2. What is your choice of anesthetic and sedation? What methods do you use? Can you use a propofol drip, midazolam and fentanyl, or dexmedetomidine? What are the advantages and disadvantages of each approach?

Given her wackiness, morbid obesity, and claustrophobia, I would not mess around with anything other than a general anesthetic. Secure the airway, have her completely anesthetized, and get her through the study as quickly as possible. Messing around with anything less risks losing the airway, having her desaturate, or having her lose it in the machine, move around, and prolong the procedure.

3. You sedate with propofol, but the patient keeps wiggling around, complaining that her back hurts, and is unable to hold still. The MRI technician says he cannot get a good study. How do you increase sedation? What are the general risks and those specific to MRI?

Look at the previous answer. Any half-baked sedation that starts "begging for more sedation" is also begging for trouble. I would stop the case, get her out of the big donut, induce general anesthesia, and restart the study.

4. The patient obstructs, and you can no longer see an end-tidal CO_2 trace. What do you do? When you pull her out, you see that she has obstructed, but by vigorous shaking, you can get her to open her own airway. Should you resedate and send her back in?

Vigorous shaking tells you that you are no longer in conscious sedation. You are dangerously close to general anesthesia. There is no way to resedate her. Go to general anesthesia now.

5. At what point would you proceed to general anesthesia? What are the risks of general anesthesia compared with sedation? Is one safer than the other? Do you induce on the MRI table or on the gurney? If she has a difficult airway, where is the safest place to intubate her? What if there is a problem with the fiberoptic intubation and MRI?

Now. General anesthesia poses the usual risks of a lost airway with an unsuccessful intubation attempt, upper airway damage (including tooth chipping), aspiration, hemodynamic instability, adverse reaction to anesthesia, and a sore throat. No study shows that general is safer than MAC, but closed claims reviews do show that MACs appear quite often as airway catastrophes. These studies have no denominator, so it is hard to draw any perfect conclusions, but it is worth noting how often MAC has gone bad. If you are concerned about her airway, put her on the gurney because you can tip her head up to help keep her oxygenated, you can put her head down in case she vomits at induction, and you can roll fiberoptic equipment close to her (do not let the metal parts of the fiberoptic gear get near the MRI) if she has a difficult airway.

6. You induce and place a laryngeal mask airway (LMA). When the patient is in the MRI scanner, the end-tidal CO_2 monitor looks funny—"partially blocked" maybe—and the oxygen saturation level drops from 99% to 83%. What is the differential diagnosis? You pull her out, and you see green fluid in the LMA. What is your next move?

Blocked end-tidal CO_2 and dropping oxygen saturation constitute respiratory obstruction, so get her out of the MRI scanner immediately. Green fluid in the MRI mandates treatment for aspiration, with the patient's head down and turned to the left. Suction, secure the airway, and provide supportive ventilatory care.

7. On removal of the LMA, you see emesis in the back of her throat. The MRI table does not have a Trendelenburg button. What do you do? If the suction pulls out of the wall, do you go ahead and intubate through the emesis? What is the remedy for aspiration at this point?

Because it is too hard to move her over to a gurney, turn her head to the side. Absent suction, you can put your hand in and try to sweep out as much as you can (a little cloth or gauze can help mop up) and then intubate through the emesis, lifting hard to pull the trachea "up out of the puddle" (easier said than done, but you do what you have to). Scream and shout for someone to get the suction working, because as soon as you intubate, you will want to suction out the ETT. As discussed earlier, treatment is supportive, using ventilation, positive end expiratory pressure (PEEP), and time to cure the aspiration.

8. You intubate, and the oxygen saturation level is 88%. Do you proceed with the rest of the MRI study? What if the diagnosis of cauda equine syndrome is not yet made? Do you use PEEP? How much? What are the drawbacks and limitations of PEEP?

This MRI was listed as an emergency, the same as an appendectomy is an emergency, so you will proceed unless it is impossible to keep this patient alive. Treat this low saturation level as you would any other. Go to 100% oxygen, listen to both sides of the chest, suction, treat bronchospasm, and use the fiberoptic equipment to suction as best you can. Go all the way to rigid bronchoscopy if you have to fish out tons of material. PEEP is *good* because it opens up alveoli, but PEEP is *bad* because it inhibits venous return and can drop the blood pressure. If the patient progresses to acute respiratory distress syndrome (ARDS), there will be a high-wire act between too little PEEP (leading do desaturation) and too much PEEP (leading to hypotension).

9. While working on the aspiration, you failed to notice the blood pressure, and now the blood pressure alarm going off. The patient is on 3% sevoflurane, and you cannot feel a pulse. What do you do? Describe the effects of high-inspired, potent inhaled agents in the setting of a cardiovascular collapse?

Turn the agent all the way off, increase fluids, and give a pressor, such as phenylephrine or ephedrine. The kicker with a high inspired inhaled agent during cardiovascular collapse is that because there is no cardiac output to "carry away" the potent agent, the alveolar concentration of the agent goes up, up, up, further potentiating the agent's cardiovascular depression. More agent means more depression, which means more agent builds up, causing more depression, and the spiral continues downward. For this reason, you have to stop delivery of that agent pronto.

10. Will you extubate at the end of the case? Would you extubate if her oxygen saturation level was 95% on 50% oxygen? A colleague suggests extubating and, if she needs it, giving her continuous positive airway pressure (CPAP) by mask. Is this a good idea? How does mask CPAP work? In what setting is mask CPAP a good idea?

Use extubation only if the patient does not need the tube. That sounds a bit jejune (love that word!), but it is the truth. If the patient meets extubation criteria in all realms (neurologic, pulmonary, cardiac stability), remove the tube. If the chest radiograph looks okay and her saturation level remains acceptable on the amount of oxygen you can give without the tube (here, 50%, which you can give by facemask, and there is no need for high PEEP), she is okay. Mask CPAP works the way "intubated CPAP" works; it recruits alveoli and supports oxygenation. The patient must have intact neurologic status, the ability to tolerate the mask (she is claustrophobic, so maybe no go here), and an ability to handle secretions. In such a setting, mask CPAP is helpful for the person who cannot keep saturated with plain supplemental oxygen. Mask CPAP is particularly helpful in the sleep apnea population.

How It Actually Happened

I hate to disappoint you, but the real case had none of the aspiration horrors described earlier. However, all this aspiration business might have happened, so I did my darndest to prevent it.

I used general endotracheal anesthesia right from the get-go. She wanted conscious sedation. Because of morbid obesity, an extremely tight fit in the MRI, a patient who was very difficult to get to and impossible to sit up, and narcotics all day long (so much for gastric emptying), I was not taking any chances. We went for unconscious sedation.

This approach allowed the study to get finished very quickly, and she was not wiggling around from back pain and not getting oversedated with us running in and pulling her out in a panic. Zoom in and zoom out. This approach shortened everyone's time there, especially hers. All went well, although in the setting of this book, you almost *want* things to go wrong.

CASE 7: EAR TUBES: WHAT COULD BE EASIER?

Preoperative Questions

1. What are normal expectations for a child with trisomy 21? What are the cardiac, airway, and gastrointestinal problems? Do you expect parental separation issues? Is line placement different?

Think "multisystem problems," and think "this could be tough." Forty percent of trisomy 21 patients have congenital cardiac lesions, most linked to endocardial cushion defects. The airway is a challenge on several fronts; a thick tongue, a short neck, and an atlanto-axial dislocation is a possibility. These patients have a higher than normal incidence of duodenal atresia and a higher incidence of reflux. At 20 months, parental separation is not a huge problem, but in older kids, this can be a curiously vexing problem. The children can be quite affectionate (so if they bond with you, they will come along fine), but they can also be quite stubborn (so if they do not want to go with you, they DO NOT WANT TO GO WITH YOU), and it can be hard to divine how this will go. Lines are difficult, because they have medialization of vasculature, more subcutaneous fat, and looser skin, all making for a tough intravenous line insertion.

2. Go into detail regarding cardiac issues for patients with trisomy 21. What is an endocardial cushion defect? What are the implications of a ventricular septal defect (VSD) repair or an atrial septal defect (ASD) repair? Should an intracardiac patch or primary repair be done? Is subacute bacterial endocarditis (SBE) prophylaxis necessary for this case?

An endocardial cushion defect sits in the middle of the heart, so it can "reach out and touch" just about anything. If this heart of the heart does not come together and separate the various compartments of the heart, you end up with incomplete walls (i.e., ASD and VSD), incompletely formed valves (i.e., tricuspid and mitral valve insufficiencies), and conduction defects (i.e., the conduction system runs in the center of the heart). If the various defects have been repaired, you need subacute bacterial endocarditis (SBE) prophylaxis for potentially contaminating procedures. If the various defects have not been repaired, you have to be careful about bubbles in the intravenous line. Primary repair of a defect implies a small hole fixed with the tissue in that location. If you have to put a patch in, it implies a bigger defect, and more likely, the conduction system is involved. This is not a contaminating case, so you do not need SBE prophylaxis.

3. Is sedation appropriate for this child? If so, which sedative should be used? What if the child were younger? What if the child were older? What if the child did not have trisomy 21? When would it be appropriate for the parents to be present at induction? What if the parents are inappropriate in the holding area?

No sedation is necessary at age 20 months. Younger children also do not need sedation. I would also hesitate to sedate an older trisomy 21 patient because their response to sedatives is unpredictable (they may become agitated), and their airways are more likely to obstruct because of the redundant tissue.

I would give an older child without trisomy 21 oral midazolam as a preoperative sedative. More important than all these sedatives is a good preoperative visit and building trust and confidence with the parents. Keep the mother happy; keep the kid happy.

Some people have parents in the room for induction; I choose not to. When the child hits the excitement phase, I do not want to be looking out for mom and the kid. If the parents behaved inappropriately in the holding area, all the more reason for keeping them out of the OR. However, many people may disagree with this position and defend having the parents in the room.

4. Is laboratory work necessary? If so, which studies should be ordered? Do you need a chest radiograph, C-spine film, abdominal film, or MRI scan? The child has had corrective heart surgery; do you need a baseline ECG?

No laboratory work is necessary, nor is a chest, C-spine, or abdominal film; MRI; map of no-longer-a-planet Pluto; or any other crazy stuff. You could go nuts and get every neck study known to man, but you are not going to do anything differently. You will still exercise caution in extending the neck, and you are not about to do an awake intubation on a 20 month old—(I would like to see that!).

A baseline ECG is a good idea because of the endocardial cushion defect and corrective surgery (a stitch can nail the conduction system). It is good to have an ECG in case trouble arises intraoperatively or postoperatively.

5. Discuss the management of the patient's NPO status? Is there any difference for a patient with trisomy 21? Is there any difference if the child is on reflux precautions? Discuss clear liquids versus regular food. If the child's body mass index (BMI) is greater than 35, would that change your NPO management?

At this age, the patient gets clear liquids up to 2 hours preoperatively. Trisomy 21 patients have more reflux, so you could consider going longer. If the kid were on reflux precautions, I would go with clear liquids up to 4 hours preoperatively. Clear liquids pass through the stomach faster than food (like that hoagie Philly cheesesteak fried onion monster you are eating and dribbling all over this book). I am guessing about extending the NPO time (and would admit so on the exam). If the child were morbidly obese, I would also extend the NPO time. Patients with a higher body mass index (BMI) empty their stomachs at the same speed as patients with lower BMI, but they have more reflux, so it is a mixed picture.

Intraoperative Questions

1. Do you perform an intravenous or a mask induction? Why or why not? Which agent would you use and why? What if you have difficulty placing an intravenous line? Do you even need an intravenous line for this case? A colleague suggests you skip it.

Perform a mask induction. This is a quick case, and it will be over before you can get an intravenous line in! Breathe down with sevoflurane (works quickly, pleasant odor). I would not even bother trying.

2. You do a mask induction with sevoflurane, nitrous oxide, and oxygen, and the child goes into laryngospasm at a 3% sevoflurane end-tidal level. What do you do? Should you increase or decrease the level of sevoflurane? Should you

adjust the nitrous oxide level? Should you awaken the patient or give something intramuscularly?

Off with the nitrous, up on the sevoflurane, and call for help. You are better off going "deeper and getting control" than "surfacing." I would not give anything intramuscularly unless the laryngospasm did not break with conventional measures.

3. Laryngospasm was not broken with earlier maneuvers (e.g., increasing sevoflurane, turning off the nitrous oxide, maintaining 20 cm H_2O positive pressure). How do you break the laryngospasm? The patient's heart rate is 80 beats/min, and the oxygen saturation level is 35%.

Administer intramuscular rocuronium. I do not want to give succinylcholine because it may trigger hyperkalemia, and suxamethonium chloride can further worsen the bradycardia.

4. Laryngospasm resolves, and the patient is stable. The surgeon is anxious to proceed. How will you manage the rest of the case? Will you use a mask, LMA, ETT, or intravenous line? Should you cancel the because of airway complications?

This kid has proved he is a player and may give more trouble, so I would go with the Full Monty: Place an intravenous line, and intubate. I would not cancel the case, because this kid needs his ears drained, and it might as well get done now. We are here now, so let's fix it now.

5. You choose to intubate. What is your choice of blade and ETT size? You place the 1.5 Wis-Hipple laryngoscope and you see redundant pharyngeal tissue; how do you manage this? A second look with a different blade reveals the same view. Now what do you do?

Use a Miller 1 straight blade. If you are having trouble with the Wis-Hipple laryngoscope, change to a different blade, such as the Miller 1 I wanted in the first place.

Because the straight blades have not been satisfactory, I would go to a curved blade. Sometimes, the flange on a curved blade gives you a little better ability to push tissue out of the way.

6. Do you need neuromuscular blockade for intubation? The procedure will require 15 minutes of surgical time according to the surgeon. Can you use suxamethonium? Why or why not? Is rocuronium a better choice? What is the dosage?

No. You can intubate off breathing deep alone. Suxamethonium is not suggested in children because an undiagnosed case of muscular dystrophy (you cannot tell in little kids) could result in a fatal hyperkalemic response. I would not use rocuronium either because you do not need it to intubate. If you give it, you have to reverse it later. Simplify, simplify! Do not use it in the first place.

7. On 4% sevoflurane, the heart rate drops from 120 to 4 beats/min (yes, 4). You have no intravenous line. What is your treatment plan? Will you use cardiopulmonary resuscitation (CPR), intramuscular atropine, or intramuscular epinephrine? Will you place a line? Will you administer epinephrine or bicarbonate through the ETT? Should you consider intraosseous placement for line access?

Start chest compressions immediately, give intramuscular atropine, and give intramuscular epinephrine if there is no response. Place a line, intubate, and give epinephrine through the ETT. Do not use bicarbonate down the ETT. If you cannot get a line, place an intraosseous line.

8. Several attempts at intravenous access have failed. How many times should you "go peripheral" before you "go central"? Discuss the intraosseous option. What if the child were 10 years old? Where is the best place to establish central access?

Try three times, and then go central. Intraosseous access works, but people usually are hesitant to do it, because it is just not done that often. As the child gets older, pushing through into the bone becomes more and more difficult. You could place one intratibially in a 10-year-old child, but because it becomes harder as a kid gets older, I would gravitate toward placing a central line. I would go femoral. You can place an internal jugular or a subclavian line in a 10-year-old child, but I would choose a femoral line to avoid the risk of dropping a lung.

9. The surgeon cannot visualize the tympanic membrane, and the case is now of indefinite length. You have been doing the case by mask for 30 minutes. Do you change? Do you place an LMA or ETT?

This child is at increased risk for reflux, and this case could go on and on. To simplify things, I would put the case on hold for a second, secure the airway with an ETT, and then let the surgeon proceed. An LMA places the child at risk for aspiration, so I would not use it.

10. You did the entire case without an intravenous line by using mask ventilation. How do you manage post-emergence delirium? How do you manage pain control? Do you need to give anything for ear tubes? Would you use rectal Tylenol, intramuscular ketorolac, intranasal fentanyl, intramuscular morphine, intramuscular Demerol, or intramuscular ketamine?

Make sure delirium is not hypoxemia or hypercarbia. Then, reassure the patient, and get the parents nearby to help calm the patient down. This case does not need a lot of pain control, so I would opt not to give Tylenol, intramuscular ketorolac (the injection may hurt more than the tubes), or intranasal fentanyl; you do not want to give narcotics to a young child who is sensitive to them, and the airway is liable to occlude. The same advice applies to the rest of the proffered goodies. You do not need them, and they may cause respiratory distress—do not give them!

How It Actually Happened

The day looked pretty good, spring was in the air, and there was even a fresh scent wafting through the ambulatory center. Someone had put Renuzit air fresheners in all the plugs, and we were all high but did not know it.

Then this happened. The kid had no cardiac history. We sedated the child with 0.5 mg/kg of oral midazolam. Parents were not allowed in the OR (both got hives from the Renuzit). A calm child was induced by mask with nitrous oxide, oxygen, and sevoflurane. So far, so good. At an end-tidal sevoflurane level of 3.5%, the heart rate dropped (no kidding) from 120 beats/min to the sub-basement of 4. Count them, 4 beats.

A great hue and cry went up from the assembled care team, and much help was sought in a high-decibel manner. Cardiopulmonary resuscitation (CPR) was immediately initiated, sevoflurane and nitrous were turned off, and intramuscular atropine (0.2 mg) was given, but there was no change in the heart rate. Intramuscular atropine (0.4 mg) was given, and the heart rate went up to 40 beats/min. CPR was continued because that heart rate in a 20-month-old child is insufficient for cardiac output.

Attempts to place an intravenous line were fast and furious, without success but with much cursing and gnashing of teeth. Intramuscular epinephrine (100 μg) was given. The heart rate rose to 110 beats/min, and an intravenous line was placed. The child was awakened, the case was cancelled, and everyone stepped out of the room and had a nervous breakdown.

I should have continued loading trucks for Nabisco. Stuff like this never happened at the Oreo factory.

CASE 8: UNRELENTING MISERY

Intraoperative Questions

1. Should you use invasive monitors? Why or why not? If you decide on an arterial line, would you place it before or after induction? If you decide on a CVP line, would you place it before or after induction? Why?

Place an arterial line after induction. You do not need beat-to-beat blood pressure measurement during induction (no critical arterial lesions in her coronaries or valves or carotids to worry about). However, a femoral shaft repair is fraught with blood loss and problems during drilling, and you will need access then for beat-to-beat blood pressure measurement and blood gas analysis. A CVP line is a good idea. You will need volume access, and a patient with cancer at this stage is unlikely to have any good peripheral access left.

2. You attempt a left radial arterial line, but you create a hematoma. The patient is groaning and complaining that her entire life consists of needle sticks and nausea from chemotherapy. Do you continue? Do you go to another site? Which site? If you "end up having to go femoral," do you first induce, or do you "topicalize better" and proceed. What are the risks of a femoral arterial line?

Re-evaluating the actual need for extremely close blood pressure measurement during induction, you realize you do not need it. I would stop torturing her. I would go femoral if the radials were not happening. A femoral arterial line has risks:

- It is the same as other sites regarding infection.
- If you go too deep, you can spear the bowel. Not good!
- It is a little more cumbersome to keep a femoral arterial line when you sit the patient up the next day.

3. Just as you are about to induce, a medical student (going into anesthesia) asks whether you consider her to be a "full stomach." Do you perform an RSI? What are the risks of RSI compared with modified RSI and with regular induction?

I consider her a full stomach. Effective gastric emptying requires a complicated interplay of the gastrointestinal tract and autonomic nervous system. This woman is completely out of balance because of her cancer "load" and cancer treatment. I would perform a modified RSI.

For an RSI, if you truly do not put one breath into the patient and wait until the suxamethonium has caused complete relaxation and only then do laryngoscopy, you run the risk of the patient desaturating. The biggest problem from a practical standpoint is the state of your head as you put the laryngoscope in. If the saturation monitor reading is already dipping, your laryngoscopy is more likely to be panicky. You are more likely to see what you want to see in your rush to get the tube in.

A modified RSI runs more risk of putting air in the stomach and therefore more risk for aspiration. However, this is the technique I prefer. Putting in the laryngoscope with a dipping saturation monitor puts you in a scared state. It is better to do a few hand ventilations (gently, with cricoid pressure) and have the blade go in with the patient well saturated. (NOTE: The author is NOT a fan of cricoid pressure, but you'll note some contributing authors are.)

Regular induction runs the risk of aspiration. The highly vaunted cricoid pressure maneuver has never been proved to be effective, so it is hard to quantify the various risks!

4. You induce with propofol and rocuronium. Just before intubating, you see the blood pressure is 60/40 mm Hg. Do you intubate right away? Do you give her a pressor? If you "release fluids wide open," how much fluid gets in over a minute through a 20-gauge peripheral line? After intubation, the blood pressure is still 60/40 mm Hg. What is your management plan? What is the effect of putting her head down?

I would intubate right away. My hope is that the "heavy metal poisoning" of the laryngoscope will provide enough sympathetic stimulation to raise the blood pressure. Opening an intravenous line wide open (e.g., the 20-gauge line mentioned in the question) does not put a ton of volume into the patient very fast. In a minute, you may get 20 mL in, tops. If you have persistent blood pressure problems, give a pressor (100 µg of phenylephrine) to buy time while you give more fluids. Putting the patient's head down helps to increase venous return and helps to increase the blood pressure. Alternatively, you can have an assistant lift the legs. Putting her head down may increase the ICP, whereas lifting her legs can increase her blood pressure without increasing her ICP. Lifting the legs is better in terms of increasing the cerebral perfusion pressure.

5. With incision, the patient moves. Your twitch monitor showed no twitches with train of four and none with tetanus. How does a twitch monitor work? How could the patient move with no muscle twitches? Do you give more relaxant? Does an allergic reaction to the relaxant explain the earlier hypotension?

The twitch monitor works by sending a direct current to the skin that conducts through the skin to the underlying nerve, causing a muscular contraction. (Note: Direct current causes strong muscular contractions, but alternating current does not.) Because the patient is clearly not paralyzed, the twitch monitor is malfunctioning, probably caused by a dead battery. The fact that you did not check it means you have a dead battery powering your brain. I would give more relaxant now, get a new twitch monitor, and continue to monitor the twitch closely, because this weak, debilitated patient will need complete muscle strength at the end of the case. An allergic reaction to muscle relaxant could have explained her earlier hypotension because neuromuscular blockers are a common cause of allergic reactions in the OR.

6. With the patient's poor nutritional status, what problems can you anticipate with your anesthetic? What does a low albumin level mean to us? Is there any effect on the volume of distribution? What is the volume of distribution?

Volume of distribution is an *apparent* volume into which a drug distributes. It is described as *apparent* because some drugs have a volume of distribution greater than the entire body! Lipophilic drugs, in general, have large ones; they distribute more widely to all the tissues, and they get "soaked up" by all the fatty tissues and proteins. Hydrophilic drugs, in general, have small ones; they do not distribute throughout the tissues but tend to "stay" in the blood. This woman, with her poor nutritional status, does not have much fatty tissue or proteins around to interact with the drugs, and her drugs will have a smaller volume of distribution. From a practical standpoint, we get more "bang for the buck" with every drug we give. The narcotics, muscle relaxants, sedatives, and induction agents have no place to "distribute to." For this reason, you will have to "give less and wait longer" for everything you give. The low albumin level means her wound healing will be poor. Extremely poor albumin correlates with poor outcome.

7. As the surgeon drills through the femoral shaft, the end-tidal CO_2 wave suddenly disappears. What could explain this? How can the monitor malfunction? Can it be explained by a kink, pathophysiologic reason, or embolus?

Dropping CO_2 values means less CO_2 is being delivered to the monitor. Barring a kink or a disconnection, that translates into less CO_2 being delivered to the lungs. Something in the circulatory system is blocking flow to the lungs; consider an embolus ("cork in the pulmonary circulation"). Because the surgeon is drilling through bone marrow and tumor mass, I suspect a ground-up puree of tumor and bone marrow is entering the circulation, causing a combined tumor and fat embolus in the pulmonary circulation.

8. You see yellow fluid filling the end-tidal CO_2 sampling line, running all the way back up into the Defend container, and snaking its way up and into the guts of your machine. What effect will this have on your equipment? How did this happen? Explain the possibilities of a fat embolus, regular embolus, and congestive heart failure (CHF). How will you make the diagnosis?

If the goop gets in the delicate guts of the machine, it may ruin it, so try to stop it before it overflows. The fat and tumor embolus has caused a catastrophe in the lungs. Right ventricular outflow is plugged, causing acute right heart failure, and the lung itself, in response to the embolus, is injured, and fluid is pouring into the alveoli, causing pulmonary edema. All the Starling forces are now out of whack, with fluid leaving the circulatory part of the lungs and entering the respiratory part of the lungs. Regardless of the source of the embolus (e.g., fat, tumor, amniotic fluid, blood clot), the hemodynamic and respiratory effects are the same, with a right heart that cannot empty, a left heart that cannot get full, and a distressed lung between them. The timing of this event argues against CHF. With TEE, you would see the difference quickly. CHF would be shown by an overfilled, poorly functioning left ventricle. This embolus would be demonstrated by a dilated right side and an empty left side of the heart.

9. The blood pressure drops to 70/45 mm Hg, you lose the saturation waveform, and ST-segment depression occurs. What explains these hemodynamic findings? How will you manage this situation? Explain your choice of hemodynamic support and monitoring.

You are close to code status, with a nearly impossible situation. Everything hinges on the glob or globs of stuff plugging up the outflow from the right ventricle to the lungs, and short of miraculously pulling that out (few surgeons do this kind of heroic procedure, let alone in this patient with metastatic cancer), all you can do is support as best you can. Use 100% oxygen and some PEEP (although it is difficult with the hypotension) to try to maintain oxygenation. Hemodynamic support can be offered with inotropes such as epinephrine and milrinone or norepinephrine. Guide your support by TEE in the OR.

10. The ETT keeps filling with yellow fluid. Should you use suction? Explain your choice in terms of Starling forces. What if fluid dries and obstructs? She has a 7.0-French ETT in; should you change the tube? If the instability continues, do you cancel the case? What do you tell the surgeon?

Do not suction the ETT; it just sucks more pulmonary edema fluid into the lungs. However, if it is so bad that the ETT obstructs, you have to. I would not change the tube in the middle of this nightmare on Elm Street. Starling forces "hold" fluid in the "right place" by a combination of hydrostatic pressure and interstitial pressure, laid against a background of capillary permeability. Higher hydrostatic pressure (from the right heart failure) favors fluid going into the lungs. Lower interstitial pressure (from her poor nutritional state and low levels of proteins in the blood) favors fluid going into the lungs. Capillary permeability can increase in response to an embolus, which also favors fluid going into the lungs. Everything is working against you! I would tell the surgeon to get done as soon as possible (he cannot leave an open femur hanging in the breeze), and I would say it in a high, distressed voice.

Postoperative Questions

1. During transfer to the bed to go to the ICU, the patient goes from a right lateral decubitus position to supine. What physiologic alterations occur with this change? Is there any chance for hemodynamic worsening with this move? Will oxygenation worsen, or will it improve—or can you tell?

Going supine may help your oxygenation, but in the setting of this embolus (which went God knows where), anything can happen. In general, the supine position provides better $\dot{V}/\dot{Q}$ matching than the lateral decubitus position. It also has the distinct advantage that it allows you to "get at everything." I would keep my eyes peeled because the move could dislodge an embolus and make everything come crashing down.

2. On arrival to the ICU, the patient arrests. Describe how you proceed through advanced cardiac life support (ACLS) protocol in the setting of the patient's fat embolus. At what point do you open the chest and attempt surgical removal of the embolus from the pulmonary artery?

The ACLS protocol emphasizes fast and hard chest compressions at the rate of 100 per minute. These compressions may be of particular benefit in this case, because they may "break up" the embolus and improve things. I would give drugs according to the protocol (1 mg of epinephrine every 3 minutes), would shock any shockable rhythm immediately, and would use amiodarone if pharmacologic help was needed for rhythm control. I would not encourage opening this woman's chest and fishing out the embolus. It may not be a single embolus, and her overall situation is grim.

3. The patient is successfully resuscitated, and TEE is called for. What would you expect to see if an embolus is the correct diagnosis? What would you see if CHF is the diagnosis? What other findings on TEE could help with her management?

TEE in the case of regular CHF would show left ventricular or biventricular failure, with a poor EF as demonstrated by little difference between end-diastolic and end-systolic volumes. TEE shows a distinctive pattern, consistent with a "cork" in the right ventricle. The right side is dilated, and the left side is empty. In guiding therapy, TEE can show you exactly what the volume situation is, rather than getting a set of numbers and hoping you can "divine" what is really happening.

4. In the ICU, the patient's blood gas assessment shows a Po_2 level of 55 on 100% oxygen. How can you improve her oxygenation? You institute PEEP, and things get worse. Explain this result. Using TEE, could anything explain this refractory hypoxemia? Can anything related to West's zones 1, 2, or 3 explain this?

Standard treatment for poor oxygenation is 100% oxygenation, PEEP, and tube maintenance (e.g., making sure it is in the right place, not blocked or kinked). A paradoxical response to PEEP may indicate a previously undiagnosed patent foramen ovale. As you increase the PEEP, you increase the shunt, pushing blood across to the left. Alternatively, high PEEP may push more blood to West's zone 3, where blood flow is rich but aeration is poor. Invoking this West stuff is pretty theoretical and may be a myth that comforts us. I am sticking with the patent foramen ovale, which I will check with TEE.

5. The husband comes in the ICU and is alarmed at the turn of events. "But she's a no-code!" he yells. She did not want to end up on a ton of tubes and stuff. "Let her go!" How do you respond to this new information? Is she a no-code? What are the ethics of letting her go now?

This is a beast. In general, no one is a no-code in the OR. You can argue that a code in the OR is usually iatrogenic. We cannot just kill them and say, "Oh well, it was meant to be." However, at this stage and with family input, you can re-assess, and if all are agreed, you can take the next step and withdraw therapy. This whole situation is controversial and not written in stone.

How It Actually Happened

This was a case that scared me out of my wits! Misery was the right name for this encounter, because it was miserable from start to finish. Moving the patient was difficult, because she hurt everywhere, and her eyes had such a "when will this end?" look that you almost could not look at her. The orthopedic specialist knew the score on the whole deal and was doing this "prophylactic pinning" because he did not want her last days compounded by the agony of a femur snapping.

When the end-tidal value disappeared, I went through the standard motions when I saw the fluid in the line and knew just what had happened. I told the surgeon right away, called for help, and we had to go the whole nine yards with resuscitation, right up to floating a Swan-Ganz catheter (this was before the era of "TEE über Alles") and starting epinephrine and dobutamine drips.

The brain killer in all this was our sense of uselessness at this resuscitation. Why bring her back from the brink when her life was unending agony and she had a life span measured in weeks or months? However, "in for a penny, in for a pound," and we treated and "saved" her, if that word even applies here. Truth to tell, it would have been better the other way.

CASE 9: WHAT WAS THAT POPPING SOUND?

Intraoperative Questions

1. Discuss the risks inherent in placing a tracheostomy, including the possibilities of an airway fire and subcutaneous emphysema. Should you intubate first and then do the tracheostomy, or do the tracheostomy with the patient awake? In what situation would you do the tracheostomy first?

A tracheostomy can go in the wrong place, in which case, it is called a subcutaneous emphysemotomy, because that is what it would cause. Of particular concern in a tracheostomy is the proximity of surgical cautery with an oxygen-containing tube (i.e., trachea), and there is always the risk of a fire. In this case, the man's airway is okay, and you can do the intubation in regular fashion and then do the tracheostomy while he is anesthetized. If his airway was compromised (e.g., fungating tumor on the epiglottis) and a routine induction or an awake intubation ran the risk of losing the airway, you should do the tracheostomy first.

2. Before induction, consider the blurred vision complaint. Is it evidence of increased ICP? What does it mean in the absence of other signs? Are there any risks with "assuming increased ICP" and proceeding "as if he has it for sure"? How do you induce a patient with increased ICP?

Blurred vision is probably caused by the aneurysm pressing on his optic chiasm. I would seek other signs of increased ICP (e.g., headache, nausea) and ask the neurosurgeon if he suspected increased ICP (funduscopic examination shows increased cup to disk ratio or papilledema; I certainly would not trust *my* funduscopic examination). You may see oculomotor or abducens palsy (again trusting the neurosurgeon, who does better neurologic examinations than I do). There is a risk of assuming ICP and just going for it, because the real problem here is this monster aneurysm. If you do an RSI with big swings in pressure, you could rupture the aneurysm, ending the case before it even started. This case requires blunting the sympathetic response to intubation and preventing a big shear force from forming across the aneurysm. You want to give a narcotic with lidocaine, and you want to maintain normocarbia as you ventilate before induction. In a regular case of increased ICP, you assume "full head, full stomach" and perform a modified RSI with the same goals in mind: blunt the sympathetic response to intubation, guard the airway against aspiration, maintain normocarbia, and try not to screw up everything.

3. Which invasive monitors will you use for this long, complicated case? Is there any need for specialized CVP if you are concerned about an air embolus? What are the complications with placing such a CVP line? What constitutes the best placement for a central, internal jugular, external jugular, subclavian, or femoral line?

A monster blood loss could occur if the aneurysm ruptures. Place an arterial line and a big central line. I would place a Cordis line in the femoral vein. An arterial line is used for beat-to-beat blood pressure measurement. The Cordis is used for volume replacement. A femoral site is used because this will not impair venous drainage of the head (as a jugular or subclavian would), and you can get at and troubleshoot a femoral line during an intracranial case. It is hard to check a jugular or subclavian line when the patient is up in pins and the head is far, far away from you.

Unless the patient is going to be in a sitting position, you do not need a multi-orifice CVP line situated at the superior vena cava (SVC) and right atrial junction. If the patient is sitting, you will need such a line, as well as a precordial Doppler, to be able to detect and treat an air embolism.

4. The surgeon performs a fantastically complicated dissection through the face. What are the dangers with dissection around the eye? The heart rate drops to 35 beats/min while pulling on the eye. What is the mechanism, and what is the treatment? How will you paralyze and maintain paralysis to ensure the patient does not buck at the absolute worst time?

The oculocardiac reflex is a danger during dissection around the eye. If the heart rate drops to 35 beats/min, the traction on an extraocular eye muscle is sending information to the brain, and the vagus is sending a response to the heart to slow down. Tell the surgeons to stop, and treat only with atropine if the bradycardia does not respond to this release of tension. Because this patient must be kept absolutely still, keep a twitch monitor where you can see it (you may have access to one arm), make sure it works and has fresh batteries (if necessary, test it on a friend, using tetanus, just for laughs), and is closely watched throughout the case. Keep the patient at one twitch and just barely at that.

5. A bulging brain is a problem as dissection continues. How do you assist the surgeon? Do you use mannitol? What is the mechanism and what are the shortcomings of mannitol? Should you use Lasix? Should you employ hyperventilation? What are the problems with hyperventilation?

Make sure venous drainage of the head is optimal. You may have to adjust the pins to make sure the head is not so acutely flexed that drainage is impossible. Mannitol and furosemide can provide short-term help in decreasing brain water, but both have inherent problems; for mannitol to be completely effective, you need an intact blood-brain barrier, and surgery violates that barrier. Furosemide increases fluid loss, and that can lead to a decrease in blood pressure, forcing you to give more fluids, so you can end up chasing your tail. You can also keep the inhaled agents below 0.5 minimum alveolar concentration (MAC), because potent inhaled agents can increase cerebral blood flow. Because hyperventilation can lead to cerebral ischemia, it is no longer recommended. In the short term in an absolute crisis, you can do it in a desperate attempt to "unload" the brain, but long-term hyperventilation is not the answer. You eventually have to stop hyperventilating, and you can get rebound intracranial hypertension. You must keep the patient well oxygenated (duh!) because hypoxemia causes an increase in cerebral blood flow, until hypoxemia causes *no* flow, when the patient dies. If you have a cerebrospinal fluid drain in place, you can drain some off (about 15 mL, aiming at keeping ICP about 12 cm H_2O).

6. The surgeon is nearing the base of this monster and asks for "the most hypotension you can possibly give." How do you manage this? Do you use potent inhaled agents? What are the problems with that approach? Do you use

narcotics, vasodilators, nicardipine, or pentathol? What are the advantages and disadvantages of each?

This is a very tense time in this kind of a case. Should you use potent inhaled agents to get the pressure down? That high of a MAC of agents can cause increased ICP. Narcotics can take the pressure down only so far, but you cannot really keep going up and up on narcotics such as a vasoactive drip; the blood pressure will most likely remain stable. Vasodilators such as sodium nitroprusside and nitroglycerin can also increase cerebral blood flow. Because nicardipine drops blood pressure but does not increase cerebral blood flow, it is a good choice. Pentathol is good at reducing cerebral metabolic rate, but there is hell to pay at emergence because the pentathol in high doses prevents rapid emergence. I would use a half-MAC of vapor, make sure I had a good amount of narcotic on board, and run a nicardipine drip until the systolic blood pressure is about 70 mm Hg.

7. The blood pressure is 70/50 mm Hg, and there is no ectopy or ST-segment change. The surgeon says, " I need lower pressure, or this guy is going to die." How much lower can you go? What problems do you anticipate? Are there any options at this point other than going lower and lower?

How much lower in this case is unclear. If the surgeon says he really needs it much lower, you should suggest going on CPB and doing it under circulatory arrest. You can lower the blood pressure with more nicardipine, more of everything, but once you get below a mean pressure of 50 mm Hg, you are in an area for which there is no research to tell you what is safe.

8. A faint "pop" is heard. The blood pressure increases to 280/150 mm Hg, and the heart rate drops into the 30s. What could explain this—syringe swap or infusion of a wrong inotrope? What is the pathophysiologic mechanism? What is your response? What is the best way to control "absolutely out of control hypertension"?

When the pressure soars, make sure your drips and syringes are all in the right place. This could be a vial of norepinephrine given by mistake or a wide-open phenylephrine drip. Give a vial of propofol or pentathol, whichever you pick up first, to get that blood pressure out of the stratosphere. This is most likely an extreme Cushing's triad response, with bleeding in the field leading to increased ICP, followed by adaptive hypertension (i.e., body's attempt to maintain cerebral perfusion pressure) and a reflex bradycardia (i.e., response to the extreme hypotension). Because the cranium is already open, this must be a horrific intracranial bleed to register as increased ICP.

9. The surgeon says, "Oh, damn!" You look over the field, and you see the brain bulging up like a basketball from the skull. The sulci are flattened, and the normal gray of the brain has become fiery red and looks hemorrhagic. What caused this? What options do you have at this point? Should you accept electroencephalographic (EEG) silence or resort to hyperventilation as a desperation maneuver?

The bulging is from a bleed into the center of the brain. You can try anything you want at this point; it probably will not make much difference. You can use large amounts of pentathol to silence the EEG, hyperventilation (this is a time for desperation maneuvers), and a quick re-evaluation to make sure you are not doing something stupid, such as not ventilating or blowing a tuba into the cerebrospinal fluid drain.

10. The organ donation consultant is called. How do you manage the hemodynamics and intracranial issues as preparation is made to transfer the patient to the ICU? What hemodynamic changes can you anticipate in the brain-dead patient?

This is not what you were planning on, but pros adapt. At this point, you make sure as much "good" is happening to the soon-to-be-donated organs as possible. Send for an ABG analysis, maintain hemodynamic stability, and if you suction the ETT, use careful aseptic technique (they may want the lungs). Maintain urine output. The main *wrong* thing to do is to say "Oh, the hell with it," and let the patient deteriorate through lack of vigilance. This, for example, is a perfectly good heart. Should you let the fluids drift down, put the guy into a hypotensive state, and flog the heart with dopamine to keep the pressure up? It is not good for the heart or for anything else. The brain-dead patient will not have a normal adaptive hemodynamic system, so close blood pressure monitoring and quick responses to dips and jumps are important.

Postoperative Questions

1. In the ICU, the patient starts putting out 1.5 L of urine each hour. What could be causing this? Is it diabetes insipidus? What is the mechanism? What about mannitol infusion? What is the mechanism of diuresis with mannitol? What is the treatment if the patient has diabetes insipidus?

Intracranial injury can cause diabetes insipidus. The body is excreting excess free water. Alternatively, this could be polyuria from mannitol infusion. Mannitol causes an osmotic diuresis in the kidney itself, whereas diabetes insipidus has a central cause (i.e., brain is releasing inadequate antidiuretic hormone [ADH]). Because of the patient's injury, this looks like he has central diabetes insipidus. Treatment is replacement with isotonic crystalloid solution, infusion of aqueous ADH (this may be hard to get in your pharmacy), or vasopressin. You have to monitor the volume status closely to make sure you keep up with the fluids. You should also monitor sodium because the patient can become severely hypernatremic.

2. An air leak develops around the cuff, and the patient cannot be ventilated adequately. How can you change the tube? Is the intubating stylet ready? What about fiberoptic access, a tube changer, or direct laryngoscopy? What if the patient is extremely swollen?

Take a good, long look at everything about this airway before you make a move. Was the patient easy to intubate the first time? Has he swollen up a lot with all these shenanigans? Did they do a tracheostomy on him? (Life is much easier if they did that already.) After you have looked things over, change the tube after suctioning the mouth, placing a tube changer as a back up and under direct vision. Do not place blind faith in the tube changer, because you can do everything right but still end up somehow getting the tube in the esophagus, as many of us can attest to.

3. Plans include harvesting the heart. As you are planning to go back to the OR, the patient becomes hemodynamically unstable. How can you stabilize the patient but not endanger the heart and keep it viable for another organ recipient?

The main protection for the heart is to make sure that common sense and fixing what you can fix take precedence over starting a bunch of inotropes to save the day. All inotropes flog the heart in one way or another. Use them only if you have fixed everything else. Are there blood gas problems? Fix the oxygenation. Is there a low hematocrit? Transfuse. (Yes, you can transfuse an organ donor.) Do for this donor what you would do for anyone else who had hemodynamic instability. Fix what you can fix, and if you need to, start inotropic support after you have fixed everything you can fix.

4. During the organ harvest, how do you manage the anesthetic? Do you use muscle relaxants, narcotics, or potent inhaled agents? If the patient is brain dead, do you need to do anything at all? Why or why not?

The brain-dead patient feels nothing, but because reflexive responses to noxious stimuli are still present, anesthetize with potent vapors, and give neuromuscular relaxation. Keep it simple, and do what you always do. Anesthetize the way you know how as you would for anyone else.

5. The surgeon asks for heparin as he is about to clamp the aorta and dissect out the heart. You give 3 mL of heparin, thinking it is the 10,000 U/mL concentration of heparin. As the surgeon clamps, you look down and see you gave the 1000 U/mL concentration of heparin, thereby severely underdosing. What do you do?

Yell STOP at the top of your lungs! With inadequate heparinization, the heart and everything else can develop clots while waiting for transplantation. Do the right thing, admit your mistake, give the additional heparin, and give those organs the best possible chance for a successful launch. A lot of organ recipients are counting on you!

How It Actually Happened

I again found myself on the hot seat in a catastrophe. Words cannot describe what I felt when that blood pressure went through the upper reaches of the stratosphere after that aneurysm popped. Being raised in the "it is always my fault" of anesthesia-ness, I thought I had given a syringe of phenylephrine or epinephrine by mistake. Then I thought the patient had gotten superlight and driven his blood pressure skyward.

I had the sequence turned around. The attempt at clipping popped the aneurysm, and it bled into the brain, giving the horrific view of this brain popping a mile out of the skull. The poor guy's circulatory system shifted into Cushing's triad gear, and that was that. After hours of painstaking dissection, the whole thing went up the spout in about 10 seconds. The next day, we harvested his organs.

Reminder: THIS IS NOT A NOVEL TO BE PERUSED. Make sure you are answering everything *before* you look at the answers. Keep in mind, *your* answers may be different, they may be *better*. This is not a textbook, this is a workbook.

CASE 10: A GUSHER

Intraoperative Questions

1. A colleague suggests you place the Swan-Ganz catheter before induction. Is this necessary? Why or why not? What is the value of pre-induction "numbers" in the setting of cardiac surgery?

No, it is not necessary. Getting a set of preoperative numbers does nothing to help you manage intraoperatively. In days of yore, we thought this was the case, but evidence-based medicine does not bear it out. For that matter, a Swan-Ganz catheter has not been shown to improve outcome *at all*, let alone after snagging a set of "before we start" numbers.

2. Would TEE and a CVP line serve just as well to monitor the patient? How about a TEE and a Cordis, a TEE and several big peripheral lines, or a CVP with no TEE? Are there any special considerations for the HIV-positive patient and the use of TEE?

TEE and a Cordis are the best bet. That provides you adequate volume access, a dependable line (peripheral lines tucked to the side could infiltrate or get blocked by surgeons leaning in), and all the information you will need to guide you during the case. Even an imperfect knowledge of TEE can serve you, because you are looking for a few key things:

- Full or empty
- Ventricle functioning well or not
- Perivalvular leak after the valve is replaced

Placing the Cordis catheter allows someone later on (who *does* believe in Swan-Ganz catheters or somehow cannot manage without one) to place it without having to stick the patient again.

Caveat: Remember, these are the boards, and you do not have to agree with any of the previous information. You can say, "I want a Swan-Ganz catheter," as long as you can justify it. To be able to adjust inotropes and vasopressors, I will need cardiac output, pulmonary artery pressures, and systemic vascular resistance. Without a wedge, I do not know what is really going on, so I need a Swan-Ganz catheter." There is no *right* answer on the boards; there are *justifiable* answers that a consultant in anesthesia can defend.

3. Which induction agents should you use? Do you "have to use etomidate" because you are in the heart room? Should you use pentathol, ketamine, or propofol? Describe the pros and cons of each. Does any outcome study show a difference?

It is not the wand that does the magic; it is the magician wielding the wand. There is no proof that any induction agent has an advantage over any other. Etomidate has the advantage of maintaining hemodynamic stability, but it has the disadvantage of not really blunting the tachycardic response to intubation if you use it alone. Ketamine keeps you stable but can also lead to tachycardia, which is not a huge problem in this young patient, but then again, maybe he has damaged his myocardium with injectable cocaine through the years and he cannot tolerate tachycardia so well, so why risk it? Propofol and pentathol can drop the blood pressure if you use a lot and are careless, but we are not careless! The world's first heart transplantation was induced with pentathol; they used a reduced dose, like any careful anesthesiologist knows to do. You can use whatever you want.

I would use etomidate with fentanyl to blunt the tachycardic response to intubation. I would not push for a severe slowing of his heart rate, because he has regurgitation, and a slow, slow heart rate favors backward flow.

4. With laryngoscopy, his heart rate drops into the 30s. What is the mechanism, and is treatment necessary? What should be done in the setting of aortic

regurgitation? Should you forge ahead and intubate, or should you treat before you intubate?

Narcotics plus a vagal response to instrumenting the pharynx might have led to this bradycardia. This is the wrong way to go with a regurgitant lesion, because you prefer a faster rate to favor forward flow. The longer the diastole, the more time there is for regurgitation to occur, and that is not desirable.

If I had a good view of the cords, I would go ahead and intubate, because intubation should stimulate the sympathetic nervous system and get that heart rate up. If the bradycardia persisted, I would treat with ephedrine. If it got severe, I would give atropine and CPR if necessary to make sure the atropine gets mixed around in there.

5. With sternotomy, the surgeon says "Oh, damn!" What are the implications of such a statement? What are the dangers during sternotomy? What could have gone wrong? Is there any difference when this is a repeat operation?

When a surgeon says, "Oh, damn," it is like hearing the pilot on your flight saying, "Assume emergency landing positions." Not good.

During a sternotomy, the saw can go through lung (a headache but fixable with some stapling) or through the "stuck to the sternum heart," which is somewhat more problematic. Particularly with a repeat operation, the heart can be closely applied to the back of the sternum and therefore "sawable." Blood loss will be massive, and the surgeons may have to place femoral-femoral bypass while they hold a finger in the dike of the torn heart. All you can do is hang blood as fast as you can and support the blood pressure as best you can.

6. The left arterial line dampens and registers a blood pressure in the 20s and 30s. That is the differential diagnosis for a severely damped arterial line? With retraction, you see bright arterial blood shooting above the level of the screen. What is your management plan at this point?

Believe bad news is bad news. Never assume it is a problem with the transducer. There *may* be a bubble in the line, a surgeon leaning on the arm, or some other innocent explanation, but more likely, the blood pressure is that low because of blood loss. I guess you could imagine the saw going so far left it sawed off the subclavian artery feeding the left arm, but I cannot imagine such horror even on the boards.

Call for help. Get a rapid infuser. Get the perfusion people in the room. Hang blood. Get extra surgeons to get you femoral-femoral access. Pray.

7. The aorta and left subclavian are torn open by the saw. How do you manage this catastrophe? Address the issues of the anesthetic level, resuscitation, muscle relaxation, rapid transfusion, and dangers of rapid transfusion. When do you get a rapid infuser? Do you use the cardiopulmonary bypass machine to transfuse?

They *did* tear open the left subclavian! (This book is full of *cases that actually happened*, not just crazy stuff we dreamed up.) You are now in full resuscitation mode:

- Turn off all potent inhaled agents (cannot afford the cardiac depression).
- Call for everyone within a hundred miles to lend a hand.
- Use muscle relaxation (cannot afford to have the patient move).
- Use care with what is said because recall is a distinct possibility.

- Consider massive transfusion, with its attendant dangers: hypothermia, hypocalcemia, and a dilutional effect on coagulation and platelets.
- If the vital signs support it, use something to decrease memories, such as midazolam.

8. You place the patient on femoral-femoral bypass. What is the difference between this approach and conventional bypass? What are the problems with femoral-femoral bypass? What are the advantages? What if the perfusionists say they cannot get enough flow? How would a blood gas measurement reflect inadequate flow?

Femoral-femoral bypass sometimes causes problems with flow. You do not have access to a huge "vessel" for drainage (the femoral vein is just not as big as the right atrium), and you do not have access to a completely physiologic vessel for infusing (infuse the aorta, and blood flows in the "usual way" to all the arterial bed; when you infuse through the femoral artery, you have a curious reverse of flow up the aorta). It can be hard to adequately perfuse, and concerns arise over whether the flow will be adequate to, for example, the spinal cord. The perfusionists may see a low mixed venous oxygen value on their machine, indicating inadequate output. An ABG determination may show metabolic acidosis, another indicator may show inadequate perfusion in some vascular bed. The best cure is to make sure the lines are lined up, not kinked, and doing okay. With time, if the surgeon can get control in the chest, he or she can transfer to chest lines, at least for venous drainage.

9. A blood gas determination shows a pH of 7.03 on bypass. How will you manage this? Will you use bicarbonate or just let adequate perfusion take place? What are the problems with using bicarbonate? How about using trishydroxymethylaminomethane (THAM)? The blood gas determination also shows a hematocrit of 17%. Should you transfuse? Should you wait until you come off bypass and then transfuse?

First, do what you can to increase oxygen delivery to the tissues, such as treating the hematocrit of 17%. Transfuse up to the mid-20s. It is better to improve perfusion to fix acidosis than to throw base in the form of bicarbonate or THAM at the acidosis in the hope of making the numbers better. It is a noble goal to avoid giving blood on bypass, because the cardiopulmonary bypass (CPB) machine beats up blood, but anytime the hematocrit is below 24%, evidence-based medicine supports transfusion. In this case, we have additional reasons to transfuse, including severe blood loss from a saw wound (cue the soundtrack to *Texas Chainsaw Massacre*) and acidosis, indicating you need to improve oxygen delivery *now*.

10. As you are coming off bypass, a TEE examination shows a perivalvular leak. What is the implication? What if the TEE study shows a small amount of central regurgitation? How would a tissue valve look compared with a prosthetic valve?

A perivalvular leak indicates the valve is seated poorly or sewn in imperfectly. You have to go back on bypass and fix this. A small amount of central regurgitation is a normal finding. Artificial valves need a little regurgitation to make them close. (Our original valves do not need this regurgitation. Call it *intelligent design*, if you like.) Tissue valves throw little shadows from their metallic stents (they are like little poles that the valve leaflets hang from). A completely prosthetic valve throws a big shadow from its big metal leaflet. It may also click!

Postoperative Questions

1. Concern is raised about the patient's neurologic status. How do you evaluate this in the immediate postoperative period? Would you use muscle relaxants, narcotics, or sedatives? Do you go to CT right away? Would bispectral (BIS) index monitoring be helpful? Would an EEG study help? What is the timing for each of these methods?

   To get a good evaluation, you have to first eliminate the following:

   - Pharmacologic causes of delayed awakening (e.g., sedatives, relaxants, narcotics)
   - Metabolic causes of delayed awakening (e.g., hypothermia, hypoglycemia, electrolyte derangements)

Oh, yeah, you have to make sure the patient is not dead. That is a real confounder when it comes to wondering why the guy is not waking up? After you have ruled out pharmacology, metabolism, and death, it is worth getting a radiology study to see what is going on. A BIS value can be useful, because it gives you a processed view of what is going on:

   - BIS value of 70 is helpful.
   - BIS value of 5 argues that you have got a problem.

A genuine EEG with real live neurologic evaluation is preferable to our awake-o-meter. I would get these studies as soon as the patient was stable the next day. If the patient is really brain dead, you'll want to know early on to guide treatment, aggressiveness, and family communications.

2. The patient's lactic acid level is progressively increasing. What could be causing this? Something in the gut or leg? What if the patient has an IABP? What if the amylase level rises? Does this indicate pancreatitis? What is the treatment? What is abdominal compartment syndrome, and how do you treat it?

When the lactic acid level is rising, something, somewhere, is dying. After a big hit like this, with big blood loss and hypoperfusion, the list of potential candidates includes just about everything (e.g., gut, liver, pancreas [amylase rise]). The intra-aortic balloon pump (IABP) adds the possibility of leg ischemia, with dead tissue in the hypoperfused leg. The balloon could also be impeding perfusion in the gut or to the kidneys.

   Abdominal compartment syndrome is just like compartment syndrome elsewhere (e.g., lower leg). Increased pressure in the abdomen leads to abdominal distention, which can get tight enough to cut off circulation to the gut. Treatment includes exploratory laparotomy to open the abdomen, relieve the pressure, and see what caused the pressure rise in the first place (often, dead gut).

3. Bleeding is noticed in the chest tubes. How much bleeding is acceptable? When would you need to re-explore? The surgeon says to give more fresh-frozen plasma (FFP). Do you agree? Why or why not? How would you diagnose tamponade?

If a chest tube is putting out enough blood to make you uncomfortable, send for a thromboelastogram (TEG). If the TEG result is normal, get the surgeon, and tell him you need to explore. Stalling and hanging more factors are a waste of time. This is a battle that will go on forever, but the key element has to be common sense. If the coagulation tests do not show any medical cause of bleeding, it must be surgical bleeding.

The reverse is not necessarily true. If the coagulation tests show a medical cause of bleeding, surgical bleeding can still be occurring. A high PT does not exclude a loose stitch. I would re-explore if there is more than 200 mL/hr and no sign of slowing.

Tamponade is a clinical diagnosis, supported by a TEE finding of a pericardial effusion and strongly supported by TEE showing atrial collapse during systole or ventricular collapse during diastole, or both. The clinical signs are hypotension, tachycardia, increased need for inotropic support, and equalization of filling pressures.

4. Two days later, the blood pressure is 70/60 mm Hg, the heart rate is 130 beats/min, and the cardiac output is 8 L/m. What is your diagnosis? Is something other than sepsis possible? What is the treatment? The surgeon is horrified when he sees what you are doing. Explain the rationale for the use of any vasoactive drugs.

With high output and low blood pressure, tachycardia is sepsis until proved otherwise. These are the classic parameters of a severely vasodilated state. Theoretically, this could be an allergic reaction with massive vasodilation, but given the history, I would go with sepsis. Treatment includes treating the source of the sepsis and supporting the patient in the meantime. Support centers on norepinephrine to raise systemic vascular resistance and fluid replacement. The patient also needs ventilatory support.

Why? The treatment for not enough systemic vascular resistance is to provide systemic vascular resistance, and norepinephrine does just that. If the patient does not respond to norepinephrine, you could try vasopressin because it sometimes works when norepinephrine does not.

5. The neurologic workup shows no brain activity after 1 week. What are the criteria for brain death? Do you need blood flow studies? Is a clinical examination alone sufficient? Do you need a CT scan or EEG study? Do you try carbon dioxide and see if that stimulates breathing?

Brain death means there is no blood flow to the brain. That is the definitive study. All the other things (e.g., EEG, cold calorics, CO_2, anything else you can dream up) are just supplements to this simple fact.

How It Actually Happened

Death stalks the OR in this one. This case looked routine, and no one suspected the aorta was stuck so close behind the sternum. The chest radiograph and CT scan did not throw up any red flags. However, the saw went right through the aorta and sheared off the subclavian as well. Blood loss was brisk, and that is an understatement.

We started transfusing, and one surgeon put his hand in the field and tried to do the Dutch boy with his finger in the dike routine. A second surgeon went with a femoral-femoral bypass. We went on bypass as soon as possible. Then we did circulatory arrest to replace the aortic arch. What a mess.

The valve was replaced, as was the aortic arch. We came off bypass with just epinephrine and got to the unit okay. In the OR and the ICU, the patient got a massive transfusion. Lucky for us, he did not come back for bleeding. Later on, no brain activity was detected, and the patient eventually died.

CASE 11: GUMMING UP THE PULMONARY WORKS

Intraoperative Questions

1. What monitors do you want to use in this patient and why?
Hook up her triple-lumen line and monitor the CVP from there. Place an arterial line for beat-to-beat blood pressure measurement and blood gases (e.g., asthma, diabetes).

2. Do you want an arterial line before or after induction? Why or why not?
The arterial line is needed after induction. Unless you are an absolute moron and overdose her on induction, you are unlikely to need beat-to-beat blood pressure measurement then. (When you say *moron*, try to avoid looking either examiner in the face.)

3. How would you induce this patient? What is your induction agent of choice? Why?
Use ketamine. You can get tachycardia from this, but with some narcotic preinduction, this should be controllable. My primary concern is not inducing bronchospasm, and the sympathomimetic effect of ketamine will prove useful here. Because she has been immobile in bed, I would avoid succinylcholine but would do a modified RSI using vecuronium.

4. On induction, the patient desaturates to 88%. What is your response?
Place an oral airway, turn the head to the side (it helps in mask ventilation, no kidding!), put her in reverse Trendelenburg to get some weight off her abdomen, and then intubate. Even if she is not completely relaxed and coughs a little, you will be able to overcome this. She is edentulous and should be easy to intubate.

5. The blood pressure is 90/40 mm Hg. Her oxygen saturation level is 77%, and the saturation level is slowly declining. What are your first reflex thoughts and actions?
Do the hypoxemia drill:

- Believe the bad news; do not blame it on the monitor.
- Use 100% oxygen (with a glance at the oxygen analyzer to make sure you are actually on 100% oxygen).
- Hand ventilate and listen; make sure the tube is in the correct place.
- Suction.
- Use bronchodilators if it sounds like bronchospasm.
- With the pressure low, turn off all potent inhaled agents, give fluids, and put the head down.

Note: This is the classic question "where you put yourself in the OR and do what you would do in the OR."

6. What are you going to do with the ventilatory settings? Would you use positive end expiratory pressure (PEEP)? If so, how much PEEP?
After I had done everything possible to improve oxygen delivery, I would start PEEP at 5 cm H_2O, checking to make sure this did not make the blood pressure drop. I would work my way up on the PEEP. If it got past 10 cm H_2O of PEEP, I would get some help in the room and would get an ICU ventilator.

7. The surgeon opens the peritoneum and finds bile spillage throughout. After a while, as he retracts the first part of duodenum to look for any possible perforation, the heart rate drops to 40 from 89 beats/min. What is your first response?

Ease up on that peritoneum! The surgeon's tugging is causing a vagal response. If, when he lets up, the bradycardia persists, I would see if it was symptomatic (hypotension) and then treat with atropine.

8. One hour into the procedure, the peak airway pressure rises to 44 from 31 cm H_2O. What is the differential diagnosis, and what is your response?

Something is making it harder to push air into this patient. Go geographic, starting from the circuit and tube (e.g., kink, clogged) and then going from the outside of the patient to the inside: musculoskeletal (e.g., scoliosis, but not in this case), pneumothorax (possible, she has a central line; listen to the chest if you suspect pneumothorax, decompress, and then place a chest tube), and the airways themselves (highly likely, an exacerbation of bronchospasm).

9. Would you extubate this patient in the OR? Why or why not?

No. She has had hot "chitlins" shoved back into her, which is very much like having a gastroschisis repair, if you think about it (God forbid you should think during this ordeal). With bile spillage, she is sure to become septic, so plan ahead, and have her airway secured for the postoperative storm. ARDS and sepsis are better handled in an intubated patient!

Postoperative Questions

1. You decide to keep the patient intubated. What type of ventilatory mode would you prefer in this patient? Why?

Although there are myriad options, it is hard to find proof that pressure support is better than volume control, let alone the alphabet soup of inverted I:E ratios all the way up to exotic things such as rotating the patient all the way around.

Stick to basics: 6 mL/kg at 12 breaths/min, get a gas determination, and go from there. To play it safe, start at 100% oxygen and 5 cm H_2O of PEEP, and then make adjustments. As a final crowning glory, call in a board-certified ICU specialist, because he or she will know the latest and preventing lung injury with different modes. Later, when things go to hell, you have got someone to share the blame with. Of note, smaller tidal volumes seem to cause less pulmonary damage than the higher tidal volumes (10 mL/Kg) we used to recommend.

2. The surgical ICU resident tells you that the heparin drip needs to be restarted. What is your response?

You have just completed surgery, and restarting heparin can restart bleeding. I would wait at least 12 hours, make sure there is no sign of bleeding, and then restart the heparin and follow coagulation study results.

3. As you are about to leave the ICU, the nurse calls you and shouts, "Her oxygen saturation is 95%." What is your response to the nurse?

Check the ventilation settings. Maybe you are titrating to "best PEEP," are down to 40% oxygen, and this 95% is fine. However, if this is a change, go back to the hypoxemia drill. This may include using CT to see if the patient has a pulmonary embolus adding to the woes.

4. You take care of the situation in the previous question, and then you go down to the OR to set up for another case. The same nurse calls and tells you, "The patient's saturation is now 85%." What is your response, other than exclaiming *damn* again?

That *is* a problem; I do not care what kind of best PEEP-ing you are up to. Go to the bedside, send a sample for a blood gas determination, go to 100% oxygen, ventilate with an Ambu bag, do fiberoptic bronchoscopy, and see if there is something down there. Paralyze the patient, because you do not need her fighting the ventilator and eating up valuable oxygen in the fight.

5. What is the difference between low-molecular-weight heparin (LMWH) and unfractionated heparin?

Plasma half-life and bioavailability are higher for LMWH compared with generic unfractionated heparin. This comes into play when neuraxial procedures are in the offing.

How It Actually Happened

This one is heavy on explanations, so read carefully! I was actually walking down to the main desk in the OR when the coordinator called me and said that I needed to do this emergency case. I asked my resident to quickly set up the room, including a transducer set up for a possible CVP and arterial line.

The patient arrives. She looked tachypneic and I asked her few questions. I saw that the heparin drip has been off. I quickly browsed through her chart, and the most important factor that I had in mind in this particular situation was the "saddle embolism" physiology of dead space, anticoagulation, and so on.

The patient comes to the room, and I hooked up the ECG, blood pressure cuff (activated the cuff at the same time), and pulse oximetry. Her preinduction blood pressure was 170/100 mm Hg, and heart rate was 88 beats/min. She got pre-oxygenated, and I induced her with 1.5 mg/kg of propofol and 1.2 mg/kg of rocuronium (rapid sequence). My resident puts the tube in, goes to the right position, and I see end-tidal CO_2—wow, what a relief! Oops! She starts desaturating to 88%. Her blood pressure now is 90/40 mm Hg. My resident adds PEEP and increases the tidal volume because the airway comes first. He also auscultates the lungs. They are clear. The tube is not kinked. She is on 100% F_{IO_2}. The saturation keeps dropping; now it is 82%, 78%. I asked my resident to administer 10 mg of ephedrine. Saturation is now 99%, and the blood pressure is now 150/98 mm Hg. The blood pressure cuff gave very reliable readings. Even though she was obese, the cuff size was appropriate, and we did not put an arterial line until the middle of the procedure, when we decided to keep her intubated,

What do you think happened here? *Dead space* is the answer. The patient needed a high blood pressure to bypass the iceberg (i.e., pulmonary embolism) and perfuse her lungs. If the lung does not get a certain reasonable relatively high blood pressure, the clot is not going to be bypassed. In this case, we are talking about circulation, breathing, and airway (CBA) instead of airway, breathing, and circulation (ABC). In rare instances, the heart gets priority. (Remember the CPR protocol for ventricular fibrillation in the ACLS guidelines: Get a damn defibrillator first!)

The sudden bradycardia during the middle of the procedure was a result of vagal response. The increased peak airway pressure was a result of a "tight chest" resulting from her asthma. The former improved on commanding the surgeon, and the latter improved with an albuterol puff through the ETT.

I decided to keep her intubated because she is very likely to become septic from probable peritonitis. In these instances, it may be worthwhile to have her on the appropriate antibiotic therapy, optimize, and then consider extubation. Why worry at all because it is the job of the intensivist to wean her off the vent? The board wants you to know about ventilatory modes and weaning techniques.

There is no study to indicate that one mode of ventilation is better than another. Whether it is assist-control (AC) ventilation or synchronized intermittent mandatory ventilation (SIMV) does not matter. I put her on SIMV at an FIO_2 of 100% to start (the FIO_2 has to be weaned).

When to restart the heparin is a question of clinical judgment that has to be extensively discussed with the surgical team. Most likely, if there is no clinical indication of bleeding, most surgeons would not mind restarting the heparin drip within 12 to 24 hours. Some may delay it. Remember, pulmonary embolism is a killer, too. Bleeding into the belly could be catastrophic too. Use good clinical judgment, please.

What do you think will be your first response when you see saturation going down in the ICU? You learned your lesson in the OR. *Get that damn blood pressure right! Remember ABC!*

LMWH is a relatively recent addition to the list of anticoagulants for treatment and prophylaxis of deep venous thrombosis (DVT). As a prophylactic, LMWH is as effective as standard heparin or warfarin (Coumadin) and does not require monitoring of the activated partial thromboplastin time (aPTT) or the international normalized ratio (INR). LMWH is used for other conditions, such as atrial fibrillation and orthopedic procedures. LMWH is a commonly used option in patients with documented DVT, no risk factors for bleeding, and the ability to administer injections with or without the help of a visiting nurse or family member.

CASE 12: TRAUMATIC DISORDER DURING PREGNANCY

Preoperative Questions

1. What are the initial steps for evaluating a pregnant trauma patient?
The ABCs of resuscitation should be followed in the pregnant trauma patient as in any other patient. The mother's condition must be evaluated first, and after it is established that she is stable, the fetus should be assessed.

2. How should the patient be positioned during the evaluation?
Pregnant patients should be evaluated with left lateral tilt after about 20 weeks' gestation to avoid or minimize aortocaval compression. Initially, maternal blood pressure may not be affected, but uteroplacental blood flow may be compromised, and fetal distress may be the first sign for aortocaval compression or maternal hemodynamic instability. Placental abruption is a big concern after intra-abdominal or pelvic trauma, and continuous fetal heart rate evaluation is recommended for 2 to 3 hours after the accident.

3. What, if any, radiologic procedures should be performed on this patient? Why or why not? Would your choice of radiologic evaluation be affected if the pregnancy were at 8 weeks' estimated gestational age? What about 17 weeks' estimated gestational age?

In an emergency situation, especially with multiple trauma or intra-abdominal emergencies, radiologic evaluation should proceed as if the patient were not pregnant. The following question should be asked: "Would you want this radiographic study if the patient was not pregnant?" If the answer is yes, the study should be done. Delay in diagnosis of intra-abdominal conditions is common in pregnant patients and often results from unjustified concerns regarding appropriate radiographic evaluation and physical examination. No single radiologic test exposes the fetus to dangerous levels of radiation; most are in the millirad range. Even if the pregnancy is still in the first trimester, there is insufficient evidence to support termination of the pregnancy because of exposure to radiation from common radiographic procedures. This is even less of a concern when the pregnancy is well advanced into the second or third trimester, because all fetal organ systems are well past the period of organogenesis (8 to 56 days).

Intraoperative Questions

1. How will you proceed?
A cesarean section should be performed in shock trauma only if the patient is in extremis and if there is a viable fetus. Otherwise, the patient should be quickly moved to the OR while all necessary personnel, including the neonatal intensive care unit (NICU) staff, anesthesiologist, obstetrician, and trauma surgeons, are assembled. Fetal distress alone is not an indication for an emergency cesarean section in shock trauma, and performance of an emergency cesarean section in this situation may further compromise the mother. This patient should not have a cesarean section in shock trauma. She has many injuries, most of which have not been fully evaluated (i.e., there is no cervical spine film—and there is a real possibility of intra-abdominal trauma and hemorrhage).

2. What are the anesthetic considerations in this situation?
Pregnant patients can lose up to 40% of their blood volume before becoming hemodynamically unstable, and fetal distress (in this case, probably from placental abruption) may be a warning sign that the mother's hemodynamic profile is not as stable as you may think based on the vital signs. It cannot be stressed enough that the pregnant patient at 20 weeks' estimated gestational age or further along should be positioned with left uterine displacement.

3. What are the indications for an emergency cesarean section in the shock-trauma department?
Cesarean section is indicated only if the patient is in extremis and there is a viable fetus.

4. What is the CPR protocol for pregnant women? What is the optimal time from the start of cardiac arrest to delivery of the fetus in terms of maternal-fetal morbidity and mortality? Is CPR effective in the pregnant patient?
CPR usually is ineffective in the pregnant patient, especially if the pregnancy is well advanced. The gravid uterus prevents adequate venous return, and positioning the patient with left uterine displacement (a necessity) makes CPR less effective. In terms of medications, the standard advanced cardiac life support (ACLS) protocol should be followed. When maternal cardiac arrest occurs, performance of a cesarean section within 5 minutes of its onset is associated with the best outcomes for the mother and baby.

5. What problems would you anticipate intraoperatively in this patient?

Rapid-sequence intubation in a term pregnant trauma patient who weighs 300 pounds and who does not have cervical spine clearance can be a nightmare. Because she has had two prior cesarean sections, there may be adhesions, and incision-to-delivery time may be delayed. The uterus is likely to be atonic after delivery of the fetus. Pitocin, Methergine, and Hemabate (prostaglandin $F_{2\alpha}$) should be available. They are often not part of the standard OR drug boxes. Intra-abdominal bleeding from other sources may have already occurred. It is a very real possibility that this patient will "crash" after induction or certainly after delivery of the fetus once the abdomen is open.

An adequate type and cross has probably not been done, so the patient will need to receive un–crossmatched O negative blood or partially crossmatched blood after a specimen is sent to the blood bank. A cell saver may be used after amniotic fluid has been cleared from the field. You will likely need lots of help, so call for help early!

How It Actually Happened

The stuff you see sometimes is enough to make you hang this up and go drive a UPS truck. The senior anesthesia resident on the obstetrics rotation was sent down to the ER to check out what was happening after the anesthesia attending covering labor and delivery (the obstetrics anesthesia director) overheard the obstetric department residents saying they were going to shock trauma to evaluate a pregnant lady after a motor vehicle accident (MVA). The obstetrics anesthesia attending is off to a meeting but is carrying her beeper. The resident arrives to find a patient with multiple trauma and a nonreassuring fetal heart rate tracing. An experienced anesthesia attending arrives from the OR. A senior maternal-fetal medicine attending arrives, evaluates the fetus, and declares that he wishes to proceed with an immediate cesarean section in the shock-trauma department. The NICU is called, and an anesthesia machine and equipment are requested from the main OR (same floor as the shock-trauma department). The anesthesia attending does not do a lot of obstetric cases and is not sure if this is the right way to proceed. He asks for the obstetrics anesthesia attending to be paged stat to the shock-trauma unit.

Moments later, the obstetrics anesthesia attending arrives to a packed shock-trauma department to find the obstetrics attending gowned and gloved with a scalpel in his hand. The anesthesia team is preparing to intubate the patient, the NICU staff are present, and the trauma and ER personnel and a host of hospital administrator types are gathered around. The patient is the wife of one of the senior-level nursing administrators.

The incoming anesthesia attending makes eye contact with the other anesthesia attending, gets a brief synopsis of the transpired events, and observes that the patient is awake and alert! Now is the moment of decision! She feels very strongly that this is not an appropriate indication for a cesarean section in the shock-trauma department. She taps the obstetrician on the shoulder and tells him she thinks this is a very bad idea because the patient will die if he performs the cesarean section here. He agrees. She confirms with the other anesthesia attending that there is an available OR and announces to all assembled, "We are going to the OR." The doors to the shock-trauma department burst open, and everyone follows to the OR. General anesthesia is induced with a rapid sequence induction (RSI), an ETT is placed on the first attempt, and particulate food matter is suctioned from the stomach. A cesarean section is performed because the neonate is in extremis. Ultimately, the patient required many blood transfusions (e.g., uterine atony, splenic laceration), but she kept her uterus, went to the SICU, and went home within a week. Unfortunately, the baby died.

What is the lesson? Do not be afraid to make difficult decisions in a crisis situation. Use the knowledge you have to make these types of decisions, and do not back down if you think the patient's status is at risk. Pregnant patients should have cesarean sections in the shock-trauma department only if there is a maternal code situation.

CASE 13: THORACO WHACKO

Preoperative Questions

1. Can you do this procedure under spinal or epidural anesthesia only?
This procedure is relatively new in the vascular surgery literature. It requires a high level of technical expertise and is relatively new at Stony Brook. With this in mind, I would perform a general technique. If I were to attempt a regional technique, I would warn the surgical team and the patient about the likelihood of needing to convert to a general anesthesia technique. As Giesecke states, "Those patients with poor left ventricular function, congestive heart failure, or significant pulmonary dysfunction may not be able to remain supine for the duration of the procedure without receiving general anesthesia. Likewise, a general anesthetic may be necessary for patients with chronic low back pain who may not tolerate lying still for the entire procedure."

The beneficial effects of regional anesthesia include *decreased blood loss,* as demonstrated in some studies. Weller and colleagues, in *Evidence-Based Practice of Anesthesiology,* states, "Neuraxial blockade induces both arterial and venous hypotension below the level of blockade, which results in diminished blood loss during surgery and as long as the block is maintained postoperatively." Extrapolating from a case study including 100 radical retropubic prostatectomies, the author goes on to say that these beneficial effects on hemorrhage may be lost if positive-pressure ventilation is employed. *Avoidance of general anesthesia itself* may also be an advantage. The surgeon rightly has expressed concerns about the ability extubate this patient with a strong pulmonary history at the end of a general endotracheal anesthesia (GETA) case (discussed later). He is probably correct in that patients extubated earlier do better in some areas.

Evidence from the Cochrane group studying fast-tracking of cardiac surgery cases has included six trials. They reported the following results. There was no evidence of a difference between early and conventionally extubated patients shown in the relative risk and 95% confidence interval for the following outcomes: Mortality in intensive care was 0.8 (0.42 to 1.52); 30-day mortality was 1.2 (0.63 to 2.27); myocardial ischemia was 0.96 (0.71 to 1.30); reintubation within 24 hours of surgery was 5.93 (0.72 to 49.14). However, time spent in intensive care and in the hospital was significantly shorter for patients extubated early (7.02 hours (−7.42 to −6.61) and 1.08 days (−1.35 to −0.82), respectively).

Increased graft survival has been shown in selected trials to occur more often with thoracic epidural compared with general anesthesia (Christopherson et al) and thoracic epidural used as a supplement to general anesthesia (Tuman et al) in infrainguinal vascular surgery and aortic or infrainguinal surgery, respectively.

Regional anesthesia has some potentially detrimental effects. In the unlikely event that an intravascular catheter is placed and large doses of anticoagulation are begun, many would recommend canceling the case. For unexpected blood loss from an arterial source, for example, peripheral vasodilatation may worsen hypotension. If you had to convert to an open procedure, this would become more complicated.

Of note: this is an example of how a *written for a book* answer differs from *how-you'd-say-it in real life*. No one has these studies and statistics in their hip pocket! Know the *ideas* and say them, don't go quoting stuff like this unless you really have it down.

2. Would it matter if the surgeon makes a horizontal chevron incision or a typical midline incision?

The added morbidity of a chevron incision significantly increases the risk of postoperative pulmonary complications and prolonged intubation, although it requires that fewer dermatomes are anesthetized for adequate postoperative analgesia. A working thoracic epidural in this case is extremely important. Combined bupivacaine with opioids has shown a reduction in postoperative pulmonary complications, likely due to the ability of patients to take deep breaths. We often see increased pulmonary complications in these patients related to the fact that upper abdominal incisions are very painful and cause patients to resist deep breathing and coughing in the postoperative period. This leads to retained secretions, atelectasis, and pneumonia.

3. Will you be able to extubate this patient?

Maybe. The Texas Heart Institute experience (where all endovascular abdominal aortic aneurysms (AAAs) are done under general anesthesia and in the catheter laboratory) found that "Despite a high percentage of patients with significant pulmonary disease, most patients are successfully extubated at the completion of the procedure, before transport out of the catheterization lab" (Giesecke). Miller (2001) states, "Extubation of the trachea is generally not attempted in patients with supraceliac aortic cross-clamp times greater than 30 minutes, patients with poor baseline pulmonary function, or patients requiring large volumes of blood or crystalloid during surgery."

Extubation Criteria for AAA repair from Yao and Artusio's *Anesthesia Management* include the following: awake and alert, vital capacity greater than 15 mL/kg, pH higher than 7.30, PaO_2 greater than 60 mm Hg at an FIO_2 less than 50%, $PaCO_2$ less than 50 mm Hg, negative inspiratory force more than -20 cm H_2O, stable hemodynamic status, and respiratory rate less than 30 breaths/min (Yao). It is uncomplicated surgery, from which most data arise. A few challenges to extubation are added in this patient with poor respiratory reserve, who likely has increased airway resistance at baseline. General anesthesia further decreases airway compliance and increases elastic resistance work, the consequences of which are at least twofold: An already enlarged A-a gradient is widened, making ventilation poor, and pulmonary reserve is lessened by atelectasis, increased secretions that usually accompany general endotracheal anesthesia (GETA), and surgical factors that further decrease the functional reserve capacity (FRC). A potential third factor in this patient (if he receives too much fluid) is an even greater increase in the elastic resistance as the pulmonary interstitial pressure approaches pulmonary venous pressure and even pulmonary arterial pressure. The net result is that patients have more rapid and shallow breathing because it requires less work, but it ultimately leads to fatigue in an already compromised patient (Miller, 2005). If the patient meets the criteria previously described, I believe an attempt should be made for extubation. Extrapolating from the data gathered from the recent increase in fast-tracking cardiac patients, Lichtenthal et al. described the safe management of a large number of cardiac patients extubated in the OR after *uncomplicated* cardiac surgery. Common ideas in those studies were the use of limited doses of opioids, inhalational anesthesia for maintenance, use of non-narcotic analgesia, and a great deal of attention to temperature control and postoperative sedation. In the studies, there were no detectable adverse effects attributable to earlier extubation, and it did not result in an increase in postoperative morbidity. Opponents to immediate extubation argue that extubation in the OR can augment respiratory and cardiac workload and potentially increase the incidence of postoperative ischemia and myocardial infarction. No study has demonstrated a statistically higher incidence of myocardial infarction in patients extubated in the OR (Montes) To be fair, our patient has undergone a different surgery, and we must consider that excess fluid given intraoperatively cannot be "adjusted by a perfusionist" and that laryngeal edema and increased work of breathing are real complications of fluid over-resuscitation.

As noted earlier, don't go wild like this quoting every possible source.

Intraoperative Questions

1. What is your detailed plan for monitoring, induction, maintenance, emergence, and perioperative pain management?

A thoracic epidural is placed preoperatively, with a load consisting of 0.25% bupivacaine in 5-mL aliquots at a T2 level. Infusion of dexmedetomidine at a rate of 0.3 µg/kg/hr is started on entering the OR. Versed (2 mg) and fentanyl (50 µg) are given as intermittent boluses titrated to effect before invasive lines are placed. Hypertension must be avoided throughout the operative course because it is a major risk factor for bleeding during anastomoses and frank rupture intraoperatively. Perioperative β-blockade is advantageous and an adjunct to prevent postoperative myocardial infarctions 6 months to 2 years after the procedure. Likewise, α_2-agonists (e.g., clonidine, dexmedetomidine) may have a role as adjuncts in the prevention of perioperative cardiac morbidity and mortality in patients with suspected or known cardiac disease, especially in vascular surgical procedures. Essentially, the benefit of sympatholysis is common to β-blockers, dexmedetomidine, and the thoracic epidural infusion. Sympatholysis is most beneficial before induction and when continued for 72 hours postoperatively. The final choice of anesthetic technique probably is not as important as the smooth application of the technique.

Routine monitoring is augmented by a two-lead ECG (II, V_5) and intra-arterial blood pressure measurement. This patient should receive a large-bore central venous catheter for fluid management and vasoactive medication infusion. TEE can provide the observer with a more timely diagnosis of ischemic myocardial dysfunction when used on an intermittent basis as needed. Intraoperative and postoperative forms of pain control are best managed with a thoracic epidural (i.e., bupivacaine plus an opioid).

2. What is your plan for fluid management?

Fluid therapy is one of the most controversial topics in perioperative management. There is continuing debate about the quantity and the type of fluid resuscitation during elective major surgery. However, there are increasing reports of perioperative excessive intravascular volume leading to increased postoperative morbidity and mortality. The evidence suggests that judicious perioperative fluid therapy improves outcome after major elective *gastrointestinal* surgery. The observed benefits may not be solely attributable to crystalloid restriction but to the use of colloids instead.

Control of blood pressure is an important goal in this patient. Hypotension can be detrimental in the setting of diseased coronaries, and hypertension can be catastrophic in its own right. The pressor of choice seems to be phenylephrine (normalizing pressure and lowering the heart rate), although this may offset some of the beneficial effects of the regional technique, and it may cause regional wall motion abnormalities and increased cardiac work. Fluid management must be strictly rationed, using enough to keep up with the patient's needs and not so much that we over-resuscitate the patient. Avoidance of deep general anesthesia and use of modified preload augmentation before the epidural is placed seem to be reasonable options.

Fluid management consists of *colloids* (Hextend, maximum of 1 L, and albumin) administered to provide hemodynamic stability and maintain urine output of $0.5 \, mL \times kg^{-1} \times hr^{-1}$ and *crystalloids* administered only for maintenance. Blood loss may be replaced with colloid on a volume-to-volume basis. Predetermined algorithms that suggest replacement of third-space losses and losses through diuresis are unnecessary. Significant reduction in crystalloid volume can be achieved without encountering intraoperative hemodynamic instability or reduced urinary output by avoiding replacement of third-space losses and preloading.

3. Should he have been given a course of perioperative steroids? If so, why, and how much of what kind? Back up your answer with evidence-based literature, please.

The issue of adrenal insufficiency causing perioperative death was sparked by a case in which a 20-year-old woman who had been taking up to 100 mg of cortisone each day for 4 months died less than 6 hours after her operation. The autopsy found bilateral adrenal hemorrhages and bilateral complete adrenal cortical atrophy. Other case reports have followed, and the syndrome has been described in animal models. Daily endogenous glucocorticoid secretion equates to roughly 20 to 30 mg of hydrocortisone per day, with stress increasing requirements to 100 mg/day. Earlier studies have used suprapharmacologic and supraphysiologic doses with varied results.

This issue has been discussed for patients with asthma or chronic obstructive pulmonary disease (COPD). For example, earlier studies reported rates of perioperative pulmonary complications in asthmatics to be 24% (compared with 14% in controls). The current rate is 1% to 2%. The study authors also recommend that patients with controlled moderate to severe symptoms may benefit from a short course (3 days) of oral corticosteroids. Any reversible obstruction should be treated with bronchodilators preoperatively and intraoperatively for patients with asthma or COPD. So give the steroids is the bottom line.

Coursin and colleagues set forth guidelines for dosage of perioperative steroids based on the degree of medical or surgical stress. According to this scheme, our patient would have undergone a moderate surgical stress requiring 50 to 75 mg of intravenous hydrocortisone on the day of surgery, with a taper over 1 to 2 days to the usual dose. Only if the patient developed hypotension or shock would higher doses be required (up to 200 mg/day), and the taper would be based on vital signs and the serum sodium level (Coursin et al). These recommendations are for patients chronically and actively taking steroids. The only way to assess the absolute need for steroids is by the adrenocorticotropic hormone (ACTH) stimulation test.

How It Actually Happened

Everything went fine. Oh, well, we cannot have a disaster every time. And don't think you have to be so "study quoting" during your oral board exam.

CASE 14: LITTLE CASE WITH A BIG CONCERN

1. What are the anesthetic goals of managing a patient with critical aortic stenosis?

A basic goal for this patient is to maintain the delicate balance between supply and demand. Maximize coronary blood flow by maintaining perfusion pressure and allow maximal diastolic time, with optimal O_2 content. The real challenge in this patient in the setting of aortic stenosis is on the demand side (coronary perfusion pressure = aortic diastolic pressure – left ventricular end diastolic pressure [LVEDP]). Patients with aortic stenosis live with an elevated LVEDP because they have to push against an obstructed valve with elevated pressures. Barash states, "Full, normal (not too fast/not too slow) heart rate, and maintain normal sinus rhythm" for aortic stenosis. Aortic stenosis is worrisome because the absence of forward flow (as when preload is decreased too much) is very hard to resuscitate with CPR due to the inability of chest compressions to provide adequate stroke volume. Effective atrial kick can contribute 40% to 50% of stroke volume in the setting of aortic stenosis. This is the reason the ASA recommends that cardioversion is available for converting *any* rhythm other than sinus if it occurs intraoperatively. Optimally, you would like to tailor an anesthetic plan that does all of these things while maintaining low wall tension but not depressing the heart.

2. What are the anesthetic goals of managing an elderly patient with CHF?

The stroke volume is fixed, and the patient is heart rate dependent. The patient is likely overloaded with fluids, and I would assess for the use of furosemide preoperatively (monitoring urine output with a Foley catheter is mandatory, regardless of case duration). The use of furosemide, as with all of our interventions, must be balanced against maintaining an adequate preload in aortic stenosis. The age of this patient is a concern. According to Stoelting and Dierdorf in *Anesthesia and Co-Existing Disease,* the elderly tolerate less anesthetic with decreased reserve. An "endogenous β-blockade is present," resulting in an increased risk of hypotension with anesthesia. The MAC of volatile anesthetics is decreased as much as 30%, the brain receptors are more sensitive to narcotics, and the risk of postoperative cognitive dysfunction is a real cause of morbidity.

3. What are the anesthetic goals of managing a patient with a recent MI?

As Barash states, "small, slow, and well perfused" are goals for patients with ischemia. We already have a conflict because aortic stenosis patients prefer "full, normal heart rate and normal sinus rhythm." A balance must be struck slightly in favor of aortic stenosis. I would keep the patient full; although this will increase myocardial oxygen demand, I believe it to be a necessary evil. The heart rate can be nontachycardic (<110 beats/min) and nonbradycardic (>60 beats/min).

These contributing authors drive me crazy! You don't need to quote various big authors on your exam.

4. What is your detailed anesthetic plan, including monitoring, induction and regional technique, airway management, maintenance, pain control, and fluid replacement?

Because of the aortic stenosis, dependence on and delicate balance of coronary perfusion (aortic diastolic pressure – LVEDP) and the need to maintain forward flow by maintaining reasonable preload in a noncompliant ventricle, an arterial line should be placed in an awake patient to maintain pressure during induction. Zoll pads should be placed for the purpose of synchronized cardioversion if necessary. I would start an infusion of dexmedetomidine early in this patient. Although power has not been achieved to show decrease in postoperative MI or ischemia, intraoperative ischemia has been decreased in more than one study with Precedex and longer-acting clonidine. Sympatholysis would prove beneficial with respect to the recent MI, possible CHF status, and elderly status. Precedex also gives some postoperative pain relief, which is notoriously undertreated in the elderly. The lowest dose (0.2 μg/kg/hr with one half of the bolus and 0.5 μg/kg/hr over 10 minutes) can be used to prevent the drop in the arterial pressure, which may result in decreased stroke volume and decreased coronary perfusion, causing ischemia in this aortic stenosis patient. I would use 0.5 mg of Versed for amnesia if necessary, 1 to 2 μg/kg of fentanyl, and low-dose etomidate just before LMA insertion.

For maintenance, volatile agents may be the best in this case, although they are not perfect. The dangers are that they produce myocardial depression, slight tachycardia, and arteriolar dilation. These problems can be decreased by using desflurane with 50% nitrous oxide, and dexmedetomidine can decrease the MAC of the volatile agent. The tachycardia is often not seen as part of a mixed anesthetic. The patient will breathe spontaneously throughout with augmentation of breathing if necessary. Absence of laryngoscopy avoids a dangerous sympathetic nervous system surge, and drugs can be titrated to effect. Positive-pressure ventilation with its hemodynamic effects also can be avoided.

Adjuvants include the following:

- Use Zoll pads as described earlier.
- Phenylephrine is better than ephedrine in avoiding tachycardia.
- β-Blockade usually is effective at 50 to 60 beats per minute. Dangers from decreased diastolic time typically occur at 110 beats per minute. The middle of the road is probably best.
- Be ready with amiodarone as rhythm disturbances can occur.

Some drugs are contraindicated. Because this is a balancing act, a few things must be considered. Aortic stenosis is of utmost concern. We would like a "small" heart in the recent MI patient, but we need adequate preload for forward flow in the aortic stenosis patient. Nitroglycerin is relatively contraindicated in patients with aortic stenosis, as are nitroprusside, potent high-dose volatile anesthetics (because of decreased afterload and perfusion pressure), and spinal anesthesia (because of decreased preload and afterload).

How It Actually Happened

I am going to throw in a little movie trivia to break up all this medical stuff. My source is the great web site moviebloopers.com. During the filming of the original cult horror classic, *Night of the Living Dead*, there was one scene in which the flesh-eating zombies were eating a body. Because it was filmed in black and white, they did not need to be too accurate with the colors. So the "body" was actually baked ham with chocolate sauce on it. The director said, "We almost did not need makeup to make them look like zombies. Eating that ham with chocolate sauce made them so sick they all looked pasty and dead as is."

By the way, the case went fine.

CASE 15: HEARTBREAK HOTEL

1. What is the incidence of pediatric cardiomyopathy?

The incidence of pediatric cardiomyopathy has been estimated to be 1.13 cases per 100,000 patients, with a slightly higher incidence in New England of 1.44 cases per 100,000 patients. When categorized by type, 51% were dilated cardiomyopathy, 42% were hypertrophic cardiomyopathy, and 3% were restrictive or other types; the remaining 4% were unspecified.[1] Estimates of 5-year mortality as high as 80% have been reported, with some variability.[2]

2. What are your concerns about this patient?

Concern for this patient is related to congestive heart failure and arrhythmias in particular. We chose the use of midazolam as a sole intravenous anesthetic combined with N_2O intermittently in a spontaneously breathing patient. The decision for this was based on the known side effect profile of many other anesthetics, the available information from the various databases on anesthesia-related cardiac complications, and the combined cooperation of the patient and surgeon.

It could be said that anesthetic goals for this patient are related to the two most alarming features of the cardiac dysfunction: a dilated, hypocontractile myocardium and severe mitral regurgitation. Further myocardial depression causing CHF is a particular concern, with the awareness that circulation time is slowed and overdose is more likely. Full, fast heart rate with a low-normal blood pressure can be a concern. The shortening fraction (SF) will be misleading, and the true contractile state is difficult to determine, warranting avoidance of myocardial depression.

Much of the study of anesthetic agents and cardiac function comes from load-dependent parameters (e.g., EF, SF) and may be misleading in a patient with complicated cardiac anomalies.[3]

3. How would you monitor this patient?

An oral dose of 10 mg of midazolam is given in the holding area, with EMLA cream applied to many sites for intravenous access. On arrival at the OR, defibrillator pads were applied, and a right radial arterial line was placed. N_2O (70%) was administered for intravenous cannulation and continued intermittently throughout the case. Versed was given as an intermittent intravenous bolus in 1-mg aliquots.

4. Would you use a volatile anesthetic in a patient with already depressed myocardial function?

I would use sevoflurane and inhalational anesthesia. The two older agents, halothane and isoflurane, have been studied most extensively. Sevoflurane has been shown to cause less myocardial depression than the two older agents. Sevoflurane did not alter the heart rate or chronotropic incompetence at all concentrations in infants, but it did significantly decrease blood pressure and systemic vascular resistance. Rate-corrected velocity of circumferential fiber shortening (load independent) decreased at 1.5 but not 1 MAC. These were healthy infants who presumably had adequate reserve, whereas the situation might be altered in critically ill patients.

Schecter and colleagues[4] reported a case of cardiovascular collapse in a patient with coexisting anomalies similar to those of our patient (SF of 15%). Their anesthetic was multimodal and included midazolam, ketamine, vecuronium, and alfentanil for percutaneous endoscopic gastrostomy (PEG) tube placement. The patient was recovered, the case delayed, and on subsequent induction, midazolam, lidocaine, glycopyrrolate, vecuronium, and etomidate were used without incident.[4] The study authors posit the cause of the inability to tolerate the first anesthetic as primary myocardial depression from ketamine, sympatholysis from the combination of opioids and benzodiazepine, or bradycardia from alfentanil decreasing cardiac output.

We chose an anesthetic consisting mostly of one agent, midazolam, with intermittent use of nitrous oxide to assist in pain control. Had an additional agent been absolutely required, sevoflurane at less than 1 MAC would have been our choice.

The safety of intravenous agents has been tested by using various software programs for heart rate variability. Heart rate variability analysis can provide important clinical information on the effect of anesthesia on the autonomic nervous system and central nervous system because cyclical variation in heart rate is mediated by central neural mechanisms and by baroreceptors and chemoreceptors.[5]. For example, Win and colleagues[6] suggested a predominance of sympathetic activity when using midazolam during conscious sedation, whereas propofol was shown to result in a predominance of parasympathetic activity. Our patient with little cardiac reserve may have benefited from the effect of the former and the avoidance of the latter. More research on the optimal combination may be necessary in this challenging and frequently encountered population.

5. As the case proceeds, the patient's blood pressure and heart rate begin to drop. What agent would you use to rescue this patient?

Standby emergency drugs included dobutamine, milrinone, and epinephrine. With respect to dobutamine, hemodynamic improvements and a decrease in chronically elevated levels of atrial natriuretic peptide and cyclic guanosine monophosphate levels may be seen within 30 minutes.[7] Phosphodiesterase III inhibitors have long had a role in our institution in patients with chronic ventricular dysfunction and cardiac β-receptor downregulation.

How It Actually Happened

This was a classic case of "bring an umbrella and it will not rain." We had everything ready and were prepared for Armageddon, and the case went smooth as silk.

Test takers often ask whether they should answer with references. Most people do not. Unless you have a Rain Man–like ability to memorize the zillions of articles, you are best off just answering the question. We toss in these references because kiddie cardiomyopathy is a little obscure for many of us.

1. Lipschultz SE, Sleeper LA, Towbin JA, et al: The incidence of pediatric cardiomyopathy in two regions of the United States. N Engl J Med 2003;348:1647-1655.
2. Schecter WS, Kim C, Martinez M, et al: Anaesthetic induction in a child with end-stage cardiomyopathy. Can J Anaesth 1995;42:404-408.
2. Arola A, Touminin J, Ruuskanen O, et al: Idiopathic dilated cardiomyopathy in children: Prognostic indicators and outcome. Pediatrics 1998;101:369-376.
3. Morray JP, Geiduschek JM, Ramamoorthy C, et al: Anesthesia-related cardiac arrest in children: Initial findings of the Pediatric Perioperative Cardiac Arrest (POCA) Registry. Anesthesiology 2000;93:6-14.
5. Malliani A, Pagani M, Lombardi F, et al: Cardiovascular neural regulation explored in the frequency domain. Circulation 1991;84:482-492.
6. Win NN, Fukayama H, Kohase H, et al: The differential effects of intravenous propofol and midazolam sedation on hemodynamic and heart rate variability. Anesth Analg 2005;101:97-102.
7. Harrison TE, Gleich SJ, Flick, RP, et al: Cardiac arrest in pediatric patients undergoing noncardiac surgery. Anesthesiology 2006;105:A356.

CASE 16: SOME CHOLECYSTECTOMIES ARE MORE INVOLVED THAN OTHERS

Readers, readers, lend me your eyes! This answer section will be one of the most historically curious of this entire book. It takes on the often-asked, important questions of β-blockade, and looks in detail at the pulmonary artery catheter question. Go over this section several times, paying close attention to the discussions about perioperative risk and who should get β-blockade. This is, in effect, a "time capsule" of how we thought *before* the new ACC/AHA guidelines. You'll see a *certainty* of who needs what that is no *longer recommended.* You may want to skip it, or, you may want to study this and contrast it with current thinking. If there is ever a section for which you want to go to the original articles and read them yourselves, this is it. The original articles mentioned have algorithms that are worth going over again and again, because they center on perioperative cardiac risk, which is a biggie on the test and in real life. *Board Stiff* is a guidebook, and it does not provide the exhaustive depth you need understand this important topic. Read more deeply than what has been provided here! You must know this stuff.

1. What are the American College of Cardiology/American Heart Association (ACC/AHA) recommendations regarding preoperative cardiac evaluation in this patient?

According to the 2002 ACC/AHA guidelines regarding perioperative cardiac evaluation, the patient is considered to be at intermediate cardiovascular risk going for an intermediate-risk procedure. (Check out the 2007 recommendations as summarized in March 2008 Anesthesia and Analgesia.)

Intermediate cardiovascular risk list (plucked straight from the guidelines) is defined by the following conditions:

1. Mild angina pectoris
2. Prior MI according to the history or Q waves
3. Heart failure (compensated or prior)
4. Diabetes mellitus (insulin-dependent form is more serious)
5. Renal insufficiency

Risk of the procedure is intermediate if any of the following applies:

1. Intraperitoneal or intrathoracic procedure
2. Carotid endarterectomy
3. Head and neck surgery
4. Orthopedic surgery
5. Prostate surgery

Note: During the test, it may be damned hard to dredge up these complete lists. In my humble opinion (and I do not have a humble opinion), you could say, "I would refer to the ACC/AHA guidelines to determine the level of risk to the patient" (available online or in your hand-held computer gizmo). You do not have to be an encyclopedia for the oral boards. You do have to know how to make decisions, and looking up stuff is one of those decisions.

The patient is going for elective, noncardiac surgery. It is unknown whether she has had coronary revascularization in past 5 years. I would follow the algorithm, which involves asking whether there has been coronary vascularization in the past 5 years, whether symptoms have returned, and whether the coronaries have had "another look" to make sure the grafts are still patent. The whole Magilla here is geared toward that all-important, guiding principle: Is the patient in optimal condition for this case?

The history continues, focusing on how much the patient can do. This is a toughie, because the patient has residual lower extremity weakness. If she reports moderate or excellent functional capacity (>4 METs), she may proceed to OR given the intermediate-risk operation.

If functional capacity is poor or unknown, further noninvasive testing may be reasonable. Given the additional cardiac demands of pregnancy, an updated cardiac echocardiogram would be useful to assess cardiac function, especially with a pre-pregnant EF of only 30%. If the patient has not had a recent stress test (within 2 years), a pharmacologic stress test (e.g., myocardial perfusion SPECT) may be appropriate, according to the 2003 ACC/AHA Guidelines for the Use of Cardiac Radionuclide Imaging (pp. 1410-1411). It is unknown whether radionuclide testing is contraindicated in term pregnancy; it is probably not an absolute contraindication.

2. Should β-blockade be instituted in the preoperative period? If so, how far in advance of surgery should it be done?

According to the 2006 ACC/AHA Perioperative Guideline on β-Blocker Therapy, the patient may be considered class IIb (i.e., benefit = risk, may be considered). The patient should also be counseled that although β-blockers have been safely used in pregnancy, fetal side effects can include bradycardia, hypoglycemia, respiratory depression, and possible intrauterine growth retardation. Infants whose mothers have been receiving β-blockade should be adequately monitored and the risks versus the benefits of β-blockade in such patients must be carefully weighed.

It is doubtful whether you will remember an entire citation in the examination, but this is worth keeping in your hip pocket, because it is the latest and greatest on β-blockade. You are sure to have a β-blockade question on the test, and you are sure to have a β-blockade question in real life, too!

Add up the whole clinical picture, apply it to this patient, and you have a class IIb reason for giving this patient β-blockade. β-Blockers may be considered for patients who are undergoing intermediate- or high-risk procedures as defined in these guidelines, including vascular surgery, for whom perioperative assessment identifies cardiac risk as defined by the presence of a single clinical risk factor.

The Metoprolol CR/XL Randomized Intervention Trial in Heart Failure (MERIT-HF) trial showed β-blockers were suitable and improved survival in patients with class II to IV heart failure and a left ventricular ejection fraction (LVEF) of 40%.

What about the Revised Goldman cardiac risk index? Goldman lists six predictors of major cardiac complications:

1. High-risk surgery (intraperitoneal, intrathoracic, suprainguinal vascular procedures)
2. History of ischemic heart disease
3. History of heart failure
4. History of cerebrovascular disease
5. Insulin-dependent diabetes mellitus
6. Preoperative creatinine level greater than 2.0 mg/dL

This guy must have been an actuarial for a life insurance company because he went on to quantify the risk of cardiac death, nonfatal MI, and nonfatal (but alarming to everyone) cardiac arrest according to the number of predictors:

1. No risk factors: 0.4%
2. One risk factor: 1.0%
3. Two risk factors: 2.4%
4. Three or more: 5.4%

That "nonfatal cardiac arrest" is the one that scares hell out of me as an anesthesiologist. Make sure the paddles are working, and make sure we have paid the electric bill!

Here is where Goldman and β-blockade get married, and this is where you really start to understand who should get β-blockade instead of following our earlier impulse to put β-blockers in the air conditioning system and pipe it into every room in the hospital, including the cafeteria. The rates of cardiac death and nonfatal MI, cardiac arrest, or ventricular fibrillation, pulmonary edema, and complete heart block can be estimated according to the number of predictors and the nonuse or use of β-blockers:

1. No risk factors: 0.4% to 1.0% versus less than 1% with β-blockers
2. One or two risk factors: 2.2% to 6.6% versus 0.8% to 1.6% with β-blockers
3. Three or more risk factors: less than 9% versus more than 3% with β-blockers

This is important stuff! Go to the source (Auerback and Goldman) on this one, and read it yourself. According to the Goldman cardiac risk index, the patient has three independent predictors of cardiac complications. Institution of β-blockers can reduce the risk of a major cardiac complication. If not already on it, β-blockers should be started up to 30 days before surgery, titrating to a target of 50 to 60 beats/min.

BUT! This has all been upended by the POISE study, casting a long shadow over the β-blocker picture.

Uptodate.com: Management of Cardiac Risk for Noncardiac Surgery

- The 2006 ACC/AHA guideline update on perioperative β-blocker therapy recommended β-blockers in patients already being treated with one of these drugs for some other indication and in patients at high cardiac risk undergoing vascular surgery. β-Blockers were also considered reasonable in other selected patients at increased risk.

- A 2006 review by Auerbach and Goldman concluded that perioperative β-blocker therapy should be limited to patients at moderate to high risk. Among patients undergoing major noncardiac surgery, β-blockers should be started or titrated to a target heart rate of 60 to 65 beats/min before anesthesia is begun.
- In patients with heart failure not treated with a β-blocker or with preexisting bronchospastic lung disease, the possibility of exacerbating these conditions must be weighed against the potential benefit.
- There are insufficient data to support perioperative β-blocker therapy in patients at low to intermediate risk (e.g., Revised Cardiac Risk Index [RCRI] score of 0 or 1). However, given the risks of sudden cessation of β-blockers, therapy should be continued in patients who are already taking a β-blocker.
- When a β-blocker is given, perioperative treatment with a $β_1$-selective agent is recommended. If possible, oral therapy should begin as an outpatient up to 30 days before surgery, titrating to a heart rate between 50 and 60 beats/min. Tight heart rate control may be an important determinant of efficacy.
- It is possible that long-acting β-blockers are more effective than short-acting agents (e.g., atenolol versus metoprolol). Options include atenolol (50 to 100 mg/day taken orally) and bisoprolol (5 to 10 mg/day taken orally).
- If time does not permit, atenolol can be given intravenously (10 mg over 15 minutes) before surgery. Atenolol is then given intravenously (5 to 10 mg every 6 to 12 hours) in the immediate postoperative period until oral intake resumes. The previous dose of an oral β-blocker should be restarted when the patient is able.
- There are no data about the duration of therapy. We suggest that b-blockers be continued for at least 1 month after surgery; they are usually continued indefinitely because most of these patients have underlying heart disease.
- Great, now read the POISE study and forget everything written above.

3. What additional cardiac stress does term pregnancy incur?

Intravascular volume increased 1500 mL (35%). Plasma volume increased 45%, whereas the erythrocyte volume increased by only 20%, resulting in relative anemia of pregnancy.

Cardiac output increased 40% above normal by the third trimester, with a 30% increase in stroke volume. At the onset of labor, cardiac output increases an additional 30% above the prelabor value. Immediately after delivery, cardiac output can be up to 60% above the prelabor value.

Each uterine contraction increases cardiac output and central blood volume 10% to 25%. Systemic vascular resistance and pulmonary vascular resistance are decreased. Uterine compression of the inferior vena cava can lead to decreased venous return and preload to the heart, resulting in hypotension.

Vaginal delivery results in a blood loss of 300 to 500 mL. Cesarean section results in a blood loss of 800 to 1000 mL.

4. What other physiologic changes of pregnancy increase perioperative risk in this patient?

Minute ventilation increases (50%), as does tidal volume (40%). With the enlarging uterus, FRC is reduced by 20% at term. Decreased FRC lends itself to rapid induction or emergence and decreased anesthetic requirements. Oxygen consumption increases by 20%; this and the reduced FRC result in a decreased oxygen reserve and potential for rapid desaturation during apnea.

Upper airway mucosa, vocal cords, and arytenoids are often edematous, creating a potentially difficult airway. Gastric changes include increased gastrin with increased gastric fluid production, lowered pH, decreased gastric motility, and partial obliteration of the esophagogastric junction. These factors lead to increased aspiration risk. Increased coagulability raises risk of cerebral vascular accident, especially in this patient.

5. What anesthetic options would you present to this patient? Which will you recommend?

Options include general anesthesia with intubation or regional anesthesia with an epidural or spinal. General and regional forms have their risks and benefits. Hemodynamic stability is the main concern in this patient. The patient should be informed that with regional anesthesia, there is a definite chance of conversion to general anesthesia if complications arise.

Intraoperative Questions

1. What perioperative monitoring do you recommend?

Use standard ASA monitors: pulse oximetry, blood pressure, ECG, inspired O_2, and end-tidal CO_2. Because of heart failure, I would add an arterial line for closer blood pressure monitoring.

2. Would you put in a pulmonary artery catheter? Why or why not?

Indications for a pulmonary artery catheter include coronary artery disease with left ventricular dysfunction or recent infarction, valvular heart disease, and heart failure. Other indications are severe pulmonary disease, complex fluid management (e.g., shock, acute renal failure, acute burns, hemorrhagic pancreatitis), cardiac surgery, aortic cross-clamping, and high-risk obstetrics (e.g., severe toxemia, placental abruption) (Morgan, et al.).

Pulmonary artery catheterization requires careful consideration of the risk to benefit ratio. The 2003 ASA Practice Guidelines for Pulmonary Artery Catheterization identify surgery risk factors, patient risks, and risks of the practice setting. Proper provider competency and training reduces technical complications from catheter placement and adverse effects from *misinterpretation* of pulmonary artery catheter data. The task force assigned an appropriateness score for pulmonary artery catheterization based on the patient and surgery risk factors and on the risk of the practice setting (low versus moderate risk) (American Society of Anesthesiologists Task Force).

Keep in mind that we are looking at guidelines put together by a task force, which took 26 pages to get around to throwing together an *appropriateness score*. If that does not sound like a soft, mushy indication, I do not know soft and mushy. Best of all, they have it on a 1 to 9 scale, and all the Xs for appropriateness are in the 5 to 7 range. No one could commit with great enthusiasm one way or another. Talk about a lukewarm endorsement!

You first assume a low-risk setting (i.e., competent, experienced personnel). According to the guidelines (according to the tepid endorsement guidelines by a task force diddling with an appropriateness scale), this patient may be categorized as a moderate-risk patient undergoing moderate-risk surgery, producing an appropriateness median score of 6 or 9. However, if echocardiographic results (e.g., stable LVEF), stress testing (e.g., no ischemia), and other data (e.g., clear chest radiograph, clinical examination results) are reassuring, adequate intravenous access may be sufficient.

3. Would you do a spinal for this case? Why or why not?

A single-dose spinal may not last long enough for the cesarean section and cholecystectomy. The spinal T4 sensory level necessary for a cesarean section is associated with significant peripheral sympathetic blockade. This may lead to pronounced hypotension, reducing an already compromised cardiac output, and fetal hypoxemia. With an epidural, maternal precipitous hypotension is less likely, and continuous dosing is possible.

4. If you choose general anesthesia, what induction agents will you use?

A combination of an opioid (e.g., fentanyl) to blunt hemodynamic responses and etomidate for hemodynamic stability would be reasonable. Metoprolol or esmolol can be used for intraoperative rate control. Succinylcholine may be used in an RSI because of the dangers of aspiration in a term pregnancy.

5. If you choose general anesthesia, what maintenance agents will you use?

A combination of 50% nitrous oxide and a low concentration of a volatile agent (e.g., 1% sevoflurane, 0.5% isoflurane, 2% to 3% desflurane) provides reasonable amnesia or analgesia and reduces the cardio-depressant effects a full MAC of volatile anesthetics alone. Ketamine (0.5 mg/kg) also may be used. After delivery of the neonate, anesthesia with nitrous oxide and narcotic techniques may be considered.

6. What anesthetic technique or techniques will you choose? Describe the pros and cons.

For general anesthesia, the pros include rapid, reliable anesthesia and control of ventilation and oxygenation. The cons are the cardiac stress of induction, potentially difficult airway, and cardiac depressant effects of volatile anesthetics in a patient with left ventricular failure.

For regional anesthesia or an epidural, the pros include preservation of maternal awareness and airway-protective reflexes. A continuous epidural may be slowly titrated for the cesarean section and then to a higher level for the cholecystectomy. It may minimize the adverse effects of the increased cardiac output of labor. Cons are the potential for incomplete anesthesia, hypotension, overdose, and migration of the catheter to intravascular or intrathecal sites.

7. If you choose an epidural, what agent or agents will you use? Would you use a local anesthetic containing epinephrine?

If this patient does not have a history of arrhythmias, proper epidural placement of the anesthetic with epinephrine would not represent an additional risk. Of the intermediate-acting agents, lidocaine (2% with or without 1:200,000 epinephrine) or mepivacaine (2%) may be used. Bupivacaine and ropivacaine are long-acting options. Ropivacaine, an analog of mepivacaine, has less potential for cardiotoxicity.

8. The infant is delivered with Apgar scores of 9 and 9. Five minutes later, the patient suffers a cardiac arrest. What is your differential diagnosis?

Cardiac arrest can be caused by pulmonary embolism, air embolism, amniotic fluid embolism, hemorrhagic shock, anaphylaxis, acute MI, and epidural overdose (i.e., migration of the catheter into vascular or subarachnoid space) (Layon and Mahla; Stoeltling and Miller). Venous air embolism occurs in 20% to 50% of parturients undergoing cesarean section.

9. What clinical signs, symptoms, or monitor readings would support the various diagnoses in your differential?

Respiratory distress and a sudden decrease in end-tidal CO_2 may suggest amniotic fluid or air embolism. Cardiac arrest caused by an acute MI may also result in decreased end-tidal CO_2 values. This diagnosis may be supported by ST changes on ECG just before arrest.

10. The patient is intubated. CPR is begun. The cardiac rhythm returns to sinus, and the patient regains consciousness. Would you continue with the cholecystectomy? Why or why not?

It would be unwise to continue with an elective procedure in an unstable patient who was just resuscitated from cardiac arrest. The patient should remain intubated and sedated, and she should be transferred to cardiac intensive care unit.

How It Actually Happened

Hold onto your hat for this one. She was scheduled for a combined cesarean section and cholecystectomy. It was decided to do the cesarean section with an epidural and then gingerly raise the level of the epidural in an attempt to do the cholecystectomy by epidural, with a backup plan of general anesthesia if it proved unworkable. The baby was delivered with Apgar scores of 9 and 9. The uterus was exteriorized before suturing, and the patient suffered a cardiac arrest. The ECG showed that she had ventricular tachycardia, and the end-tidal CO_2 value was 17. CPR was performed, and her rhythm returned to sinus. She regained consciousness but was confused. It was decided to cancel the cholecystectomy. Follow-up cardiac enzyme test results were normal. The provisional diagnosis was air embolus during exteriorization of the uterus.

American Society of Anesthesiologists Task Force on Pulmonary Artery Catheterization: Practice guidelines for pulmonary artery catheterization: an updated report by the American Society of Anesthesiologists Task Force on Pulmonary Artery Catheterization. Anesthesiology 2003;99:988-1014.

Auerbach A, Goldman L: Assessing and reducing the cardiac risk of noncardiac surgery. Circulation 2006;113:1361-1376.

Fleisher LA, Beckman JA, Brown KA, et al: ACC/AHA 2006 guideline update on perioperative cardiovascular evaluation for noncardiac surgery: focused update on perioperative beta-blocker therapy: A report of the American College of Cardiology/American Heart Association Task Force on Practice Guidelines (Writing Committee to Update the 2002 Guidelines on Perioperative Cardiovascular Evaluation for Noncardiac Surgery) developed in collaboration with the American Society of Echocardiography, American Society of Nuclear Cardiology, Heart Rhythm Society, Society of Cardiovascular Anesthesiologists, Society for Cardiovascular Angiography and Interventions, and Society for Vascular Medicine and Biology. J Am Coll Cardiol 2006;47:2343-2355.

Layon AJ, Mahla ME: Cardiac arrest during pregnancy. J Clin Anesth 2005;17:229-234.

Morgan GE, Murray MJ, Mikhail MS: Clinical Anesthesiology, 4th ed. New York, McGraw-Hill Medical, 2006.

Why do we only include references here and there in this book? This is a workbook, not a textbook. Plus, we're working to develop your "what to say" skills, and most of the time you won't be reeling off direct quotes and studies.

CASE 17: FROM RUSSIA WITH LOVE

Preoperative Questions

1. What are the implications of sepsis in this patient? What are all the hemodynamic parameters you may see? What will an echocardiogram show?

Sepsis translates into hemodynamic trouble: vasodilation to the point that hypotension threatens adequate perfusion. You see low blood pressure, tachycardia (i.e., reflex to attempt to maintain adequate perfusion), fever, and flushing (i.e., vasodilation in the skin), and if you believe in Swan-Ganz catheters, you will see a high cardiac output and low systemic vascular resistance. An echocardiogram would show an empty heart beating away furiously; it looks just like hypovolemia. You may not see every item previously listed. The patient may be on β-blockers, may have baseline poor cardiac function, or may not be able to mount a fever. If all three of these happen at once, you may see a septic patient without tachycardia; an echocardiogram may show the heart, although empty, not beating furiously (it cannot!); and the patient may not have fever.

2. Because the patient is septic, will you delay this case? Will you recommend they drain under local anesthesia in the ICU? Is it your place to tell a surgeon what procedure to do?

There should be no delay. The prime directive in sepsis is not hemodynamic juggling (although you will be doing plenty of that soon); it is stopping the source of the sepsis. Fix the original problem as soon as possible. If the patient is dying in front of my eyes, tell the patient he is too sick to move, and cobble together an anesthetic in the ICU. Secure the airway, and give a sedative and muscle relaxants. An "ICU anesthetic" is not rocket science.

The surgeon can do a more definitive job in the OR, and I have all my "toys" there, so I would go to the OR. Should I tell the surgeon what to do? Hell, yes! If a patient is being threatened by well-armed surgeon wielding sharp knives and dull judgment, I will go to the mat to protect the patient.

3. The preoperative potassium level is 7.5, but the patient has no history of renal disease. What will you do? Will you proceed or wait for a repeat procedure? How does hemolysis affect your laboratory test results?

Quickly look at the ECG to see if there are peaked Ts or ectopy or other signs of a high potassium level. As I am looking, I am sending a repeat sample from an arterial line or central line. You can get a potassium level from an ABG determination fairly quickly. Hemolysis from a difficult draw breaks open cells, spilling potassium, and it is the most likely explanation in this case. Look over what is hanging, too. An iatrogenic infusion of potassium can cause hyperkalemia, and that is the kind of thing that can and does happen in an ICU.

4. Define respiratory distress in the ICU. Would you intubate before moving the patient to the OR? Do you need an ABG determination? If the ABG evaluation shows a PO_2 of 61 mm Hg, do you need to intubate? What if the value is 51 mm Hg? Why? Should you wait for the controlled conditions of the OR?

Respiratory distress is like what the judge said about pornography: You know it when you see it. The best gauge is to stand at the foot of the bed and observe the patient:

- Check the respiratory rate. No sick patient can breathe fast for long.
- Check the accessory muscles.
- Notice unresponsiveness. When patients go from distress to no distress, they may be about to sink beneath the waves.

Laboratory results can tell you you are in trouble in terms of the O_2 saturation and blood gases. If the CO_2 level is climbing, time is short! If the patient looks scary, I would intubate right away without waiting for an ABG determination; 61 mm Hg is scary enough for me. You can always intubate with a regular tube, and change over in the OR, so it is better to intubate without delay.

5. Is a thoracic epidural a good idea? Why or why not? The surgeon says it will help with splinting, and the family wants him to be comfortable. What is your response?

"All in due time, my pretty," is my response. Right now, we have instability and a septic focus. It is not the time to be placing a sympathetomizer or foreign body near the CNS that is susceptible to seeding by bacteria. After the infection is gone and stability has returned, we can always place an epidural to help with splinting and comfort. At this point, we take safety over comfort.

Intraoperative Questions

1. What monitors will you place? Defend which side you will put the central line on. Explain the dangers of left-sided central lines. The resident says he never puts in subclavian lines. Is this a good patient to practice on?

The invasive monitors I use are a radial arterial line and a right-sided central line. Although the resident wants to practice subclavian lines, and it is best to do your subclavian lines in cases in which you cannot drop the lung (there *is* no lung); this is not a teaching case. The patient is unstable, and you want to do the thing you are most comfortable with, an intrajugular line. Left-sided lines have a few headaches:

- The lung cupola rides higher due to the heart pushing up the lung.
- You can nail the thoracic duct, leading to a chylothorax.
- You are clumsier at left-sided lines.

However, you should do some subclavian lines for practice, because you do not want the first time to be when you must do one (just like anything else we do).

2. What is the best way to isolate the remaining lung? Do you need to worry about isolating the lung because there is only one? What are the dangers of bronchial blockers in patients after recent surgery?

This whole area is rife with danger. The "dearly departed" right lung has what? at the stump site. A regular ETT going down the right side could punch a hole. A double-lumen tube or bronchial blocker going astray could cause similar trouble. Your best bet in this imperfect world is a left-sided double-lumen ETT placed with utmost delicacy to avoid going down the right side by mistake.

3. This patient is 6 feet 5 inches tall and weighs 120 kg. Are there any special concerns given the weight and the height? How do you determine how deep to place the ETT?

The average man will have the ETT in good position with the tube at about 22 to 24 cm at the teeth. This man is taller, so the tube must be deeper. The 120 kg is somewhat overweight, but it is not too terrible given his height. He is a lot closer to ideal body weight than most patients!

Note: Do not crack "ideal body weight" jokes if your examiner is, shall we say, separated from ideal body weight himself or herself. The examiner may not see the humor.

4. You notice a leak on the ventilatory circuit. What are the potential sources of leaks in the system? What devices are built into the system to detect leaks or detect line crossovers?

A leak can occur anywhere in your delivery circuit, but there are several usual suspects:

- An inspiratory or expiratory arm you knocked off (clumsy oaf!)
- A connection to the ETT
- A CO_2 absorber that is poorly sealed (e.g., granule in the O ring)

Less likely areas in the system are cracks in the manifold in the machine. The machine has low-pressure alarms, and the end-tidal CO_2 alarm will sound if you have a big leak. The only thing that would detect a line crossover is the oxygen analyzer in the inspiratory limb. Be especially aware of this when construction is going on in the hospital.

After you have ruled out something in your circuit, you have to consider a hole somewhere in the patient's respiratory system (e.g., trachea, bronchi, alveoli). Given this patient's recent surgery and infection, a spooky possibility is a blowout in the stump.

5. As you are trying to bag ventilate the patient, the leak suddenly becomes catastrophically large, and you cannot move any air. What do you do? Can the surgeon help you?

If there is any doubt that it is anything in the machine or circuit, get an Ambu bag and an O_2 tank, and take the machine out of the equation. This is a stump blowout, and you have to get a delivery mechanism past the hole. The surgeon can help by setting up femoral-femoral bypass and oxygenating that way or by opening the chest and trying to clamp the leaking bronchus. This would be a "splash and slash" procedure, with everything geared to speed.

6. Is there any advantage to a double-lumen tube in this case? How would it work in the post-pneumonectomy setting? Should it be right or left sided?

This guy is big, and you may have trouble getting a regular tube deep enough. Do not use a right-sided tube, which would push the stump open more. Place a left-sided double-lumen tube, close off all ventilation to the right, and ventilate only the left. In your rush and panic, you may place it too deep and ventilate only the left lingula and lower lobe, but for now, the main thing is to ventilate something, anything. You can always pull it back later and make sure you are not too deep and bypassing the left upper lobe.

7. While attempting to place a different ETT, you notice (how did you miss this?) that the patient has an old tracheostomy site. Can using the tracheostomy site help? How?

If the tracheostomy site is still open, you can put a tube down there. A double-lumen tube may be a tight fit, but a single-lumen tube can get in there quickly. Given his height, this shortcut through the trachea may save the day.

8. The saturation drops to 65%, and the patient develops multifocal ectopy. Do you treat with lidocaine or amiodarone? Do you not treat with anything and keep working on the saturation alone?

This ectopy is from hypoxemia, so futzing with amiodarone will not do much good. Keep working on getting the saturation level up.

9. At the end of the case, would you extubate this patient? Would you keep a single-lumen tube in? How about a bronchial blocker or a double-lumen tube? What are the problems of sending the patient to the ICU with a double-lumen ETT?

I would not extubate this patient for all the tea in China. I would secure whatever tube I had in with a battleship's anchor chains and post a flock of Pit Bulls around it with instructions to bite anyone who got within canine distance.

Whatever tube you got in you can keep in. Even a double-lumen tube is okay; you just have to tell the staff how it works and talk to the respiratory specialist about it. There is always one respiratory technician who has seen this before and does not freak out.

When you arrive with a double-lumen tube, you will always get some static, but with adequate instruction and sedation, you can keep it in. After the patient is more stable, the swelling from the OR is down, and things are cool and calm, you can change the tube over to a single-lumen tube.

10. The ICU staff members say they are unfamiliar with the double-lumen ETT. What in-service training will you offer them? What are other options? Should you change the tube the next day or in a few days? What are the problems with sedation with a tube sitting on the carina?

A hands-on demonstration takes about 5 minutes, and any ICU staff member familiar with ventilation can figure this out. A change to a single-lumen tube is best done under more stable conditions. If you do keep the double-lumen tube deep, it does sit on the carina and requires a lot of sedation to keep the patient calm (the carina is about as richly innervated a spot as we have in our bodies). One good option is to pull the double-lumen tube back, above the carina, and use it as a single-lumen ETT.

One distinct advantage of this approach occurs in case of re-exploration. You already have the tube in that you need. You reposition it under fiberoptic guidance, and voila! You are ready for the next operation. Remember, just because this operation is done, it does not mean there will not be another operation.

How It Actually Happened

Be glad you were not there! This enormous guy came down and looked like death warmed over. He was septic from the word go, and he was flying on only one lung. He goes off to sleep, and all seems well, but he then develops a little leak. I "round up the usual suspects," thinking, okay, maybe he has a small fistula. He had an 8.5-French ETT in, by the way. All of a sudden, there is a monstrous leak, and I cannot ventilate at all. I figured the stump to the right lung blew out (that is exactly what happened). The surgeon might have "helped" the blowout, by the way, but you did not read that here.

I become frantic to get that 8.5-French tube shoved down the left main stem bronchus, but in this 6-foot 5-inch guy, it will not reach! His saturation level has become that of a facultative anaerobe. Lucky for me, I grabbed a left-sided double-lumen tube (I needed something long enough to go past that useless right main stem stump). I got it in and increased his saturation level, and I collapsed in a heap, convinced that dermatology was my true calling.

CASE 18: TO LIVE FOREVER, NEVER SEE A DOCTOR

Intraoperative Questions

1. The patient is on Plavix, but the coagulation study results are normal. What are the implications of Plavix therapy? What does the Society of Regional Anesthesia say about it? Are these guidelines or standard of practice? What is the difference?

Plavix is a platelet inhibitor. You do not want to perform elective surgery or risk an epidural hematoma until the effect has worn off. Our regional anesthesia experts tell us to hold off for at least 7 days before placing a neuraxial anesthetic in any patient on this platelet-inhibiting drug. Their comments are guidelines, not the standard of practice. Continuous monitoring of vital signs is an example of a standard of practice (i.e., you have to do it).

2. An epidural is placed without problems. Which local anesthetic would you use? Why? Is there any advantage of one over another? Would you include narcotics or epinephrine? Why or why not?

I would use levobupivacaine. There is no perfect local anesthetic with a clearly demonstrated, outcome-based, proven advantage over another. In the theoretical realm, levobupivacaine is thought to be less cardiotoxic than bupivacaine in case of an intravascular injection. I would include narcotics because they help with postoperative pain relief and keep the patient comfortable intraoperatively. I would include epinephrine. Although not a perfect marker of intravascular injection, the epinephrine should alert me if the injection goes into a vessel by an increase in heart rate.

3. The patient complains of shortness of breath. How will you tell the difference between a high block resulting from CHF and aspiration? Do you need to stop the case and get a chest radiograph? Do you need to intubate? Why or why not?

For a high block, I would test the patient's sensory level with a twitch monitor, a handy device that does not leave any pinpricks and that works like a charm. Knowing his history (i.e., good EF) and by adding up the fluid balance, I would be able to peg whether CHF occurred (very unlikely here). By knowing the patient's level of consciousness and what I had given so far, I should be able to tell if he has vomited and inhaled the contents.

I would intubate only if vital signs showed instability, particularly low oxygen saturation, or if the patient looked clinically in trouble (respiratory rate, accessory muscles)

4. You give 2 L of fluid. What do you expect his hematocrit to be now? The patient is hypertensive. How does that change your interpretation of the hematocrit? When should you transfuse?

The hematocrit started at 29%. My guess is that 2 L of fluid dropped it to the mid-20s, but I would not rely on such a shot in the dark. I would get a hematocrit determination right away. Hypertension adds the patient's age to the mix; the patient's age, a hematocrit in the mid-20s, and ongoing blood loss add up to an indication to transfuse. A hypertensive patient has shifted his autoregulation curve to the right (exact numbers are hard to nail down), and oxygen delivery can become an issue in the cerebral vasculature. In terms of a "magic number" at which you transfuse, the only evidence comes from the cardiac literature, which states that hematocrit values lower than 24% and higher than 34% are associated with worse outcomes. I would transfuse the patient and aim at keeping the hematocrit at about 30%.

5. Midazolam (4 mg) is given early in the case. What are the implications of this amount in an 82-year-old man? What are the differences in pharmacology in the geriatric and younger populations? What about the volume of distribution?

A dose of 4 mg of midazolam is pretty hefty. I would have given 2 mg and watched carefully for signs of adequate sedation (e.g., slurred speech but still easily arousable). In general, the best approach to pharmacology in the elderly is to give less and wait longer, because every aspect of pharmacodynamics favors more effect and a longer effect in this age group. Midazolam may be short acting in the young, but it can be long acting in the elderly.

Volume of distribution in the elderly is increased, because older patients have decreased lean body mass and total body water and increased total body fat. Hey, why are you looking at me like that? The elderly have a decreased central compartment volume, and the initial plasma concentration after intravenous administration may have more "kick" than you would expect with their increased volume of distribution. With all the instructions to "give more because of this" (e.g., increased volume of distribution) but "give less because of that" (e.g., decreased central compartment, decreased clearance, increased sensitivity), you should still follow the advice to give less and wait longer in treating the elderly.

6. The case goes well, but the suction shows 2500 mL of reddish fluid. How will you determine the blood loss in this case? What is the difference if the red fluid is "clear enough to be able to read a newspaper through it" versus dark red? The surgeon says, "There is urine mixed in." Does that change your thinking? According to our friend the surgeon, the patient is "pissing like a horse." He does not specify whether a Palomino or an Arabian.

I do not care if the fluid in there is Veuve Cliquot champagne, 2500 mL is a lot. I would check the vital signs, looking for hypovolemia (e.g., hypotension, tachycardia), send a sample for a hematocrit value, and while those are in progress, go over how much irrigation they used, subtract that number from 2500, and try to get a feel for how much blood has been lost. Clearer liquid is encouraging, and if the fluid were dark red and obviously blood, I would start transfusing right away. The key element is to assume the worst until you have proved otherwise.

7. You transfuse 2 units of blood while the patient is awake, and the surgeon assures you. "That is enough." How will you determine whether this really is enough? The patient is on atenolol; are there any problems associated with that?

First, ignore the surgeon. Second, reassess the vital signs, send another sample for a hematocrit value, and send a sample for an ABG determination. Look for signs that something is in trouble, such as metabolic acidosis, which would indicate inadequate perfusion.

For a case with this much blood loss, I would have a central line in and would follow that CVP trend. I would not place a pulmonary artery catheter, because there is no evidence-based study showing an outcome difference, and the hassle of putting it in, tending to it, and wrestling with its complications (mainly distraction while you screw around with it) outweigh any benefit.

Atenolol, a long-acting β-blocker, can be a real hassle. Reflex tachycardia from hypovolemia or anemia is "cut off at the knees" when a β-blocker is on board.

8. You place the Foley catheter at the end of the case, and the Foley is bloody. The surgeon assures you, "It will clear." How do you interpret this? How would you determine whether there is a significant amount of blood in the abdomen? How much blood can you "hide" in the abdomen? Where else can significant amounts of blood hide?

First, ignore the surgeon. Second, lots of dark blood is scary, so tend to the vital signs, get more blood, make sure your access is adequate, and in case of doubt, transfuse. It is better to overdo it (the worst that can happen is you have to keep the patient on a ventilator) than underdo it and kill the guy.

Blood by the gallon can hide in the abdomen. Other spooky places of "blood hide and seek" are the thigh, upper arm in an obese person, and the chest. It is not possible to hide a lot of blood in the head (the patient will herniate first—small comfort) or in a tight compartment area, such as the lower leg or arm. The worst place to hide blood is on the floor! The patient can bleed under the drapes and drench the floor before someone looks down and says, "What the hell is that?"

9. In the PACU, the patient is initially stable, but the ECG shows that the patient goes from a normal rate and that the complex widens. How do you evaluate this? How could heavy bleeding cause what looks like a hyperkalemic response?

A wide complex means *get help now*. Assess the ABCs, making sure the patient has some vital signs. If the wide complex is ventricular tachycardia, follow ACLS protocol (i.e., shock synchronously if you have a blood pressure, and shock asynchronously if its pulseless). Use blood gas values to determine the cause. Secure the airway. Use chest compressions if there is no pulse. Transfuse, because the most likely cause is hypovolemia. Heavy bleeding might have led to hypotension, and the wide complex might be an ST elevation so high you are not seeing ventricular tachycardia; you are seeing a tombstone ECG.

10. Do you redose the epidural at the end of the case? What if you are concerned with ongoing bleeding? What is the effect of sympathectomy? What is the effect in the setting of β-blockade?

Do not redose the epidural. The epidural is there for pain relief and patient comfort. Our twin tasks are *safety* and comfort. Right now, the big concern is safety. Avoid giving anything through the epidural. You cannot afford the sympathectomy, and even narcotics through the epidural confuse the picture. Use the epidural later, when all is swell and groovy.

Postoperative Questions

1. Now the Foley catheter has frank blood pouring out. You are transfusing 4 units of blood. At what point do you place invasive monitors? He had none before. Do you place a triple-lumen or a Cordis line?

You place invasive monitors—arterial line and CVP line—now! Better yet, you put them in before. Look around for a handy-dandy time machine, and go back in time and place the lines an hour earlier.

I would place a Cordis. You need monster access and a triple-lumen tube is just not big enough. A bunch of long, skinny lines impede flow too much. You want all the flow characteristics to work, all the way up to using a rapid transfuser.

2. Do you start plasma component therapy? Do you use platelets, FFP, cryoprecipitate, or Amicar?

Send for a thromboelastogram (TEG) and laboratory studies to determine whether component therapy is needed. The most likely cause of "medical bleeding" (forget the gusher in the field for a second) is dilutional thrombocytopenia. While waiting for the laboratory test results to come back, I would start with platelets. This patient has lost enough blood that you can make an argument for giving FFP, too. Purists would say, "Wait until the TEG tells you exactly what is going on," but purists are not looking in the field seeing widespread oozing. If you want to be somewhat more scientific, you can go with "give FFP when the PT or PTT is 1.5 times normal."

I would ε-aminocaproic acid. It seems to help.

3. The wide complex continues. Is it related to the blood? How much potassium do you get from a bag of blood or from a bag of old blood? Should you request "young blood" for this young-at-heart guy?

The patient can get hyperkalemia from blood. Because older blood is more likely to have a higher potassium level than younger blood, it is reasonable in this case to ask the blood bank to give you blood with a shorter shelf life. However, this is mostly theoretical, because even in massive transfusions, you rarely run into hyperkalemia from the blood. Want a number? The average unit of blood has on the order of 7 mEq/L of potassium.

4. The platelets arrive and are type A positive, but the patient is A negative. Can you transfuse this bag of platelets? What are the rules of engagement regarding FFP, platelets, and cryoprecipitate and blood type?

You can transfuse the platelets. This topic is a perennial source of confusion. The American Red Cross Blood Services (they should know) has provided transfusion guidelines.

Platelet concentrate products should be ABO identical *when possible* because platelet increments may be higher. If not possible, good clinical results are usually obtained with ABO-mismatched platelets. Transfusion of large quantities of ABO-incompatible plasma (the platelets are floating in plasma, so every platelet transfusion is really a platelet plus plasma transfusion) may lead to a positive direct antiglobulin test result and, rarely, to clinically significant red cell destruction.

Rh compatibility is important but not always possible. Postexposure prophylaxis with anti-Rh immune globulin should be considered after Rh-positive platelet product transfusions to Rh-negative women who may have children in the future (not exactly this case).

What is the story for FFP? The Red Cross says that plasma product transfusions should be ABO compatible. Crossmatching and Rh compatibility are not required for plasma product transfusions.

I took a big chunk of time on this question, because a friend got creamed on his boards, largely because they asked him this exact question. When I ask around, hardly anyone knows these rules, because in the OR, we just make sure the paperwork is good, and we hang the stuff. People rarely look at the blood type or Rh and think about it. Go over the Red Cross rules or make a trip to the blood bank, and make sure you have this down pat. All this stuff is available online. I Googled *transfusion guidelines*, and got it right away.

5. His blood pressure drops as you are transfusing. There are signs of ischemia, and he is complaining of chest pain. Do you start a phenylephrine drip to increase perfusion? Even if the blood pressure goes up, have you actually increased perfusion? What is the difference between perfusion and pressure?

You are in a jam, because he could be having a transfusion reaction, but during a massive transfusion, the very things that indicate a transfusion reaction (e.g., hematuria, oozing, hypotension) are actually happening! Your best bet is to do everything you can to improve the ischemic picture:

- Secure the airway, and ensure adequate oxygen.
- Pour in the blood, checking hematocrit values and blood gases frequently.
- Check the calcium (the blood can drop the calcium, and a calcium bolus can increase the blood pressure, helping the perfusion picture).

Starting a vasopressor is a two-edged sword, because you do increase the blood pressure, but the very act of vasoconstriction may also affect the coronary supply. A higher pressure may not translate into more blood flow going to the heart. Perfusion is blood delivered. Pressure says how high the pushing is in the pipes, not how much is getting through the pipes.

I would start phenylephrine only after I did everything I could to get the pressure up by volume replacement. It would buy time while I got volume to do the real job, and I would turn the vasopressor off as soon as the pressure becomes normalized with volume resuscitation.

How It Actually Happened

Beware the "little case under a local anesthetic." This adorable 82-year-old guy was a tribute to aging well. He had a great sense of humor, but even his patience was tried when a monster intra-abdominal bleed occurred. At one point, he was white as a ghost and looked scared. Who could blame him?

Here is the sequence. With the epidural, the prostatectomy was done without too much fuss. There was a lot of red irrigation fluid, so we did transfuse him. That went well. In the PACU, he suddenly has a wide complex. We figured it was ischemia, not hyperkalemia (i.e., the potassium test result was fine). His hematocrit level was 32% (he must have been eating iron during the case), but then he went white as a ghost, and we knew he was bleeding (you can bleed to death and still have a normal hematocrit).

The surgeon comes in and says, "This is just ooze. Let's just do a little exploration under a local." Back in the OR, the surgeon tears open all the staples. What about the little incision under a local? We intubated lickety-split with etomidate alone, and they found a ton of oozing and bleeding. They emptied enough Avitene for three counties into his abdomen and eventually stopped the bleeding. He got FFP, platelets, and 4 more units of blood.

He did fine, *mirabile dictu*. Remember this the next time the surgeon says he is going to do "a little something under a local."

CASE 19: HIP CHECK

Preoperative Questions

1. What is multi-infarct dementia? Compare it with other causes of dementia? What are the implications for anesthesia and for obtaining consent?

Multi-infarct dementia is a diagnosis made when no one really knows what is going on. We do not know much about dementia, and you can say we are demented when it comes to dementia. The key element is to make sure in our rush to make the diagnosis that we do not miss a treatable cause of dementia, such as subdural hematoma, infectious disease (I know of a case of cerebral tuberculosis that manifested as a dementia!), or normal-pressure hydrocephalus.

The implications for us are many. Dementia does not kill you fast like a massive MI, but it kills you slowly through poor nutrition, immunocompromise, skin breakdown, and a progressive inability to handle secretions. All of these affect the course of an anesthetic.

Consent must come from a responsible caregiver, because the patient cannot give consent. In an emergency, a group of doctors can sign a consent (e.g., you cannot reach a relative, and the patient has a cerebral bleed).

2. The patient is debilitated and does no activity. Do you need further evaluation of her cardiac status before proceeding? Because she has a hip fracture that cannot wait too long, is it worth pursuing this further? What is the risk of waiting longer?

This patient needs her hip fracture fixed, or she will die of a pulmonary embolus or pneumonia. Further workup is a waste of time. Doing a full-court press dobutamine stress echocardiogram is also a waste of time because you are not about to revascularize her even if you do see a fixable cardiac lesion. However, to guide treatment, at least some idea of what kind of cardiac function she has will be useful. Ask for a transthoracic echocardiogram, and tell the technician, "Give me a number on her cardiac EF, and alert me about any glaring valvular lesion." You will conduct your anesthetic with close attention to heart rate and blood pressure, as you always do, so stalling for more than an easy-to-get transthoracic echocardiogram just puts off the inevitable.

3. Discuss the implications of the following in her history: arthritis, low sodium level, and low potassium level. Should you move to correct the electrolyte abnormalities before proceeding? Why or why not?

The airway is first and foremost. Arthritis can affect each "hinge" in the airway, from her neck to her jaw to the arytenoids. Do a good airway examination, and have the goodies nearby if you anticipate a difficult airway. Arthritis is a systemic inflammation, and every organ system can be involved. It can involve pericardial effusion (glad you asked for that transthoracic echocardiogram!) and a rhythm disturbance (look closely at that ECG, and make sure the external pacer is nearby and you know how to hook it up and work it in case you get in trouble). Where else can you have trouble? Name it! Kidneys, lungs, anywhere. In a practical sense, you know that arthritis can affect all these areas, and you make sure there is nothing obvious that will hurt you, such as a pleural effusion or renal failure.

An acute drop in the sodium level can cause problems (e.g., transurethral resection of the prostate [TURP] syndrome). In a chronic setting like this (e.g., debilitated patient, chronic disease), you can drive yourself crazy in an attempt to make the patient "euboxemic." Pouring in sodium is not a great idea (can cause central pontine demyelinolysis and congestive heart failure), and magically "wringing out" the free water and normalizing the sodium level that way is just as likely to get you in trouble (dry out the patient and cause hypotension when you induce). After you notice this low sodium level, you use normal saline judiciously, and you follow sodium levels during the case. In all likelihood, you will try to keep the sodium the same.

In the acute setting (e.g., after bypass in a cardiac case, mannitol causing acute hypokalemia), you transfuse potassium aggressively to prevent rhythm disturbances. In this chronic setting, you realize that the total potassium deficiency is probably enormous (hundreds of milliequivalents), and you do not want to pour that amount in the patient unless you are planning on starting a cardioplegia clinic. You follow the potassium levels intraoperatively, you may infuse some, but you do not go crazy with it. You are mainly looking at keeping the potassium level from getting much lower.

4. Her ECG shows tachycardia. What are the possible reasons? What are the problems with tachycardia? She is on metoprolol; how can she be tachycardic? Does she need more β-blockade? What are the dangers of this approach?

Tachycardia should always trigger a hunt for the reason. Is this an adaptive response to a problem that needs fixing (e.g., hypoxemia, hypovolemia, anemia, pain)? If so, those causes should be fixed first. Is this a primary cardiac rhythm disturbance (e.g., atrial fibrillation with rapid response)? What is the patient's baseline heart rate? A look in the chart will help with old vital signs. The twin dangers of tachycardia are that it shortens diastole, cutting down on coronary perfusion and places more strain on the cardiac muscle. In effect, you are making the heart sprint, which could make the heart outrun its blood supply.

How can someone on a β-blocker be tachycardic? The patient is not on enough β-blocker! Maybe she forgot to take it; drug mix-ups in the demented are common, and a nursing facility may also make the mistake.

More β-blockade will help control the tachycardia. A concern of giving more β-blockade centers on the pharmacology of β-blockade because too much blockade can cause a dangerously low heart rate. You may trigger bronchospasm. After the anesthetic is "off and running," you have cut out the patient's ability to respond if you screw up your volume assessment. You have removed one of the body's defense mechanisms—tachycardia—and the patient may need it to stay alive!

Thinking regarding β-blockade has done some back flips in recent years. For a while, it looked like β-blockade was going to take over the world, and we would give everyone and their second cousin β-blockade. We could have crop dusters with β-blockers flying over our preoperative clinics, spraying anyone coming within a mile of the OR. However, a closer look at outcomes has narrowed the recommendations. High-risk vascular cases may need β-blockers, but it is not so clear that β-blockade offers a real advantage to everyone else. And the POISE study tells us we may get more strokes and death in exchange for fewer MI's. Not a bargain.

5. A chest radiograph shows atelectasis and possible pneumonia, and the radiologist will not commit. What are the implications of atelectasis? What are the implications of pneumonia? Should you proceed with surgery? If you delay, what about the pulmonary embolism risk?

Damn those radiologists! Okay, you are stuck, so think it through. A debilitated patient who is not moving around much and cannot even be helped to move around much (a fractured hip hurts!) will not take deep breaths and is prone to atelectasis. This is bad news for us because atelectasis means a scrunched up lung that is not participating in gas exchange, leading to shunt and favoring hypoxemia. In a perfect world, you would do some deep breathing exercises with the patient and clear that up, but that is unlikely with her dementia.

If she has pneumonia, you have an infection that could seed the hardware going in her hip, as well as providing a lung infection that could bloom and go all the way to ARDS and death. Make sure she had a thorough workup and was started on appropriate antibiotics. An older, sicker person may not mount a fever and may not have a high white count. They do not "read the book" in terms of making a diagnosis of pneumonia easy. Talk it over with the surgeon, and make sure you are at least treating a pneumonia if she has one. However, sitting around forever on a fractured hip while the pneumonia is getting treated is not a great option either, because the risk for pulmonary embolism is ever present. Start treatment, and then do the operation.

Intraoperative Questions

1. Do you use any invasive monitors? A colleague suggests you "keep a finger on her pulse and use etomidate" rather than subject her to an awake placement of an arterial line. Is this approach as good? Is there any evidence to show an arterial line is needed?

Use an arterial line to start and a good central line after she is under anesthesia. No one has ever proved an arterial line prevents induction-sudden-death-from-too-much-damn-anesthetic syndrome (ISDFTMDAS), so that must be one of those things we have to accept on "our best guess" grounds. If you absolutely cannot get her to cooperate for an arterial line, you can induce carefully, and feel the pulse (it cannot tell you 140 from 120 beats/min, but it will tell you present from absent). With a non-stupid dose of etomidate, you should be able to induce her without causing cardiovascular collapse.

2. Her wrists are curled up, cutting off access to her radial arteries. Where to now? Should you use a brachial site? What are the risks? Should you use an axillary site? What are the risks? Should you use a femoral site? What if you try femoral access but go too deep and get intestinal "juice" in the needle?

A brachial site is okay, although some would quail that it is "an end artery, and you should never use it." Brachial arteries go in all the time without evidence of arms falling off left and right. I would go with a femoral site because it is easier (bigger vessel) and reliable. If I went too deep and hit intestinal contents (spooky, but such a thing can happen), I would withdraw and inform general surgery that we have violated the gut and will need to do an exploratory laparotomy and repair of an intestinal hole.

3. You cannot get a good airway examination, but she looks "arthritis scary." She will not cooperate with an awake intubation—no way, no how. How do you secure the airway? Should you try a breathe down, asleep fiberoptic, or awake fiberoptic approach with some curious concatenation of sedatives?

Dexmedetomidine is damned good at zoning out just about anybody, even the mentally challenged, as is the case here. I would give her one half of the usual loading dose, watching for bradycardia and hypotension and cutting off the drip if either appeared. If she tolerated this well, I would attempt the intubation awake, taping down her forehead (with gauze on the forehead to prevent skin damage) and having an assistant lift the chin hard to keep her from wiggling sideways, and that will keep the airway aligned so that after I am in, I can go a little anterior, and voila! Absent her cooperation, I would breathe her down, have her keep breathing spontaneously, and do a fiberoptic bronchoscopy in that manner.

4. You successfully intubate but have a hard time hearing her breath sounds. How will you make sure you do not have a right main stem intubation? Should you look at the markings on the ETT? Use a fiberoptic assessment? It is too much of a hassle?

Common sense would tell me that if I am at about 20 to 22 cm at the teeth, I should not be too deep. However, a quick look with a fiberoptic scope is no hassle, so I would put it in and make sure I saw the carina.

5. You have a triple-lumen subclavian line in on the right. The distal port does not aspirate but the proximal two do. Do you transfuse through this line? Is there any troubleshooting you can do? What could be wrong? What could be "really bad" wrong?

The third port may have curled back, preventing you from aspirating. On a more sinister note, the most distal port may have poked through the vessel and is now sitting in the pleural cavity. This has all the earmarks of a suspicious line, and the best thing to do is replace the line, pull the old line, get a chest radiograph, and keep your antennae up for anything weird that may happen later. You never want to start a case with a creepy line that you are not sure about.

6. The surgeon is unpleasantly surprised, telling you that her whole pelvic girdle is as fragile as tissue paper and falls apart with manipulation. How will this affect your management? Are there special risks? Is there need for more access? What do you do in the middle of the case?

The more the bone pulls apart, the more likely fat emboli are to enter the circulation. This is bad news in large print. Make sure there is an ICU bed for her postoperatively, and if you do not have monster access, have the surgeons put another line in for you, cutting down in the femoral region. Placing a central line with the patient on her side up by her neck or in the subclavian vein would be damned difficult.

7. Ventricular ectopy occurs. How do you tell "serious" ectopy from "harmless" ectopy? What is the mechanism of ventricular ectopy? How will you tell it from a reentrant rhythm? What diagnostic maneuvers do you employ? The potassium level is 2.8 mEq/L; is this the cause? Why or why not? What is the treatment?

Any "new" ectopy is cause for concern. Look for the cause! Run blood gas and electrolyte tests, and remember to ask for a blood glucose level. If anything is abnormal, fix it.

Ectopy is an aberration in the conduction system. Normally, the ventricle is activated "from above," with the signal starting in the atrium, taking a "stutter step" as it passes through the insulating barrier between atria and ventricles, and then spreading out through the conduction system in the ventricle.

While you are sending a sample for a gas determination and fixing anything that "feeds a happy heart" (e.g., adequate perfusion through adequate blood pressure, adequate hematocrit ensuring oxygen delivery), take a good look at the ECG. If there is a narrow complex, the signal originated above the insulating barrier. If there is a wide complex, the signal originated below the insulating barrier separating the atria from the ventricles. For some reason, an unhappy cell in the ventricle despaired of ever getting an electrical signal and started a signal of its own. Make that ventricular cell happy by correcting any chemical or perfusion abnormalities, and it is less likely to start a signal of its own.

If the potassium value was 2.8 mEq/L to start, and it has not changed, it is unlikely to be the cause for the ectopy. However, if everything else is absolutely normal, I would hang some potassium replacement as a "well, this may fix it" maneuver. Treatment, after fixing everything I could fix, consists of amiodarone if the rhythm looked threatening (i.e., more than five unifocal premature ventricular contractions [PVCs]/min, runs of ventricular tachycardia, or multifocal PVCs). The idea is to prevent a truly malignant rhythm that could cause cardiovascular collapse.

8. "Oh, damn. I forgot about doing a regional to keep her from getting deep venous thrombosis or a pulmonary embolism!" you say to yourself. The case is finishing. Do you put in a regional for postoperative pain relief and to decrease clot risk? Would such a maneuver help now? What is the thinking behind regional anesthesia to decrease pulmonary embolisms?

Regional anesthesia for hips is one of the rare things in anesthesia that has demonstrated benefit; there are fewer cases of DVT and fewer pulmonary embolisms. The sympathectomy increases blood flow in the lower extremities, lessening the chance of pooling and clot formation. Regional anesthesia at the end of the case can help pain relief, but I would wait until the patient is awake and cooperative (admittedly tough in the demented patient) before placing the regional. I know that regionals decrease pulmonary embolisms but do not know if it helps when the regional is placed *after* the case.

9. The case finishes, and the patient is on her side, fully awake and alert. Can you extubate her on the side? Why or why not? Is it safer than on her back? Could you extubate someone prone at the end of the case? How do you ventilate in such a case?

If she meets extubation criteria, with good neuromuscular, airway protection, and mechanics, she can be extubated on her side or even prone. If patients vomit, they are already in the perfect position! You can mask someone on her side and even prone, but prone is tough. If prone, I would have helpers move the patient at least on the side to make my life easier.

10. Just as you move the patient supine and are loosening the tape on her ETT, her face becomes completely gray, her blood pressure drops, the end-tidal

CO_2 gets cut in half, and she goes into ventricular tachycardia. Why caused this reaction? What is the treatment, including the ACLS protocol?

This "instant death" from "completely normal" looks like a pulmonary embolus, dislodged during her move from lateral decubitus to supine. Keep the ETT in place, go to 100% oxygen, call for help, shock, and start cardiac compressions immediately (that movement may break up the pulmonary embolus enough to restore life, but it is a desperate situation, and this is wishful thinking). With help in place, make sure you have not contributed to the collapse (e.g., anesthetic vaporizer on, line disconnected). Send a sample for a blood gas determination to make sure there is not a metabolic cause for her troubles. The keys are help, effective compressions, and continued looking.

How It Actually Happened

Yogi Berra hit it on the head when he said, "It is not over 'til it's over." This case pushed me to the nth degree as the pelvis kept falling apart (all those years of non-weight bearing in the wheelchair had caused her bones to "melt," in the words of the surgeon). The operation took longer and longer, and more and more blood was spilled, but I kept up, and all seemed well until the end.

She really did get gray as a ghost as we turned her, and I am sure a pulmonary embolus came loose. It was a classic drop in end-tidal CO_2 and loss of hemodynamics, and that was that. This occurred in the pre-TEE days, so we went all out with a Swan-Ganz catheter, people piling in the room to help out, and inotropes up the whazoo. None of our efforts worked, and she died.

CASE 20: BITING OFF MORE THAN YOU CAN CHEW

Intraoperative Questions

1. How do you do an airway examination when you cannot do an airway examination? What do you look for, without spooking the patient, that will tip you off one way or another?

Do the easy stuff first. Do his lips pucker in, showing you he is edentulous? If he is edentulous, he is unlikely to be a difficult intubation. If he does like to listen to Barney, play it! That may make him cooperative enough to open his mouth and get some kind of a look. From the outside, you can swing around to the side and get a feel for a receding chin. Although you cannot get a complete examination of the airway, you can still find out some useful information.

2. How do you obtain intravenous access in this patient? What are the intramuscular options? Should you play the Barney CD? Do Barney karaoke? Breathe down? How do you breathe down a 280-pound, uncooperative patient? Which agent should you use if you do this? Why?

The needle will freak him out, so you will not get this in any smooth fashion. Oral sedation, per rectum, and breathing down are all theoretical options, but they just plain will not work in the real world. This is ketamine dart country, and it may take more than one. Have the concentrated ketamine and lots of people around to help you after you place the intramuscular medication. Play the Barney music to assist in keeping him calm. In the theoretical world of breathing down a 280-pound, uncooperative person, you would use a rapid-acting, nonpungent agent, and sevoflurane is that agent.

3. You breathe him down but still cannot find anything peripheral. How do you get access? Are there any special tricks for placing a peripheral line?

If you cannot get peripheral access, go central. With enough ketamine, you may get him to hold still enough for an intrajugular line. Use an echocardiogram to guide you, because the patient's obesity will make the stick a difficult one. If he wiggles his head too much, go femoral.

Tricks that can help place a peripheral line include warm soaks, hanging the arm down, and nitroglycerin cream. There is an extremely expensive device that throws an eerie green light on the arm and shows veins as dark lines, but it costs about 25,000 dollars and is not likely to be available. The ultimate way to get a line stick out is to use a blood pressure cuff. Inflate to above systolic pressure; keep there 1 minute, lower it to between systolic and diastolic pressure, trapping the blood; and get your stick. In a ketamine-darted, uncooperative, morbidly obese patient, this is an unlikely stick, and I would still go central.

4. You have the patient breathing spontaneously and need to use a fiberoptic scope to place the ETT. The surgeon prefers the nasal route but understands you have issues. What do you do? Should you use oral or nasal intubation? Should you do one and then switch?

Buy the oral surgeons something nice, because you may have to impose on them. Secure the airway anyway you can quickly; if that means by mouth, get it by mouth. Now you have a secure airway and can get control of the situation; for example, you can get a better intravenous line with the patient holding still and getting vasodilation from the potent inhaled agents.

In a controlled situation, you can look through the nose by fiberoptics, see if you have got a good shot, place a tube changer down the oral tube as a backup, and place a tube by nose. Alternatively, you can keep the oral tube in and move it around as the oral surgeon works. The main idea is not to sacrifice an okay tube to try to get a perfect tube.

5. While placing the nasal tube, the patient gets light, and green liquid is seen in the posterior pharynx. What is your management plan? Should you turn the patient to his side? Should you soldier on and get the tube in? Should you then use suction, steroids, or antibiotics? Is there any case in which you would use antibiotics?

You are about to secure the airway and get the tube in right away; you inflate the cuff, preventing further aspiration. If you are not close, do the standard things you do when a patient vomits at induction: turn the head down and to the side, suction, and secure the airway as soon as possible.

Do not use steroids and antibiotics. The only time you use antibiotics is for witnessed aspiration of feculent material.

6. You have intubated the patient and suctioned out some green liquid. Do you proceed with this case or cancel? What are the risks of canceling or proceeding? If you cancel, do you keep the patient intubated? Why or why not?

A purist would say you should cancel the case, because you have a patient with aspiration during an elective case. This patient is not in optimal condition for an elective case. However, a pragmatist would first assess how bad the aspiration is. Is the saturation level holding? If so, I would proceed with the case. Whoever anesthetizes this patient will face the same daunting tasks you just faced, and sooner or later, this man needs to have his dental rehabilitation done. Theoretically, if you cancel this case, this same horror show may happen again, and he will never get his dental work done. He will end up with dental abscesses, bacterial endocarditis, or Ludwig's angina. So this is not a purely elective case, and I would do the case if his saturation level holds.

7. You proceed, and the oxygen saturation drifts from 98% down to 91%. The surgeon says there is another hour of work. How will you manage this low saturation level? Is it time to cancel? If you choose PEEP, what are the problems with PEEP? What is best method of ventilation? What would make you get an "ICU ventilator"?

Do the routine work first. Make sure the tube is in the right place, with no kinks or mucous plugs. Suction, go to 100% oxygen, and look with a fiberoptic scope. After you have done everything to "optimize the tube," add PEEP, and put the patient in a reverse Trendelenburg position. These maneuvers add FRC to the patient and should help oxygenation. PEEP always has the potential for impeding venous return and dropping the blood pressure and for posing the risk of barotrauma. You can play with the ventilator and use pressure-support ventilation rather than volume-control ventilation. Is one genuinely better than another? No. I would go to an ICU ventilator only if the OR ventilator could not do the job (inspiratory pressures were very high, and high PEEP was needed). If things were getting that bad, I would tell the surgeons to wrap it up, because we are getting into the "kill the patient" realm if you have to shift gears and roll in an ICU ventilator.

8. The patient bucks violently (the sevoflurane ran to empty, and you did not notice it) and sits bolt upright, knocking over all equipment and one person. How will you get the situation under control? How do you determine whether the patient is still intubated? If he has been extubated, then what?

An intravenous bolus is the quickest way to get the patient back down. Propofol at an induction dose can be used to get him back down. Once there, look for end-tidal CO_2 and breath sounds to make sure you have not lost the ETT. If extubation occurs, mask ventilate as best you can. Keep the patient's head up, which will keep the weight off his diaphragm and make him easier to ventilate. Get help and a fiberoptic scope.

If you have to intubate by means of direct laryngoscopy, keep one end point clear. If the patient's life depends on it, do not hesitate to break his teeth to get the tube in. No one should die of a lost airway with all of his teeth still in. The dentist is right there—blame him!

9. To get things under control, you give 150 mg of propofol. Thirty seconds later, the BIS goes to 5. What does this mean, and what are your concerns? What is the BIS? Why does propofol have that effect? How soon should it "return to normal"? What do you do if it is still low (in the teens) 30 minutes later?

A bolus of propofol will drop the bispectral index (BIS) value after a delay of about 30 seconds, so the drop to 5 is not a concern. The BIS is a processed EEG that has a proprietary algorithm built into its hardware to guide sedation. According to this algorithm, 100 is wide awake, 50 usually reflects an anesthetized state, and lower than 50 means a deeper anesthetic state. The EEG suppression (and low BIS value) from propofol should wear off in a few minutes. If, 30 minutes later, the BIS value is still low, it may indicate the anesthetic is too deep. Anything else that could cut down on EEG output (e.g., brain damage, brain death) may be indicated by such a low BIS value. As with any other possible neurologic change, you should pursue anything that could be hurting the brain and accounting for the low BIS value, including metabolic derangements such as hypoglycemia, hypoxemia (I hope to God you noticed that before now!), pharmacologic causes (e.g., too deep of an anesthetic), and intracranial pathology.

10. Do you extubate at the end of this case? The surgeon says the patient will be a wild child and that it may be best to get the tube out. Do you agree? Go back to basics, and see if the patient meets extubation criteria:

   - Can protect his own airway
   - Full neuromuscular reversal
   - Hemodynamic stability
   - Does not need the ETT for respiratory support

The biggie is the last one, because he might have aspirated. You need an ETT if you need high F_{IO_2} and PEEP (you can give both by mask, but this patient is unlikely to cooperate). If the patient will likely keep his oxygen saturation level above 93% (this is arbitrary, but you have to pick a cutoff somewhere) without the ETT, I would extubate. If, however, he needs 50% O_2 and 10 cm H_2O of PEEP to keep his saturation up, I would not extubate. Everything is tempered by the fact that this patient will likely not cooperate in deep breathing exercises or respiratory therapy and may not keep a mask on.

If the aspiration is bad, he needs the tube. If the aspiration is slight and has not shown itself within 2 hours, it is unlikely to progress more, and you can extubate.

Postoperative Questions

1. True to form, the patient is a wild child and goes nuts in the PACU. How will you sedate him? How will you know this is just "him" and not an intracranial event?

In an acute setting, with the staff and patient in danger, I would give a bolus of propofol just to keep everyone safe. If ongoing ventilation is needed, I would run a dexmedetomidine drip, because it will provide sedation, will not depress ventilation, and will cut down sympathetic outflow to prevent hypertension and tachycardia.

2. The mother goes ape when she finds out he is on a ventilator. How do you explain to her the events of the aspiration and the treatment plan? If she asks whether you did something wrong, what do you say?

Get the mother in a private setting, and then use the CONES approach in describing this event:

   Context: I would tell her who I am and why we need to talk about the events in the OR.
   Opening shot: "Your son needs to stay on the ventilator because his stomach contents got into his lungs before we put the breathing tube in."
   Narrative: Provide an objective narrative of the sequence of events as they happened.
   Emotions: At this point I would let the mother run the full gamut of her emotions.

Strategy: I would lay out the plan of keeping him on the ventilator until the aspiration resolves. Then I would leave contact information for her and make sure she was kept in the loop for all further developments.

When she levels an accusation at me, I would say, "I don't take credit when things go well, because sometimes it is out of my hands when things go well. In the same vein, I don't take all the blame when things do not go well because things are just plain out of my hands there, too. I did the best I could, and would not do anything differently next time."

3. The plan is to keep him intubated overnight. Does he need an arterial line? What if this is just for "airway protection"? What other methods besides arterial blood gases can you use to keep track of his ventilatory status overnight?

On a vent, you need an arterial line. You could follow him with O_2 saturation levels and clinical examinations, but that is lazy medicine. You have got the patient on a ventilator, so do the right thing, and give the respiratory people and ICU staff what they need—a way to get blood gases.

4. In the morning, the patient's ABG determination shows a Po_2 of 65 mm Hg on 50% oxygen and 5 cm H_2O of PEEP. Can you extubate? What else goes into the decision? How does the aspiration influence you?

The situation is too borderline. I would not extubate. You will have a hell of a time getting this patient to keep a 50% facemask on, so I would proceed conservatively and keep the ETT in. Aspiration may bloom, so check a chest radiograph, and look for signs that pneumonia has set in (e.g., fever, increased white cell count, left shift). The decision to extubate has to take in the usual parameters, but more importantly, it has to take in (corny as this sounds) the whole patient, with special consideration given to how much he can work with you after extubation.

5. The ICU nurses say that they can halve the dose of propofol if they keep playing the Barney CD. What are your options? Should you pipe Barney over the entire hospital intercom system? Should you offer headphones to the ICU staff so they do not go nuts? Should you put on a Barney suit and sing live? Why or why not?

Barney again. Hey, if you can help the kid by playing the music he likes, play the music. Just because we are applied pharmacologists who put in tubes and squeeze bags, we should not be blind to alternative methods that can help the clinical situation. So crank the Barney music!

How It Actually Happened

No one looks good in this one. Dental rehabilitation cases are the albatross around any anesthesiologist's neck. I talked with an oral surgeon who did these cases, and she absolutely loves doing them. Go figure!

This guy was tough as they get, and he had to go big time on the ketamine dart (150 mg). He did aspirate as we were intubating, but we forged ahead instead of delaying the case because he was just as likely to aspirate the next time.

We did get it done, but in the postoperative ICU, his course was rocky, requiring 4 days of ventilation. He could not cooperate, and we could not get any deep breathing out of him. We had to sedate every time he got light, and round and round we went. Mom was major mad, but not at us; she was frustrated by the whole situation. Who can blame her?

All's well that ends well. He left the hospital vertical, unlike so many of the cases I present.

CASE 21: HOW FAR CAN YOU GO?

Preoperative Questions

1. Would you treat this patient's blood pressure before surgery? Why or why not?

I would evaluate several different preoperative blood pressure measurements from this patient from both arms to determine his blood pressure range. I would treat this patient's blood pressure only if it were higher than his preoperative normal values.

2. What is your target for this patient's intraoperative blood pressure? What blood pressure do you use as a baseline when calculating intraoperative blood pressure goals? For this particular surgery, is a higher or lower blood pressure preferable? Why?

Intraoperative goals are to maintain his blood pressure at the high-normal range of his predetermined preoperative range of blood pressures. In this particular surgery, it is better to maintain a higher rather than lower blood pressure to maintain cerebral perfusion through collateral flow (i.e. circle of Willis and vertebral arteries) during cross-clamping of the carotid artery. The brain's autoregulatory function is likely to be dysfunctional in a patient with sclerotic carotid arteries. The cerebral perfusion pressure will be low because of the stenosis at the level of the carotid arteries, and the cerebral vessels will already be maximally dilated, with no further autoregulatory ability. Perfusion of the brain, therefore, is pressure dependent and not able to tolerate drops in systemic blood pressure.

3. Does this patient require a preoperative transfusion? Why or why not? Would you have blood available for this patient? Would you type and cross-match or type and screen for antibodies? How many units will you use? What hematocrit do you want to maintain in this patient and why?

It would be ideal for this patient to have a hematocrit of at least 30% to optimize the oxygen carrying capacity of the blood. It is likely that this patient has comorbid conditions, including coronary artery disease, and the O_2 carrying capacity becomes important to prevent brain and cardiac ischemia. Large fluid shifts and large blood loss are unlikely in this particular operation, but it is a good idea to transfuse him preoperatively to achieve a hematocrit of 30%. He needs a type and screen and type and crossmatch for surgery, and 1 unit of blood should be available. The need for a blood transfusion during this particular operation is low, and a type and screen would normally be sufficient. However, given his baseline anemia and anticoagulated status, a crossmatch is a good idea.

4. Does this patient need a cardiac workup before going to surgery? Why or why not? What specific information would you want? How would this information change your anesthetic management?

The gist of the new guidelines is best summarized as follows: Unless his situation would attract your attention in the ER (an MI is happening right in front of your eyes, valvular disease causing CHF), proceed with the case. So, skip the workup and proceed with surgery, following standard anesthetic practice.

Intraoperative Questions

1. The surgeon requests regional anesthesia for this patient. How do you respond? Does the LMWH alter your plan in any way? How do LMWH and heparin work?

Regional anesthesia for carotid endarterectomy (CEA) has positive and negative aspects. The positives include the ability to continually monitor neurologic function in a way superior to stump pressure, somatosensory evoked potentials (SSEPs), or the EEG and avoidance of volatile anesthetic and intravenous induction agent-induced drops in blood pressure. The negatives include the inability to protect the airway, inability to induce cerebral protection, and necessity for the patient's compliance. Regional anesthesia can be performed with a superficial and deep cervical plexus block. The block is unlikely to be affected by the use of LMWH if the last dose was administered more than 4 hours earlier.

Heparin's mechanism of action is to bind to antithrombin III and produce a conformational change that allows rapid combination with and inhibition of thrombin and prevention of fibrin formation. Maximal effects occur within minutes.

2. Suppose you are doing general anesthesia for this case because the patient refuses to stay awake during the procedure. How do you induce him? Why do you use etomidate, not propofol? Can you use propofol? Will you keep the patient paralyzed throughout the procedure? Would you give an opiate as well? If so, how much and why?

Induction is best with thiopental for cerebral protection. Etomidate is superior to propofol because it will not drop the blood pressure, but propofol is acceptable. I would keep the patient paralyzed throughout the procedure to prevent any movement at the operative site. Opiates are a good choice to protect the heart from increases in heart rate and blood pressure during induction, but more than induction doses may not be necessary or desirable because the patient needs to wake up promptly postoperatively so neurologic function can be evaluated.

3. How do you monitor this patient? When do you place your arterial line and why? Is there any difference if the case is done under general or regional anesthesia? Do you use EEG monitoring? What is a stump pressure? Why do surgeons place a shunt during some CEAs?

The arterial line is placed before induction, because induction is a time of cardiovascular lability. In addition to an arterial line, we will use pulse oximetry, ECG with leads II and V, a temperature probe, an oxygen sensor, and a capnograph. A CVP line should not be necessary. There should be no differences between the use of regional or general anesthesia, except in regard to cerebral function. If we are using regional anesthesia, an EEG, SSEPs, or stump pressure is not necessary because the patient can communicate with the OR team to determine if there are cerebral perfusion problems. EEG monitoring is an option in general anesthesia to monitor cerebral perfusion. Stump pressure is the pressure cephalad to the cross-clamped carotid artery and represents the collateral circulation from the contralateral carotid artery and vertebral artery through the circle of Willis. A stump pressure of more than 50 mm Hg denotes adequate perfusion, although studies have shown that there is poor correlation between stump pressure and cerebral perfusion. A shunt is placed by the surgeon if there are signs that there is not adequate collateral perfusion (i.e., stump pressure less than 50 mm Hg).

4. Intraoperatively, the patient remains hypertensive, with a mean arterial pressure above 100 mm Hg. How do you manage his blood pressure?

I would be cautious in lowering his blood pressure, because his cerebral perfusion depends on maintaining his blood pressure in the high-normal range. Of course, excessive hypertension needs to be treated. Nitroglycerin has beneficial effects on the coronary circulation. Nitroprusside is another choice. β-Blockade should be avoided, whereas nicardipine has beneficial cardiac effects.

5. Your treatment results in a drop in pressure to 70/40 mm Hg. How do you manage this? Does his bradycardia alter your treatment plan? Why or why not?

Hypotension should be treated with intravenous fluids and phenylephrine. If there is also bradycardia, I would be less likely to use an α-agonist. Bradycardia can be the result of the surgeon's manipulation of the carotid baroreceptor and can be avoided by asking the surgeon to infiltrate the region with 1% lidocaine, although the infiltration itself has been known to cause bradycardia. Bradycardia should be treated with atropine.

6. The patient develops ST depression and T-wave inversion during this episode of hypotension. How do you respond? If the ECG changes reverse themselves when the pressure is raised, and the surgery has not yet started, do you cancel the case and wake the patient? Why or why not?

When the patient develops ECG changes, I would respond with 100% O_2 and attempt to raise the pressure with a fluid bolus. After the ECG changes reverse themselves, the case should be canceled until a full cardiac workup can be completed. This surgery is not emergent, and the relative hypertension necessary to maintain cerebral perfusion during carotid cross-clamping can put extreme stress on the heart.

How It Actually Happened

Halfway through the case, aliens from outer space landed on the roof of the hospital, abducted the anesthesia team, probed their brains, found nothing worth emulating, and released them back into the OR with no time elapsed. All this was duly noted on the record.

CASE 22: ROAD WARRIOR

Preoperative Evaluation

1. What criteria are used to evaluate the cervical spine? What information would you want to obtain from C-spine films? How useful is a lateral C-spine film?

Patients frequently come to the OR with a C-spine collar in place, and nobody has a clue about whether the spine is clear. To clear a spine, you need cervical films (plain film or CT) that show the entirety of the cervical spine. Plus, to "clear a neck" you need a lucid patient. Given normal films, palpation of the spine can elicit ligamentous or bony tenderness, assuming that the patient is not intoxicated, heavily medicated, or suffering from pain elsewhere that can serve as a distracting injury. A single film cannot be used to clear a spine, and if the patient is drunk or medicated, you should proceed with caution, performing an intubation with inline stabilization and minimizing neck movement.

2. How would you diagnose myocardial contusion? What are the physical findings? What are the ECG and echocardiographic findings? How about getting creatine phosphokinase (CPK) and troponin levels?

Myocardial contusion can be difficult to diagnose and can remain asymptomatic for hours after an injury. A high index of suspicion is needed when examining patients suffering chest wall trauma (a broken steering wheel is a red flag). Patients with contusion can have a normal-appearing ECG, and echocardiography is not a useful diagnostic tool. CPK levels can be elevated in all trauma patients due to muscle injury, including injury to the diaphragm and tongue, both of which are associated with deceleration injury and both of which result in elevations of the MB isoenzyme, confusing the picture even more. Troponins are specific for cardiac injury, and some studies suggest that troponin levels increase with the severity of a cardiac contusion. Unfortunately, myocardial ischemia from hypotension also can result in troponin release, and a high index of suspicion is needed for patients with thoracic trauma. In this patient, the combination of chest trauma, nonspecific ECG changes, and PVCs make me concerned that he might have myocardial contusion and develop further arrhythmias and hypotension.

3. Would you order a type and screen or a type and cross of blood products? What is the difference? Would type-specific blood be adequate? What is trauma blood? What are the implications of administering trauma blood before switching to type and cross blood?

A type and crossmatch would be appropriate for this patient, considering that he has been the victim of trauma and has apparent hypovolemia and anemia. A type and screen checks the patient's blood for possible antibodies against transfused blood, and crossmatching tests the patient's blood specifically against the donor blood. It is safest to use crossmatched blood, but using screened blood is still considered relatively safe, with the risk of transfusion reaction remaining very low. Trauma blood is typically uncrossmatched type O-negative (or positive) blood given to patients who cannot wait for a type and screen or crossmatch to be completed. If a significant amount of trauma blood is given (>4 to 8 units of packed red cells), there is a risk of antibodies in the trauma blood reacting with crossmatched blood if it is given subsequently.

Intraoperative Questions

1. Is an arterial line indicated? Why or why not? How would you assess volume status? Should central venous pressures be measured? Pulmonary artery pressures?

Although open femur fractures can be associated with significant bleeding, this patient appears to be hemodynamically stable, and I do not anticipate significant fluid shifts during the operation. If the patient did not have a history of cardiac disease, I would not place an arterial line (or use other invasive monitoring) for this case. Given the patient's apparent cardiac contusion, however, an arterial line can help me to monitor beat-to-beat blood pressure changes and alert me to sudden hypotension from ventricular dysfunction. I would assess volume status using urine output, blood pressure, pulse, and arterial line or respiratory variability. Although a central line could be useful, I would not place one in a patient with apparent cardiac injury with PVCs because I would be concerned about malignant dysrhythmia developing during wire and line placement. A pulmonary artery catheter may be helpful in detecting early ventricular dysfunction, but I would not elect to place one for similar reasons.

2. How will you manage the airway? Does anesthetic management include C-spine considerations? If awake intubation is chosen, how would you anesthetize the airway? What induction agent and muscle relaxant would you select? What agents will you use for maintenance? Would you use a BIS monitor?

Assuming the patient does not have a cleared airway, I would opt for a rapid sequence intubation (RSI) with in-line stabilization. This assumes that the airway appeared otherwise normal. If it did not appear to be an easy airway, I would opt for awake fiberoptic intubation. To topicalize the airway, I would anesthetize the oropharynx with benzocaine spray, the hypopharynx with nebulized lidocaine, and the glottis with transtracheal cocaine or lidocaine. If the patient had a difficult airway, had a noncleared spine, and was uncooperative for awake fiberoptic intubation, I would be an unhappy anesthesiologist! I would try to balance the need for a secure airway, an immobile neck, and an RSI in any way possible.

Assuming I am doing in-line stabilization and an RSI, I would use ketamine or etomidate (in an attempt to avoid cardiovascular depression) and succinylcholine. I would use opiates and low-dose volatile agents for maintenance (also to avoid cardiovascular depression), and I would like to have a BIS monitor, because trauma patients are at high risk for intraoperative recall.

3. Ten minutes after intubation, peak airway pressure increases to 45 cm H_2O. How do you respond? What is the differential diagnosis? How do you diagnose and treat tension pneumothorax?

Elevated peak airway pressures immediately make me think of one-sided intubation, a circuit kink, bronchospasm, and tension pneumothorax. I would quickly switch to 100% oxygen and bag-ventilate the patient to get a feel for the respiratory compliance. I would simultaneously examine the circuit to ensure that it is not kinked, and I would then auscultate the lungs to check for wheezing or unilateral breath sounds. Tension pneumothorax and one-sided intubation can manifest with unilateral breath sounds, but other signs such as tracheal deviation (and a high index of suspicion given this patient's chest trauma) would make me more concerned about a collapsed lung. To treat this condition, I would first notify my surgical colleagues about my concerns, and I would then place a 14-gauge angiocatheter into the second intercostal space in the midclavicular line in an attempt to relieve the tension. Assuming that this fixes the problem, I would then ask the surgeon to place a chest tube before performing the scheduled operative procedure.

4. Two hours into the operation, the patient's blood pressure is 80/40 mm Hg and heart rate is 120 beats/min. How do you respond? The estimated blood loss is 1 to 2 L. After transfusing 3 units of packed red blood cells, the patient continues to bleed. The surgeon requests FFP. How would you proceed? Would you consider obtaining a thromboelastogram (TEG)? What information can you obtain from a TEG? What other tests can you do to assess coagulation?

Hypotension and tachycardia raise concerns about hypovolemia, which in this case would most likely be caused by perioperative blood loss. Given the blood loss of 1 to 2 L and the continuing bleeding, I would ensure that I have a continuing supply of blood products available. If the bleeding is described by the surgeons as "oozing" in nature, I would consider empirically giving FFP according to the surgical request. Massive transfusion (although not necessarily a 3-unit transfusion) can result in coagulopathy, but so can hypothermia (which is common in trauma patients) and disseminated intravascular coagulation (DIC). Although I do not routinely perform a TEG, it can be used to differentiate the causes of nonspecific oozing. The TEG can test for platelet dysfunction, fibrinolysis, or the presence of DIC. Other tests that are typically more readily available include platelet count, PT (which tests the extrinsic coagulation cascade), and PTT or activated clotting time (both of which test the intrinsic system).

5. During closure, tachydysrhythmia ensues as the heart rate increases from 105 to 150 beats/min. Rhythm appears to be a narrow complex. How would you respond? What are the causes? Suppose the blood pressure is 70/40 mm Hg; how would you respond? If the blood pressure is 120/80 mm Hg, what pharmacologic agents would you consider? A medical student suggests adenosine. What is your response?

Tachycardia and hypotension initially makes you think of hypovolemia, but a heart rate of 150 beats/min with a narrow complex rhythm is more likely to represent a supraventricular tachycardia (SVT). A low blood pressure indicates unstable SVT, which requires synchronized cardioversion. A normal blood pressure instead allows for the option of pharmacologic intervention. Adenosine is a good option, with an excellent chance for conversion. I would pat the student on the head and give him a gold star for the day.

How It Actually Happened

We made this one up, just like the last one, but you probably figured that out.

CASE 23: TREATING LEUKEMIA AT HOME

Intraoperative Questions

1. Why is the child listless? What is the differential diagnosis? Do you need a diagnosis before you can induce?

Causes include fever, dehydration, acute exacerbation of leukemia, homeopathic herbal therapy, bleeding, and metastatic disease to the brain. The differential diagnosis includes infection due to neutropenia, immunosuppression due to bone marrow suppression caused by leukemia, septic and cardiogenic shock, and increased ICP due to possible brain metastases.

In an emergent situation, act first, and ask questions later. There is no time to ponder. In an elective situation, I would like to see the patient better optimized, meaning that we treat the cause if possible before induction.

2. Comment on the platelet count and its implications. Explain the implications of the hematocrit. Do you need to transfuse right away in the OR?

If the patient is hemodynamically stable, and there is no evidence of bleeding, a level of 50,000 platelets is acceptable for minor procedures. However, if the patient has dysfunctional platelets or shows signs of bleeding, I would want the platelets in the range of 80,000 to 100,000. If the patient is bleeding actively, I would transfuse immediately. If there are no signs of bleeding, a hematocrit of 21% is acceptable in a hemodynamically stable child. The possible causes include bone marrow suppression due to chemotherapy or leukemia. In this case, I would transfuse immediately with leukocyte-reduced, irradiated packed red blood cells.

3. You need an intravenous line, but you are doing this operation to get an intravenous line. How do you handle this dilemma? What if you cannot get peripheral placement? Is there any technology to help get a peripheral line? Will ultrasound help?

In this case, if I could not place a peripheral intravenous line after one or two attempts or if the child is hemodynamically unstable, I would go straight for intraosseous access. Ultrasound is a great tool if it is available immediately. It is also operator dependent. Even in skillful hands, it will take longer to place an ultrasound-guided, peripheral intravenous line than to gain intraosseous access. The answer is do not bother with ultrasound; pay attention to the patient's vital signs instead.

4. You need to place a central line. How do you place a central line in a child? Is it any different from placement in an adult? What are the special problems with a central line in a child? What are the problems with placement of intrajugular, subclavian, and femoral lines?

Children are more likely than adults to pull lines, and several things need to be considered. The central line has to be out of reach of the child. A femoral line is the least favorable in the long term, because kids are mobile, and femoral lines have the highest risk of thrombosis. For this reason, subclavian and intrajugular lines are better. Broviac catheters are preferred. They are more cosmetically acceptable. There are fewer limitations on activity, there is less chance of dislodgement, and they require less care.

5. How will you induce? Is a sick kid with leukemia considered to be a "full stomach"? You breathe him down, and he vomits while in phase 2. What do you do?

If the kid has intravenous access, I would use intravenous medications. Depending on the patient's history, I would decide on an appropriate agent. In case of an elevated ICP, I would use thiopental; if the patient is hemodynamically unstable, I would use etomidate; and I would use propofol for other situations. Otherwise, I would have to use inhaled anesthetics.

I would definitely treat the kid as a full stomach. Sick equals decreased bowel motility, and the kid is on chemotherapy (even if it is homeopathic) and therefore more prone to nausea and vomiting.

If the patient vomits while in stage 2, I would suction the mouth first, intubate immediately (pray that he does not develop bronchospasm), and use bronchoscopy.

6. The surgeon places the line and tries to flush it. Just after he flushes it, the technician notices that concentrated heparin was given by mistake and that the patient just got 10,000 units of heparin. What can you anticipate will happen in this patient with a low platelet count and hematocrit? Will you reverse? Is "waiting it out" an option?

There are two scenarios: You get lucky and nothing happens, or the kid will bleed excessively. I would not take my chances and try to reverse the patient with protamine (1 mg/100 units of heparin). Patients who received protamine in the past had a 1% chance of anaphylaxis. Waiting it out is an option; the half-life of heparin is 30 to 60 minutes. If you like thrills, the patient has no history of heart disease, and you have a good malpractice insurance, you can try.

7. As you get ready to extubate, you notice bright red blood in the mouth. Will you extubate? The patient is bucking, and the surgeon says, "Come on, get the damn thing out!

It depends on how brisk the bleeding is and the source. If the bleeding is minimal and the source is identifiable (e.g., traumatic intubation by the medical student), I would extubate. However, if the bleeding is profuse, you must protect the airway first and try to control the bleeding. Ask the impatient surgeon for assistance if you have to.

Postoperative Questions

1. You are called emergently to the ICU to intubate this patient that night. Do you use suxamethonium in this emergent situation? Why or why not?

If the patient is listless and hemodynamically unstable, I would try to intubate without any drugs. There is no clear contraindication to using succinylcholine in an emergent situation in the pediatric population, except for kids with a known history of muscular dystrophy or family history of malignant hyperthermia or in kids who are burned, paralyzed, or bedridden (the usual contraindications).

2. You arrive, and the patient is covered in blood. The ICU staff attempted extubation several times to no effect. What problems do you anticipate, and how will you handle the problems? You look in and see only blood. What are the options?

Suction, and see if the view becomes better. If you see the cords, intubate. Otherwise, the following are the plausible options: a blind attempt, using a bougie, fast-track LMA through which you can blindly intubate, retrograde intubation, and a surgical airway. Much depends on whether you can ventilate the patient. Fiberoptic intubation is challenging if there is an active bleeding in the oropharynx.

3. What are the options regarding a surgical airway? Are they different for a child? Can you place an LMA and perform a tracheostomy later?

A surgical airway would be the last resort. In kids, there is a higher chance of tracheal stenosis. The goal of intubation in this kid is control of ventilation and airway protection. An LMA would not be the best choice in the kid with active bleeding.

4. You intubate, but the face is covered in blood. How do you secure the ETT? Do you use tape or string? Do you sew? How? What are the dangers of accidental extubation, and how will you prevent it?

Try to clean the face, dry the area around the mouth, and use some benzoin tincture before applying the adhesive tape. If this is impossible, make sure that the kid is sedated enough before considering suturing the tube.

5. How do you sedate this 4-year-old child? What are the long-term problems with infusion of propofol or etomidate? Does the child need stress-dose steroids? Does he need an infusion of platelets?

The first choice is benzodiazepine, especially if the patient will be intubated for several days. There are no long-term side effects.

Propofol should not be used for more that 3 days. It increases triglyceride levels, which may lead to pancreatitis. It lowers blood pressure more than benzodiazepine, and if the kid is unstable, it is definitely a bad choice.

Etomidate is no longer used in the ICU for sedation because of evidence of adrenal suppression if it is used for more than 24 hours. Some report that even one induction dose is enough to cause adrenal insufficiency.

If the patient was on steroids during the past year (prednisone equivalent of more than 10 mg) for more than 2 weeks, definitely yes. Otherwise, do a cosyntropin stimulation test to determine whether the patient qualifies for steroids.

If patient has no bleeding, I would continue to monitor. I would transfuse if the platelet level were less than 20,000 because of the increased risk of spontaneous hemorrhage. If the patient were bleeding as in this case, I would not hesitate to transfuse.

How It Actually Happened

All of the bad stuff that could happen, happened. Happily, all the responses to the bad things also happened. This combination of happen, happened, and happening led to a miraculous salvage of this patient, although whether it was attributed to our skill or happenstance is up for debate.

CASE 24: HARD TO SWALLOW

Preoperative Questions

1. What type of history is typical for a foreign body in the airway?
The child may present with acute respiratory symptoms, such as coughing, stridor, and cyanosis. Some children undergo a workup for new-onset asthma, and some children have a history of recurrent pneumonia and present for a workup.

2. Who are at risk for foreign body aspiration? What is the natural history of most choking episodes?
There is a bimodal age distribution, with children between 1 and 3 years old and those in the seventh decade of life (because of dementia) at higher risk for foreign body aspiration. Aspirated objects may subsequently change position or migrate distally, particularly after unsuccessful attempts to remove the object or if the object fragments.

3. Does the absence of symptoms in the ER or absence of radiographic abnormalities exclude an airway foreign body?
No. The most important diagnostic tools are the patient's history and a high index of suspicion.

4. What are the most common objects aspirated?
In children, the primary factors leading to aspiration are underlying curiosity about the world and the oral phase of the toddler. Loose, small objects and food found around the household increase risk. An older sibling feeding younger

children is an important historical clue. Objects that tend to stay in the mouth for prolonged periods, such as gum, sunflower seeds, or hard candy, also increase the risk.

5. What types of foreign bodies are most dangerous to the lung tissue? Which ones are the most lethal?

Vegetable material may swell over hours or days. Organic foreign bodies, such as oily nuts (commonly peanuts), induce inflammation and edema. Small batteries may cause acid spills into the lungs.

6. What interventions can be tried before arrival in the OR if the patient is rapidly deteriorating?

The most important intervention is keeping the child as calm as possible to reduce the risk for foreign body dislodgement. Supportive treatment, which includes O_2 supplementation, a dose of steroids or antibiotics, and bronchodilators, may be indicated. Continuous SpO_2 monitoring and clinical supervision are mandatory!

7. When should the case be done? Are there any risks associated with waiting or with not waiting?

This is an airway emergent case and should be done as soon as possible. Rarely, when the OR or the surgeons are not available, the child should remain under continuous monitoring in an ICU setting. NPO status should be treated as in an emergent situation, balancing between aspiration and airway compromise risks. In this case, there is no reason for delay.

8. How would you treat the patient's current symptoms?

The best treatment is removal of the foreign body in the OR as soon as possible.

Intraoperative Questions

1. Should this patient be premedicated? Explain.

Maintaining a calm patient is important. If needed, a small dose of midazolam can be given. Narcotics should be avoided in these cases, because they increase the risk for hypoventilation.

2. What technique would you use for induction of anesthesia? Discuss RSI and inhalation induction.

The procedure should be performed in a well-equipped room with a pediatric anesthesiologist in attendance. Most experienced anesthesiologists prefer inhalation rather than intravenous induction of anesthesia and a ventilating bronchoscope rather than intubation. Good results have been reported with spontaneous ventilation or positive-pressure ventilation. We prefer a smooth, calm mask induction and spontaneous ventilation through the bronchoscope.

3. How would you manage a complete airway obstruction during induction?

Rapid airway intubation and ventilation should be done immediately; it can be done by placing an ETT or a bronchoscope and pushing the foreign body into one of the main stem bronchi while ventilating through one lung.

4. How would your anesthetic management and the risks change between an acute and a chronic foreign body presentation?

Basically, the anesthetic management in the OR is the same in both scenarios, but with a chronic foreign body, the risk for requiring postoperative mechanical ventilation is higher.

5. Describe the options for removal of airway foreign body (e.g., rigid bronchoscopy, bronchotomy).
From the simplest to the more invasive, the options are rigid bronchoscopy, flexible fiberoptic bronchoscopy, bronchoscopy with removal through tracheotomy, bronchotomy, lobectomy, and pneumonectomy.

6. Are you going to intubate after the foreign body removal?
In most cases, postprocedural mask ventilation and spontaneous breathing are preferable because there is less airway stimulation during the emergence from anesthesia.

7. What are the expected postoperative complications after the foreign body removal? What would you prepare?
The most common side effect is vocal cord edema and stridor as a result of bronchoscope trauma. Bronchospasm and the accumulation of airway secretions also are common. Make sure you have suction bronchodilators and racemic epinephrine available, and consider "deep extubation" when appropriate.

How It Actually Happened

This little kid caused lots of tension in the ER. When we were called to see him, he was already tired from all the activity around him, which started a new cycle of crying along with escalating wheezing and coughing.

Because this was an emergent procedure, we proceeded to the OR as soon as possible. The little guy was lightly sedated (1 mg of midazolam in the holding area) to avoid the crying experience and then quickly brought into the OR. General anesthesia was induced by mask using a sevoflurane and oxygen mix. Spontaneous breathing was maintained throughout the procedure, avoiding positive pressure as much as possible.

Minutes after, a Lego piece was located and carefully removed (by rigid bronchoscope) from the right lung. We then continued mask ventilating with oxygen to an uneventful emergence. The patient was safely transferred to the recovery room, and the precious Lego piece was sent to the pathology department and then returned to his older brother.

You can see many Lego pieces at Legoland, just north of San Diego.

CASE 25: DONUT INTERRUPTED

Preoperative Questions

1. What are the criteria for outpatient surgery in children, infants, and former preemies? How old is this baby in terms of postgestational age?
There should be no intracranial, intrathoracic, or major abdominal surgery in the outpatient setting. There is minimal risk of anesthetic or surgical complications. Simple nursing can be provided by parents, and simple postoperative medication, such as analgesics and antiemetics, can be administered. There are no major limitations on the child's activities. Other restrictions guided by the comorbid conditions of the individual patient.

Preemies are at increased risk for apnea of prematurity, and it is recommended to wait until 50 to 55 weeks' postconceptional age for performing surgery as an outpatient. This child is approximately 48 weeks' postconceptional age.

2. What about the neonatal intensive care unit (NICU) course is critical? What about airway management and length of intubation?

The patient's NICU course suggests other comorbid conditions that may affect anesthetic management. Length of intubation may suggest the presence of tracheomalacia and the severity of preexisting lung disease, such as bronchopulmonary dysplasia. It is important to know whether the patient has a history of gastroesophageal reflux disease (GERD), cardiac problems, or neurologic complications of prematurity.

3. What is the significance of airway and breathing issues, home oxygen delivery, current home monitoring, and the child's medications?

The existence of airway and breathing issues and the need for home apnea monitoring suggest the continued apnea of prematurity. A home O_2 requirement and need for albuterol and prednisone indicate more severe, unresolved lung disease as a result of this patient's prematurity or complications in the NICU. The patient should receive a stress dose of steroids as part of his anesthetic management.

4. What would be a normal weight and vital statistics for a child with this history? What preoperative laboratory test results do you want, if any?

A weight of approximately 5 kg is in the 50th percentile for a child of this developmental age. Blood pressure should be about 90/50 mm Hg, and the mean heart rate should be 120 beats/min for the 50th percentile. Measurement of the hematocrit can be useful in this patient because there is a relationship between anemia and an increased incidence of apnea. However, given this patient's existing need for postoperative apnea monitoring and the low potential for blood loss with the proposed surgical procedure, this value is unlikely to change the management.

5. What are the NPO guidelines for this patient? Is outpatient surgery a good choice? The surgeon wants to do his easy cases first and this one last. Is this a good decision?

Children younger than 6 months should have solid food (e.g., breast milk, milk, and formula) restricted to later than 4 hours preoperatively. Clear liquids can be continued up to 2 hours before surgery.

6. How long does it take for you to tell the mother *no way* for day surgery and book the child as the first case of the day in the main OR?

This patient will need postoperative respiratory monitoring and is not a good candidate for outpatient surgery. Given the patient's age, prematurity, and coexisting diseases, it would be wise to perform surgery on this patient early in the day to minimize delays in start time and the need to maintain the patient's NPO status.

Intraoperative Questions

1. Can mom come to the OR? Does this child need midazolam? What is ⅛ L of O_2?

This patient is unlikely to have separation anxiety, and not having the mother come to the OR will allow the anesthesiologist to focus on the safe induction of anesthesia. Infants of this age usually do not need premedication for anxiety.

The ⅛ L of O_2 is a setting for low-flow oxygen supplementation. It allows for predictable administration of F_{IO_2} at a wider range of ventilatory rates without the drying effects of higher-flow oxygen delivery.

2. Should you use straight regional anesthesia? Where and when will you get intravenous access? Can you use spinal, caudal, or caudal with or without a catheter? Which local anesthetic will you use? Will you add epinephrine, clonidine, or a narcotic? When was the last time you did one of these? What the heck is a sugar nipple?

Intravenous access can be obtained in the OR. Given the stability of pediatric pressure with a neuraxial block, it is common to place the intravenous line in the numb limb after the block is placed. This allows vasodilatation due to block onset and removes the movement issues related to obtaining intravenous access in a NICU graduate. Alternatively, the intravenous line can be placed before the block, but you should anticipate a difficult intravenous line placement. Spinal and caudal forms of anesthesia as the sole anesthetic technique have been shown to reduce the incidence of postoperative apnea in previously premature infants.[1-3] The presumed length of this procedure allows for the use of a single-dose technique and should not require repeat dosing through a catheter. For a spinal anesthetic, bupivacaine or tetracaine provides an adequate duration of anesthesia. A caudal anesthetic combining 1% lidocaine and 0.5% bupivacaine can give approximately 60 minutes of surgical anesthesia. Epinephrine prolongs the duration of analgesia from single-shot caudal anesthesia. Clonidine provides improved analgesia and increased duration of the block, but it carries the risk of prolonged sedation at doses higher than 1 µg/kg, which may be a disadvantage in this patient, who is already prone to apnea and respiratory insufficiency. Although neuraxial opiates do have the potential to improve analgesia, there are disadvantages to their use. Morphine carries the risk of delayed respiratory depression, and the shorter duration of action of fentanyl may not add significantly to the analgesia of a straight local technique. Both medications may lead to other familiar side effects of opiates (e.g., nausea, vomiting, pruritus, urinary retention).

Sucrose has been used as an analgesic for minor pain in infants and newborns. The action of sucking is also calming to the hungry infant. A "sugar nipple" (historically, a whiskey nipple) consists of 4 × 4 gauze stuffed into a standard bottle nipple and soaked with a dextrose-containing solution. It should be wet enough to deliver drops when sucked on by the baby.

If you go for the whiskey option, take a good belt form the bottle before you start the case. It'll steady your nerves.

3. Can you use mask induction? What induction agent will you use? What is the risk of mask induction in a patient this age? What are the advantages of sevoflurane in this age group and with this lung pathology?

Inhalation of sevoflurane can provide rapid induction with relative cardiovascular stability. The advantage of sevoflurane is low blood solubility, providing quick onset of anesthesia and a nonirritating odor. Risks of mask induction in this age group include upper airway obstruction, which can be alleviated with the use of good mask technique or the addition of an oral airway if there is sufficient depth of anesthesia. Laryngospasm is also a potential risk if the patient is stimulated during light anesthesia. Depending on the severity of the patient's lung disease, there may be a need for prolonged postoperative ventilation if you place an ETT for the operation.

4. Can you use intravenous induction? What access will you use? When and where will you induce? Will you even be able to get an intravenous line in this infant? What are the hourly fluid needs for this child and this operation? Which fluid will you use?

Access can be obtained in the OR. Although it may be difficult to obtain intravenous access in this patient as a result of the previous stay in the NICU, it should still be possible to obtain at least a 24-gauge intravenous line, which should be sufficient for this case. An alternative is interosseous access for induction with subsequent intravenous access after the patient is asleep. Fluid management involves replacement of fluid deficits and maintenance fluid requirements. The patient will require 4 mL/kg of maintenance fluid for a total of 28 mL/hr. Insensible losses should be minimal for this type and time of procedure. Maintenance should be done in part with a 5% dextrose solution of normal saline or lactated Ringer's. The risk of a sole fluid being a glucose-containing solution is the possibility of hyperglycemia if the fluid is allowed to run open.

5. For airway management, will you use an LMA, ETT, or mask? The surgeon expects to be 35 minutes at the most.

This patient appears to have significant respiratory pathology and may have GERD given his history of prematurity. If general anesthesia is selected, the wisest course may be to secure the airway with an ETT, accepting the risk that the patient may need postoperative intubation.

6. For postoperative pain control, will you use a narcotic or caudal block? What would you use for a single-shot caudal block? What is an ilioinguinal block, and is it better or worse than other methods? What other medications would help with postoperative pain?

It should be possible and would be preferable to avoid narcotics in this patient, who is predisposed to apnea and respiratory insufficiency. A caudal block should provide adequate postoperative analgesia. Bupivacaine (0.125% to 0.25%) with epinephrine (1:200,000 or 1:400,000) will allow decreased amounts of general anesthesia and increase the duration of postoperative analgesia. The dose should be 1 mL/kg.

The ilioinguinal nerve provides sensory innervation to the inguinal area. Its blockade has been used for pain control during inguinal herniorrhaphy. This type of block provides improved pain control over general anesthesia alone, but it has not been shown to improve pain control over caudal anesthesia or to supplement general anesthesia.[4] Because this patient is having a bilateral procedure, a caudal block may be simpler and more reliable. For postoperative pain control, the patient can additionally receive rectal or oral Tylenol or Toradol (0.5 mg/kg), or both.

7. You decide to intubate so as not to lose the airway during your block and the operation. What size tube should you start with? What is a leak test, and how do you do it? Do you use a cuffed or uncuffed tube? Does the history of a 3-week intubation in the NICU worry you?

For a patient of this age and development, a 3.5-mm tube is recommended, but a size up or down should be available considering this patient's history of prolonged intubation and possible abnormalities in the airway. A leak test should be performed to determine the appropriateness of the ETT size. The leak test is performed by applying positive pressure and listening for an air leak. The leak should occur at about 15 to 25 cm H_2O. An uncuffed tube is preferred in this patient.

The history of a 3-week intubation in the NICU may suggest that the patient suffered from bronchopulmonary dysplasia, and as a result of the length of the intubation, he might have acquired subglottic stenosis.

8. What are the extubation criteria for this infant? Is a deep extubation advisable? What are the risks and benefits of a deep extubation?

If not breathing during the procedure, spontaneous respiration should be re-established. If neuromuscular blockers were administered, the adequacy of reversal should be determined because TO4 is unreliable in this group. A hip flex, lifting the legs off the table, is the standard for reversal. With this patient's probable history of bronchopulmonary dysplasia and possible reactive airway disease based on his preoperative medications, deep extubation is warranted. The risks of deep extubation include loss of the airway and laryngospasm. The ability to mask ventilate the patient during induction is reassuring as far as being able to maintain airway patency, and laryngospasm is unlikely if the extubation is done at an adequate depth of anesthesia. The benefit is a smoother emergence while minimizing the chance of aggravating the patient's reactive airway disease.

9. Give this baby a latte! What are the data regarding intraoperative caffeine in preemies having general anesthesia? What the heck does caffeine do? What is the right dose? What is the right caffeine? How much caffeine is in a cup of coffee or a shot of espresso?

Caffeine can reduce the number of apnea episodes and bradycardia events in postoperative preterm infants who require general anesthesia.[5] Caffeine is a xanthine oxidase, as are theophylline and aminophylline. Caffeine acts as a central nervous system and respiratory stimulant. A dose of 10 mg/kg has been recommended to achieve therapeutic blood levels while avoiding an increased incidence of side effects.[6] Caffeine is usually administered in the form of caffeine citrate. The average cup of coffee in the United States contains 75 mg of caffeine, but it varies widely with the type of preparation and size of cup. The average espresso contains 100 mg of caffeine.

Postoperative Questions

1. What monitors should be used in the PACU and for how long? Should this child be monitored over night? If so, which monitors should you use? Should the patient be transferred to the pediatric intensive care unit (PICU)?

The patient should be monitored by pulse oximeter and be monitored for adequate respirations with the apnea and bradycardia monitor that is used at home. Monitoring should continue throughout the hospital stay. Regardless of the type of anesthesia used, this patient is still at risk for apnea and bradycardia.

The patient should be monitored overnight with an apnea monitor and with continuous pulse oximetry. As long as adequate monitoring can be provided at a lower level of care, admission to the PICU should not be mandatory.

2. The infant is screaming in the PACU, and the nurse wants to give fentanyl. What do you want? Does all screaming indicate pain? What are the advantages of nursing and sugar for soothing infants? What are the advantages of a parent in this situation?

Assuming this patient had some form of regional anesthesia for the procedure, narcotic analgesics should not be needed and would be ill advised given his history. Irritability in this patient may reflect hunger or lack of attention. Attention by the staff may be sufficient to soothe the patient. Sugar has an analgesic effect in infants and would be appropriate in this situation. Early involvement of the parent has the advantages of a caretaker who knows how to calm the infant thereby freeing the nursing staff to attend to other needs.

3. The infant is breast-fed and will not take sugar water from a bottle. Mom wants to feed in the PACU. Now what?

Give the mother some privacy, and let the baby have what it wants, assuming that everything else is stable.

How It Actually Happened

The infant's procedure was done in the main OR with mask induction; a saphenous, 24-gauge intravenous line; and a 3.0-French ETT that leaked at 12 cm H_2O. Intravenous management was 5% dextrose in lactated Ringer's solution on a pump at 10 mL/hr, leaving about 15 to 20 mL/hr for drug delivery. A single-shot caudal was done with 7 mL of 0.125% bupivacaine and with 5 µg/mL of epinephrine (1:400,000). The baby breathed spontaneously on 2% sevoflurane, oxygen, and air for the 50-minute case. He was given 70 mg of caffeine gluconate 15 minutes before the planned extubation, which was done deep on the 2% sevoflurane. The baby was supported on 100% O_2 in the OR until awake and then transported to the PACU. He settled down without medications as soon as the mother was there, and he was allowed to breast-feed without taking clear liquids first. He spent an uneventful night in the step-down unit with an airway and breathing monitor and a pulse oximeter.

1. Somri M, Gaitini L, Vaida S, et al: Postoperative outcome in high-risk infants undergoing herniorrhaphy: Comparison between spinal and general anesthesia. Anesthesia 1998;53:762-766.
2. Coté CJ, Zaslavsky A, Downes JJ, et al: Postoperative apnea in former preterm infants after inguinal herniorrhaphy. Anesthesiology 1995;82:809-822.
3. Bouchut JC, Dubois R, Foussat C, et al: Evaluation of caudal anesthesia performed in conscious ex-premature infants for inguinal herniotomies. Paediatr Anaesth 2001;11:55-58.
4. Splinter WM, Bass J, Komocar L: Regional anesthesia for hernia repair in children: Local versus caudal anesthesia. Can J Anaesth 1995;42:197-200.
5. Welborn LG, Hannallah RS, Fink R, et al: High-dose caffeine suppresses postoperative apnea in former preterm infants. Anesthesiology 1989;71:347-349.
6. Aranda JV, Gorman W, Bergsteinsson H, Gunn T: Efficacy of caffeine in treatment of apnea in the low-birth-weight infant. J Pediatr 1977;90:467-472.

We threw in references here because some people are a little rusty on kiddie things. Caveat emptor: These references are a little old, so Medline search some more recent stuff if you have questions.

CASE 26: HELLP, I NEED SOMEBODY

Preoperative Questions

1. What is HELLP?
HELLP syndrome is a subclassification of preeclampsia and is characterized by hemolytic anemia, elevated liver enzymes, and low platelets. The incidence is 1 case in 1000 pregnancies, and it affects about 10% to 20% of severely preeclamptic women. It is a sign of severe disease and an indication for prompt delivery.

2. Is the fetal heart rate normal?
Normal fetal heart rate falls within a range of 120 to 160 beats/min, so 110 is a little slow (technically fetal bradycardia), but the poor beat-to-beat variability and the frequent late decelerations are more concerning.

3. What are late decelerations? What is their significance?
Late decelerations are classically described as the nadir of fetal heart rate deceleration occurring after the peak of contraction. This phenomenon occurs when there is uteroplacental insufficiency.

4. What is the number one determinant of fetal well-being?
The number one determinant of fetal well-being is the presence of fetal heart rate variability.

5. Should the case be delayed until the patient is NPO for 8 hours? Why or why not?
This particular case should not be delayed, and prompt delivery should occur because this fetus is already showing signs of distress with the late decelerations and poor beat-to-beat variability.

6. Is there any information from the history and physical examination that you need to obtain before proceeding with the cesarean section?
As with any delivery, a history should be obtained and physical examination should be done before administering any anesthetic. In this case, a focused examination should take place, and it should include the medical history, surgical history (including anesthetic-related problems), medications, allergies, illicit drug use, history of easy bruising or prolonged bleeding, ability to lie supine, height, weight, *airway*, heart, and lungs.

7. What is your anesthetic plan and why?
I would plan to perform a spinal anesthetic using 12 mg of hyperbaric bupivacaine, 10 µg of fentanyl, and 2 mg of Duramorph, (morphine) for postoperative analgesia. Although the platelet number is abnormally low because of the HELLP syndrome, I think a spinal anesthetic would be safer given her edematous airway and full stomach. I would have ready all the necessary items for managing a difficult airway in case the spinal fails.

8. Suppose you had chosen to perform a spinal anesthetic. Describe your preload fluid management.

Despite preeclampsia being a state of exaggerated fluid and sodium retention, these patients tend to be hypovolemic because of the shift of fluids and proteins to the extravascular compartment. Judicious fluid boluses are necessary, and colloids rather than crystalloids are probably more appropriate for achieving this. I would carefully titrate fluid to maintain urine output.

9. Would you treat the patient's blood pressure listed above preoperatively, and if yes, how?

Regional anesthetic techniques are expected to lower the blood pressure of the recipient as the sympathectomy ensues. I would not lower the blood pressure with antihypertensive agents before the spinal.

10. What monitoring would you use for this patient and why?

I would apply standard ASA monitors.

Intraoperative Questions

1. A spinal anesthetic is performed. Brisk bleeding occurs at the spinal insertion site after the needle is withdrawn. What would you do?

I noticed this brisk bleeding on withdrawal of the needle after administering the intrathecal anesthetic. In this case, the most likely cause of the bleeding is from a subcutaneous blood vessel, and it is unlikely to be tracking all the way from the dura to the skin. Prompt application of a pressure dressing would be appropriate because prolonged point compression would be unlikely to tamponade any epidural bleeding, and any delay in lying my patient flat may result in a saddle block, rendering my risky regional technique useless and putting me one step closer to choosing a general anesthetic in this unpleasant setting.

2. Three minutes after the spinal anesthetic is placed, the blood pressure drops to 70/40 mm Hg. What do you do?

I would initially treat the hypotension with ephedrine boluses and carefully administer additional intravenous fluid. I would follow this with boluses of phenylephrine if no effect was observed.

3. There is no improvement in the blood pressure after several boluses of ephedrine, phenylephrine, and fluid. What do you do?

I assume that the parturient's uterus is already being displaced to the left, but if possible, I would defy any laws of gravity and attempt to further displace with more leftward rotation of the table. If the parturient's abdomen were open at this point, I would ask the obstetrician to lift the uterus in an attempt to take more pressure off the inferior vena cava and further increase the patient's preload. The patient is most likely not prepped at this point, so I would attempt to lift up the fetus manually or ask the obstetrician to do so to relieve any inferior vena cava obstruction from the gravid uterus.

4. As the obstetricians are closing the uterus, the patient suddenly complains of chest pain. Her respiratory rate is 24 breaths/min. Pulse oximetry shows a level of 95%, but it was 99% earlier. There is a 2-mm ST depression in leads II and V_5. What is your differential diagnosis and the most likely diagnosis? How do you respond?

Chest pain in this setting can be attributed to a multitude of different causes. The most likely is venous air embolism. The differential can include venous thromboembolism, amniotic fluid embolism, pulmonary edema, myocardial ischemia or infarction, aortic dissection, or referred pain from exteriorization of the uterus. In any event, the ABCs are always the first approach to management. The first step is to administer 100% F_{IO_2} and maintain the airway.

5. After 50 minutes, the obstetricians are still operating and the patient complains of incisional pain. What do you do?

At this point in the case, the baby should be delivered and appropriately handled by the NICU team. If the mother is feeling pain, small doses of analgesics can be titrated to improve her comfort level. Fast-acting opiates such as fentanyl can achieve this. Ketamine can also be used as an adjunct, and it has the advantage of not suppressing respirations. Forty percent nitrous oxide can be used for analgesia. My analgesic plan would include keeping her awake to minimize the risk of aspiration.

Postoperative Management

1. After 1 hour in the recovery room, the patient has had no urine output. Urine output was only 50 mL intraoperatively. What do you do?

Causes for decreased urine output are prerenal, renal, and postrenal. If a Foley catheter has been placed, it is easy to rule out potential causes of obstruction such as a kinked catheter. Renal failure may be attributed to this patient's relative hypotension after the spinal anesthetic was administered. Prerenal causes are probably most likely. Initially suspecting hypovolemia, I would treat the oliguria with fluid boluses. Colloid would probably be better than crystalloid because of its better ability to remain intravascular.

2. The urine output does not improve after fluid boluses. What is your differential diagnosis? How do you respond?

After aggressive fluid management, intrinsic renal failure should become higher on your differential diagnosis list. It can be a complication of the patient's severe preeclampsia or a result from prolonged hypotension. At this point, an assessment of the patient's volume status is appropriate, and I would place a central line. Because there is a poor correlation between central venous pressure and pulmonary capillary wedge pressure (PCWP) in patients with preeclampsia, I would place a Swan-Ganz catheter. If a cardiologist was readily available, I would obtain a bedside transthoracic echocardiogram.

3. You place a Swan-Ganz catheter, and the PCWP is 48 mm Hg. What do you do?

A PCWP measurement of 48 mm Hg is severely elevated. Initially, I would attempt to diurese this patient with a loop diuretic. If it fails, the patient may need emergent hemodialysis to relieve the volume overload. I'd also make sure the transducer hadn't fallen on the ground.

4. The patient becomes very lethargic and weak. What is the differential diagnosis, and how do you respond?

The differential diagnosis for being lethargic and weak is just about endless, but items on top of this list include congestive heart failure and magnesium toxicity.

Lower on the differential list are hypotension, hypoxia, hypothermia, sedative medications, and stroke. I would check the patient's vital signs, looking for extremes in blood pressure and hypoxia. I would confirm that there is no magnesium sulfate infusion running, and send a sample for measurement of the magnesium level. I would also review the medications that the patient has received. If the patient developed respiratory weakness, I would administer calcium chloride. If the patient still had no urine output, I would call for immediate dialysis.

5. List the systemic magnesium levels at which a patient will lose the deep tendon reflex, have respiratory arrest, and have cardiac arrest.

At a magnesium level of 10 mEq/L, deep tendon reflexes are lost. Respiratory depression occurs at 12 to 15 mEq/L, respiratory arrest can occur at 15 mEq/L, and cardiac arrest occurs at 20 to 25 mEq/L.

How It Actually Happened

The patient looked as if she would be quite difficult to intubate and ventilate. Although her platelet level was 71,000, she did not have any signs or symptoms of prolonged bleeding. We thought there would be less morbidity and less delay with a spinal, and that is what we did. We planned to closely observe her neurologic function postoperatively to detect an epidural hematoma if one occurred. She received approximately 700 mL of lactated Ringer' solution before spinal placement, but we did not delay just to have that preload infused.

When we saw the brisk bleeding from the spinal site, we did become more anxious about development of a spinal hematoma. Our plan to closely monitor her postoperatively, even if it meant staying awake and checking her every 15 minutes, was unchanged.

The hypotension that was unresponsive to vasopressors (i.e., ephedrine and phenylephrine), fluids, and exaggerated tilt position suddenly improved by lifting the gravid uterus manually. The inferior vena cava must have been severely obstructed despite the left tilt. We considered inaccurate drug preparation because our vasopressors are made daily by the residents. However, this would be unlikely with two types of drugs. Our plan would have been to give a small bolus of epinephrine (maybe 2 µg) if the severe hypotension continued. Luckily, she did not have hypertension after the obstruction was relieved and the vasopressors were able to circulate.

The chest pain looked like a venous air embolism because it occurred with exteriorization of the uterus and was treated effectively with 100% O_2 and intravenous fentanyl for the pain. The ECG changes promptly normalized. We gave additional intravenous fentanyl and 40% N_2O for the incisional pain, and we asked the attending to finish closing to expedite the case. The patient was still awake but comfortable.

The postoperative oliguria was treated with intravenous fluids. Her level of magnesium sulfate decreased. After 2500 mL of lactated Ringer's solution, we heard faint crackles on lung examination. We gave Lasix (10 mg), with no response. We then placed a Swan-Ganz catheter and saw the huge PCWP. Additional Lasix and dopamine were started, with no response. She began getting shortness of breath, and the pulse oximeter reading was 92% on 100% oxygen by nonrebreathing mask. She said that she felt weak and had minimal or no deep tendon reflexes. We called for a fiberoptic scope just in case we needed to intubate her. Her airway was now Mallampati class 4; her lips, tongue, and face were extremely swollen. A renal specialist was called for immediate dialysis, and the magnesium level was 12. The patient was given intravenous calcium chloride and then underwent dialysis. She did well but remained in acute renal failure for 2 weeks.

CASE 27: OBSTETRICS AND A BAD AIRWAY

Preoperative Questions

1. What other laboratory tests or history would you like?
The history and physical examination should determine how well the patient's asthma is controlled (well or bad) and whether there have been recent PFTs. You should find out whether this is chronic or pregnancy-induced hypertension and whether it has been controlled well.

Symptoms, such as headache, visual changes, urinary symptoms, or HELLP, should be sought. You should know the history of previous pregnancies (e.g., HELLP syndrome, other complications) and her history of previous exposures to anesthesia and whether there have been complications. Determine whether the patient has allergies and her NPO status (because of the cesarean section). Obtain vital signs, including pulse oximetry and orthostatic blood pressure.

Examine her airway, and perform focused physical examinations (e.g., cardiac, pulmonary). Laboratory tests should include blood type and crossmatch, a chem-7 panel, complete blood cell count, PT, PTT, and INR.

Regarding the asthma, you want to know when the last asthma attack was and how often she takes the albuterol. Has she ever been to the ER, or has she ever been intubated because of her asthma? Has she taken any steroids in the past year for her asthma? Most parturients do better with their asthma during pregnancy. Progesterone relaxes the bronchial smooth muscle. I do not think she needs PFTs.

Another important point in this scenario is why this patient had a cesarean section. Was this a repeat cesarean section, was it failure to progress, or was it preeclampsia becoming severe?

2. How would you premedicate this patient?
The patient is obese, pregnant (just had a cesarean section), and postoperative (i.e., ileus). I think I read somewhere that parturients are considered to be full stomachs up to 14 weeks after delivery. I would consider her to have a full stomach and to be at risk for pulmonary aspiration. I would give her prophylactic Bicitra (increases the pH of existing gastric content but also slightly increases the gastric volume), an H_2-blocker (reduces gastric volume and pH but has no effect on the existing gastric content), and metoclopramide (increases gastric emptying, decreases volume, and increases lower esophageal sphincter tone). Considering her potentially very difficult airway, I would minimize the use of sedatives to maintain her airway.

3. Would you do regional or general anesthesia for this case?
According to question 4, she still has the epidural from the labor and cesarean section. If it is still working properly, I would go with a regional using the epidural. This patient is very obese and pregnant, and she probably has a very difficult airway. She is also at risk for aspiration. If she can maintain her own airway and gag reflex, I think that would be best. However, this patient is also

at risk for moderate to severe blood loss and other complications (e.g., DIC) intraoperatively, and she may need general anesthesia, depending on the course. I would make sure to have an LMA, a cart ready for a difficult airway, and extra hands in case I need help!

Most epidurals after delivery or a cesarean section come out, unless the patient is going to have a tubal ligation shortly after the delivery. There is no correct answer to this. You can do a regional or a general as long as you can back it up. You can argue that because the patient has a difficult airway, you could consider securing the airway right up front because you do not want to have to intubate emergently. You could do a spinal and epidural, but your regional may not work, and you may get a high level. You also can argue that this is a dilation and curettage (D&C) and you may want to stay away from the airway.

4. If you choose regional, would you do a spinal or an epidural? The patient did have a labor epidural, which was used for the cesarean section.

Can we use the epidural that she already has (assuming it is still working properly)? Spinal anesthesia has more rapid onset and more solid anesthesia, but if we can wait to confirm the adequate anesthesia from the epidural, I would go with it. However, you can do either. If the patient had an epidural and still had a residual block, you may want to stay away from a spinal. If there is still some local anesthetic left in the epidural space, it may find its way into the subarachnoid space when performing the spinal and result in a high spinal block. Because this patient had 18 hours in between her last operation and this one, I do not think that is a concern.

5. Is this patient considered NPO?

No. Regardless of the time of the last oral intake, pregnant patients should be considered to have a full stomach and to be at risk for pulmonary aspiration. This patient is morbidly obese (BMI = 48) and postoperative (possible ileus); both increase the risk of aspiration.

Intraoperative Questions

1. You chose to do a spinal. What local anesthetic are you planning to use? What are the downfalls of using lidocaine?

Either 5% lidocaine (75 to 100 mg) or 0.75% bupivacaine (10 to 15 mg) in 8.25% dextrose would usually be sufficient for this type of procedure (D&C). Epinephrine (0.1 mg) can enhance the quality of the block and may prolong the duration of bupivacaine. Adding 12.5 to 25 µg of fentanyl or 5 to 10 µg of sufentanil to the local anesthetics enhances the intensity of the block (requires a lower amount of local anesthetics) and prolongs its duration. The downfalls of lidocaine, especially 5% lidocaine, would be transient neurologic symptoms and cauda equina syndrome.

2. You decided to do spinal anesthesia. It worked beautifully, but the surgeon cannot control the bleeding with a simple D&C. The surgeon must open the belly and possibly do a hysterectomy. Do you continue the spinal or convert to a general anesthesia?

I would convert to a general anesthesia at this point. She is bleeding profusely, which could later compromise her hemodynamics, the case may go on for the next few hours, and the spinal may wear off. However, be careful because this patient has a difficult airway. The safest thing to do is an awake fiberoptic procedure, although it may not be easy. This case occurred at 2 AM, when there was minimal help around, and this may not be easy to do on a patient who is bleeding and when the surgeon cannot wait for 30 minutes while you are fooling around with the fiberoptic scope.

3. You decided to continue with the spinal. The surgery is taking more than 3 hours, and the patient is starting to feel the pain. What is your next move?
Convert to general anesthesia if the case is going to be longer. If the surgical team is closing, you can use 10 to 20 mg of intravenous ketamine (also good for asthma). While they are closing, you can ask the surgeon to be generous with the local anesthetic.

4. You have to put the patient to sleep. How do you do it?
You have two options: an awake fiberoptic intubation or RSI. RSI (propofol and suxamethonium) with cricoid pressure was chosen for this case. In anticipation of a difficult airway, I would have a difficult airway cart available in the room. I would also make sure to have an LMA, be able to do transtracheal jet ventilation, and have extra hands for help.

5. You did an RSI with propofol and suxamethonium tube. You cannot intubate. You could barely ventilate with two people. What is your next step?
Secure the airway with an LMA, and call for more help. Try to intubate through the LMA. After the patient is awake, do an awake fiberoptic intubation. If you can ventilate through an LMA, you can secure the airway by means of the fibroptic scope through the LMA. A regular 5 LMA takes a 6.0 ETT; a 4 LMA takes a 5.5 ETT. You go through the LMA with a fiberoptic scope into the trachea and guide the ETT over the fiberoptic scope.

6. While you are attempting to intubate the patient, she is bucking. The surgeon wants you to paralyze her right away. What do you tell the surgeon?
I would tell them to stop the procedures for now and say that we have not been able to secure the patient's airway and therefore cannot paralyze the patient at this point. I would tell the surgeon there is no point in operating on a dead human being.

7. The surgeon tells you that the patient is oozing. He wants you to give FFP. What is your response?
I would say, "Okay, let me talk to my attending." Try that just once for laughs with a real examiner! While everyone is busting a gut, go online and book a flight to next year's exam.

If you do not have any laboratory tests results (e.g., PT, PTT, INR, hematocrit, platelets) at this point, obtain them. The patient may be oozing because of coagulopathy, DIC, thrombocytopenia, or platelet dysfunction. This patient has received regional anesthesia before, so I assume her laboratory test results were normal preoperatively. Transfusing FFP may be a good idea, but the patient may also need platelets and cryoprecipitate (if she has DIC).

How It Actually Happened

This case was the talk of the town the next morning when the patient came down with the LMA still in and a skinny ETT sticking out. All were glad they had not been there when it happened, but everyone expressed admiration for the quick thinking that saved the day! Of course, it happened in the middle of the night with no one around.

She survived, and the next day, they changed the tube over a changer with the ear, nose, and throat specialist standing by, sword in hand. Whew!

CASE 28: ON CALL IN LABOR AND DELIVERY

Preoperative Questions

1. Do you establish a mutually agreed on plan for anesthesia with the obstetrician and the patient?

Yes and no. General anesthesia has a higher death rate (16 times, but who's counting?) than regional anesthesia. Throw in a horrific airway and a truly enormous patient, and you are heading into the land of no return. This is one case in which I would steer the patient toward a regional.

2. If so, how do you proceed? The obstetrician is waiting and wants to start the pitocin.

This is so bad and scary that I would take up the largest epidural needle in the world and give it another go myself.

3. There is an incomplete preoperative chart written by the day team. What do you do to evaluate the situation?

Round up the usual suspects, looking for signs of coagulopathy and heart or lung disease. Do all the things you usually do preoperatively. Given her size, you should also look for signs of sleep apnea; she is a candidate.

4. Epidurals are usually done with a 17-gauge, 3.5-inch Tuohy-Schliff needle. Would you want an alternative?

Yes. I want a longer one.

5. Would you want any additional equipment in the vicinity? If so, what items?

I want every airway gadget imaginable and the most important piece of equipment, another anesthesiologist with good hands, even if that meant getting someone from his or her home.

6. After the patient is in labor for about 15 hours, the obstetrician plans to do a cesarean section because of failure to progress. There is still no epidural. What do you do?

Try again, and get someone else to try again. You really do not want to do this under general anesthesia.

7. You have been attempting for about 2 hours without success? What do you do?

Proceed with an awake intubation.

8. After 2.5 hours and many attempts, cerebrospinal fluid flows out of the Touhy. Do you place a spinal anesthetic or still try for an epidural?

Well, that is not the end of the world. Slip the catheter in and use it as a continuous spinal.

9. The obstetrician is getting very impatient; it is the wee hours of the morning now, and she would like to get started. What do you do?

Tell her to cool her jets and read *Plaintiff Quarterly* if she wants to know what is in store if we rush.

10. The fetal heart rate should be checked how often?

It should be checked continuously after she is on the floor.

11. What are the two components of the fetal heart rate monitor?

The components are rate and pattern. You are always keeping an eye on the absolute rate (lower than 100 is the same as asystole to a baby!), and you are looking at the heart rate's relation to contractions.

12. Is it better to have a Doppler transducer or a Fetal Scalp Electrode?

Doppler is noninvasive and tells you what is going on all the time. A scalp electrode is invasive (has caused intracranial hemorrhages in babies!). Better to go with the Doppler.

13. What is the normal baseline fetal heart rate?

The normal rate is between 120 and 160, with baseline variability.

14. What is the difference between an early and a late deceleration?

Early decelerations are U-shaped depressions in the fetal heart rate pattern, usually not going below 100 beats/min, and are associated with the onset of contractions. This is usually associated with head compression and is "no biggie."

Late decelerations are also U-shaped depressions, but they occur 20 to 30 seconds after the onset of uterine contractions. They are associated with uteroplacental insufficiency and are cause for concern. Fix bayonets! Time for a normal spontaneous cesarean delivery!

15. Describe the management for fetal distress.

Management includes left uterine displacement and fluid and pressor resuscitation to restore flow to the pressure-dependent placental bed. If this does not work, supplemental O_2 is used, and the mother's position (knee to chest) is changed. Turn off anything that may be increasing contractions (e.g., pitocin), and give terbutaline to relax the uterus and re-establish flow. If none of this works, cut!

16. The obstetrician begins to worry about neonatal apnea. Can you state the difference between primary and secondary apnea?

Primary apnea occurs after the initial attempts to breathe (stimulation or tapping the feet can cause resumption of breathing). Secondary apnea occurs with continued oxygen deprivation; the baby gasps several times and then enters secondary apnea (stimulation does not restart breathing).

17. Define Apgar score.

Apgar is a scoring system for evaluating a newborn. It was developed by our very own Virginia Apgar! Go anesthesia! It gives a 0, 1, or 2 score for the following:

- Heart rate
- Respiratory effort

- Muscle tone
- Reflex irritability
- Insurance status (just threw that in to make sure you are paying attention)
- Color

How It Actually Happened

The patient was actually much larger than 450 pounds, which was an understatement. One area of the chart stated 600++. A mutually agreed on plan is of the utmost importance. The chart also mentioned that the day team had tried many times to get an epidural and place an intravenous line.

The first concern is to check the patient's airway in case she does have a cesarean section. Although multiple attempts for an epidural were made, I felt it necessary to try and get an epidural in this morbidly obese patient, as well as obtain large-bore intravenous access. This was discussed with the obstetrics department attending. The obstetrics attending then left, and a new attending took over. The plan for an epidural was discussed again. Communication is important among team members, especially because they must understand the possibility of a difficult airway or difficult intravenous access.

Attempts were made again without success. Damn! The difficult airway box was checked along with the availability for the fiberoptic scope. You should use what you are most comfortable with and have that available in the OR. The other attending in house was made aware but stated that he was unable to help if there was a need for a cesarean section. Many hours later, the obstetrician stated that this woman would need a section for failure to progress. Persistence truly paid off after about 2.5 hours of attempts for an epidural.

A pearl for obese patients: The excess soft tissue was taped up to help visualize the back. This was a much-needed intervention. It made a world of difference compared with attempting without the tape. Do not underestimate the importance of this taping. A crisscross "v" with tape was made, and the area was prepped with povidone-iodine. There was not a bed able to accommodate her weight, so this attempt was done on her bed from the labor and delivery department.

It was also necessary to have the longer Touhy needle. We had various sizes available, and the one that was successful was almost harpoon-like according to the nurse who was assisting me. The fetal heart rate was checked many times, and it was fine. A Doppler transducer was used at first, and then because it was taking a while to obtain an anesthetic, a fetal scalp electrode was placed. The fetal scalp electrode is most accurate. The cervix does need to be dilated 3 cm for its use, and membranes must be ruptured for use.

A cardiotachometer uses the peak or threshold voltage of the fetal r wave to measure the interval between each fetal cardiac cycle. There was good fetal heart rate baseline variability (fluctuations in the baseline of 2 cycles/min). The normal baseline fetal heart rate remained 140 to 150 beats/min. This gave me the leisure to continue epidural attempts. A spinal was purposefully done with the epidural needle because the epidural space was unable to be located.

The case began with our slowest obstetrician in the hospital. At the 1.5-hour mark, I suggested that we get another obstetrician to help, or my anesthetic would run out. This was a serious worry because the patient had a class

3 or 4 airway. The patient was operated on a regular bed that did not go up and down and managed to have an anesthetic that did last.

She did not even get a post-dural puncture headache. The baby girl had Apgar scores of 9 and 9. The Apgar scores signify the heart rate, respiratory effort, muscle tone, reflex irritability, and color. Measurements are made at 1 and 5 minutes (<7, then continue every 5 minutes up to 20 minutes). There are limitations to our magnificent Apgar. It is useful in predicting short-term mortality for groups of infants with low birth weight, but it has a low predictive value for the survival of an individual.

This baby was not in distress and did not have any apnea. As one of the senior anesthesiologists who trained me stated, "It is better to be lucky than good."

CASE 29: WINDOW TO MY SOUL

Preoperative Questions

1. What is a therapeutic range for an INR? Why do heart valve patients have to take anticoagulants? What happens if they do not take their anticoagulants? What if they take medications that interfere with their anticoagulants or potentiate them?

Patients with prosthetic heart valves require anticoagulation because of increased risk for thromboemboli after valve replacement. According to the ACC/AHA guidelines, antithrombotic therapy for heart valve replacement should be individualized based on the patient's clinical status and risk factors. Patient risk factors include atrial fibrillation, left ventricular dysfunction, previous thromboembolism, and a hypercoagulable state. All patients with mechanical heart valves require anticoagulation. The INR should be maintained between 2.0 and 3.0 for aortic bileaflet and Medtronic Hall valves and maintained between 2.5 and 3.5 for mechanical mitral valves, aortic disk valves, and Starr-Edwards valves. In patients with mechanical aortic valves who are at high risk for thromboembolic complications, the INR should be maintained between 2.5 and 3.5. For bioprosthetic valves, medications should be given to maintain an INR between 2.0 and 3.0 for the first 3 months in low-risk patients and lifelong therapy (INR between 2.0 and 3.0) given for high-risk patients. For patients taking medications that interfere or potentiate anticoagulants, the INR should be monitored closely to make sure that it is in the appropriate range.

2. What are the potential sources of pericardial effusion? What other conditions manifest like this? What are the physiologic effects of a rapid fluid buildup or a slow fluid buildup? What other physical signs will you look for?

Potential sources for this pericardial effusion include infection (viral or bacterial), idiopathic causes, uremia, dissecting aortic aneurysm, acute MI, recent cardiac surgery, drug-induced conditions (including anticoagulant therapy), and air. The speed of accumulation of a pericardial effusion determines the physiologic importance; slow buildup of a large effusion (>1000 mL) may produce no hemodynamic effect. However, a small effusion that develops rapidly may cause tamponade. Other physical findings of fluid buildup include friction rub, hypotension, tachycardia, tachypnea, narrow pulse pressure, pulsus paradoxus, and jugular venous distention due to increased central venous pressure.

3. The transthoracic echocardiogram (TTE) shows a pericardial effusion. What "windows" does TTE have? Compare it with TEE? Do you need TEE before you begin? Why or why not? What will TEE add?

Echo windows are standard positions on the chest wall for transducer placement that allow good ultrasound penetration without significant interference from ribs and lung tissue. Windows for a TTE include suprasternal, right parasternal, left parasternal, apical, and subcostal positions. A TEE has esophageal and upper gastric windows. In this patient, a TEE done before the surgery can provide more information about the prosthetic valve. It can help determine the adequacy of valve replacement, evaluate flow characteristics across the valve, and diagnose thrombus on the valve that may not be seen on a TTE.

4. This man had a heart operation 3 weeks earlier. Can you anticipate any problems related to his recent surgery? What will you look for in the anesthetic record? What will you do if you cannot find the old anesthetic record?

Complications related to recent aortic valve replacement include thromboemboli formation, infection, bleeding, stroke, arrhythmia, and MI. Old anesthetic records are useful if a TEE was done during the procedure to evaluate the prosthetic valve after its placement. Old anesthetic records can give information about other cardiac and anesthetic complications during the procedure.

Intraoperative Questions

1. The man talks in complete sentences and can lie flat. Do you need an arterial line before induction? Why? Are there other options for beat-to-beat blood pressure measurement? What are the advantages and disadvantages of each?

This patient presented with symptoms of shortness of breath and inability to sleep flat at night, which suggested left ventricular dysfunction. Anesthetic induction can lead to significant changes in the hemodynamics. An arterial line should be placed before induction to monitor beat-to-beat changes in systemic arterial pressure and for obtaining blood gases. Arterial tonometry produces tracings similar to an arterial line waveform, but it is limited by sensitivity to movement artifact and the need for frequent calibrations. A central venous catheter can be placed to monitor CVP, which approximates right atrial pressure, a major determinant of right ventricular end-diastolic volume, and it can be used to guide intraoperative fluid management. However, the range for normal values is large, and small changes in CVP can mean significant changes in blood volume. A pulmonary artery catheter can be used to estimate left ventricular preload and cardiac output, sample mixed venous blood, and detect air embolism and myocardial ischemia. Pulmonary artery catheters can cause arrhythmia, ventricular fibrillation, heart block, and pulmonary artery rupture. There can be misinterpretation of data obtained from the pulmonary artery catheter. ECG and TEE are also useful in the assessment of hemodynamic status.

2. You have a 20-gauge intravenous line in that runs pretty well. Do you need more volume access before induction? Can you wait and "put in a 16"

after induction? How about a central line? Which kind will you use? The surgeon says, "This will be real quick." Will his statement affect your actions?

Even though the patient has a 20-gauge intravenous line, a large-bore intravenous line should be placed. After another intravenous line is placed, a central line can be placed after induction. If you decide to have a central line, an introducer should be placed so that, if needed, a pulmonary artery catheter can be placed for cardiac monitoring. Even if the surgeon says that the surgery will be quick, a second large-bore intravenous line (besides the 20-gauge intravenous line already in place) should be placed.

Note: You can always "debate and disagree" as you read these answers. For example, you may argue against a Swan.

3. Can you do this case under local anesthesia with sedation? How? In what cases would you prefer to do this under local? What physical findings tip you to "really bad tamponade physiology" compared with "this is no big deal"?

Local anesthesia may be used in a patient who is undergoing simple drainage through a subxiphoid approach. However, patients who are undergoing a left thoracotomy or median sternotomy require general anesthesia with endotracheal intubation. Findings suggestive of "really bad" tamponade physiology include difficulty lying flat, tachycardia, tachypnea, and narrow pulse pressure.

4. You go with sedation, but as the surgeon progresses, he "drifts left" and causes a pneumothorax (you can see the lung). What physiologic changes can you anticipate? Because this is "open to air," will the patient be any worse off? Compare a tension and a nontension pneumothorax.

Physiologic changes associated with pneumothorax may include decreased vital capacity and tidal volume, decreased venous return to the heart, increased peak and plateau pressures, and hypoxia. In this patient, a tension pneumothorax could develop and lead to further deterioration in the cardiopulmonary status (e.g., hypoxemia, hypotension).

Tension pneumothorax is a pneumothorax in which intrapleural pressure is positive throughout the respiratory cycle. Positive pleural pressure can be life-threatening because ventilation is severely compromised, and the positive pressure is transmitted to the mediastinum, which results in decreased venous return to the heart and reduced cardiac output. A spontaneous pneumothorax occurs without antecedent trauma to the thorax. Primary and secondary spontaneous pneumothoraces occur in the absence or presence of an underlying pulmonary disease. A traumatic pneumothorax results from penetrating or nonpenetrating chest injuries. Treatment modalities are based on the type of pneumothorax.

5. How will you induce in this "not so bad" pericardial window patient? How would this differ from the patient who is in "a bad way"? Would you use ketamine, etomidate, or propofol?

Ketamine should be considered for induction for this patient in a "not so bad" or a "bad" situation. Large doses of ketamine should be avoided because of myocardiac depressant effects. For a situation in which general anesthesia with endotracheal intubation is required, pancuronium's circulatory effects make it a useful muscle relaxant. However, succinylcholine can also be used for intubation. Etomidate has minimal effects on the cardiovascular system but causes a mild decrease in mean arterial pressure due to a decrease in peripheral vascular resistance. Etomidate should be avoided in a severely hypotensive patient. Propofol should be avoided because it can decrease blood pressure, cardiac contractility, preload, and cardiac output, and it can cause bradycardia.

6. You induce without an arterial line and are surprised that the cuff is taking so long to cycle. How does a blood pressure cuff work? How long will it take to let you know there is no pressure or a pressure of 300 mm Hg? Is there any other way to "get the pressure faster"?

The blood pressure device used in the OR monitors the oscillating signal generated in the cuff by changes in arterial pressure. Initially, the cuff inflates to above systolic pressure, which leads to a loss of signal and oscillations. The cuff then deflates gradually in a stepwise manner. The pressure at which the original signal reappears is systolic pressure, and the point at which the signal amplitude is the largest is the mean arterial pressure. Diastolic blood pressure is calculated mathematically from the systolic and the mean arterial pressures. The time needed to get the blood pressure reading depends on the size, location, and proper placement of the cuff. An arterial line monitor measures pressure in real time and gives faster results.

7. The cuff gives you a pressure of 74/40 mm Hg, but the heart rate is still 53 beats/min. How will you treat this? Will you use splash and slash and get in right away? Will you use Neo-Synephrine, ephedrine, or epinephrine?

Hypotension and bradycardia should be treated with ephedrine. Ephedrine, with cardiovascular effects similar to epinephrine, can lead to an increase in blood pressure, heart rate, cardiac contractility, and cardiac output. Neo-Synephrine (phenylephrine), a predominantly α_1-receptor agonist (causes peripheral vasoconstriction with increase in arterial blood pressure), should be avoided because it can cause reflex bradycardia and decreased cardiac output. Epinephrine, an α_1-, β_1-, and β_2-receptor stimulant, can cause decreased systemic vascular resistance with an increase in heart rate and myocardial contractility. This leads to increased cardiac output with no significant increase in arterial blood pressure.

8. You give Neo-Synephrine, and the heart rate falls to 29 beats/min. What is your response to this? What is the reason for the drop? What is the interaction with β-blockers?

The patient's heart rate decreased most likely because of reflex bradycardia as a result of peripheral vasoconstriction caused by Neo-Synephrine. The patient should be given an anticholinergic such as atropine or glycopyrrolate in this situation. The onset of atropine is faster than glycopyrrolate, and it may be a better choice in this scenario. Patients taking β-antagonists may require higher doses of anticholinergics. Atropine is the initial drug recommended for treatment of signs of excessive blockade by β-antagonists.

9. While the surgeon is digging his finger under the sternum, you see unifocal ectopy. What is the reason for this? Do you need a blood gas determination? If a test showed a potassium level of 3.4 mEq/L and you have only peripheral lines, should you replete the potassium? How? How fast? Should you give antiarrhythmic therapy in the meantime?

Causes of unifocal ectopy include hyperkalemia or hypokalemia, hypomagnesemia, hypercarbia, hypoxemia, and myocardial irritation. A blood gas test would be helpful in determining whether hypercarbia or hypoxemia is responsible for the unifocal ectopy. If the patient has only peripheral lines, potassium can be supplemented at 10 mEq/hr. With a central line, the rate of supplementation can be increased to 20 mEq/hr. At this time, requesting the surgeon to stop the stimulus may be adequate. If ectopy continues despite lack of stimulation, antiarrhythmic therapy may be considered.

10. The surgeon says he needs to do a small left thoracotomy to get at the effusion. How do you respond? Do you add more lines? What are your postoperative ventilation plans now? What if the surgeon asks for lung isolation?

General anesthesia with endotracheal intubation is required for this procedure. If the patient already has an arterial line and large-bore intravenous lines, no further lines may be required before induction. Postoperative ventilation plans should be based on the patient's cardiac and pulmonary stability. For lung isolation, a double-lumen endobronchial tube or a single-lumen ETT with a movable endobronchial blocker may be used.

How It Actually Happened

I must live wrong because I see cases like this one. Talk about the immediacy of this book! Here I sit at 7:20 AM on Halloween morning in the middle of writing my portion of *Board Stiff Three*. This case happened last night at 6 PM. This morning, I bolted awake in a cold sweat at 1:56 AM, reliving the reflex bradycardia that scared the bejeebers out of me during this case. This is a scary profession!

This guy came to us looking the best I have ever seen for any pericardial window. He was joking around and talking in full sentences. He had a fit, "still does a lot of work" physique. When we moved him to the table, he was able to lie flat and keep talking. Pretty good!

The surgeon was around (always a good idea with a window, just in case things get spooky). We induced with a 20-gauge line and used etomidate. His blood pressure was 120/86 mm Hg before induction and 117/75 mm Hg after induction.

I had a tough time getting the arterial line, but while struggling with that, I put in a 16-gauge line. The pressure dipped a little with some "anesthetica imperfecta" to the 70s. I gave a little Neo-Synephrine, and sure enough, monster bradycardia arose. Reflex bradycardia resulted from the Neo-Synephrine, and his on-board β-blockade was not helping much. At a rate of 29 beats/min, you damn near see entire screens of flat line! Stupid me; I should have given ephedrine, especially with the "full, fast, forward" mantra of tamponade.

In no time, I gave ephedrine, pushed some glycopyrrolate, and things straightened out. However, it was one of those scary things (and dumb things!) that happen when you do this crazy thing called anesthesia. Maybe I should have kept my old job as an exotic male dancer.

CASE 30: A MASSIVE PROBLEM THAT SNUCK UP ON US

Preoperative Questions

1. What is the differential diagnosis for the causes of widening of the anterior mediastinum?

- Recurrence of thymoma (would be number one on my list)
- Aortic aneurysm
- Esophageal rupture
- Chagas disease (*Trypanosoma cruzi*)
- Pericardial tamponade
- Inhalation anthrax

2. How do you proceed?

Obtain a CT scan with intravenous contrast.

3. The CT scan shows compression of the tracheobronchial tree in the region of the carina. There is possibly a 40% compression. What else will you do?

Because a plain CT scan is not very sensitive in terms of picking up obstruction, I would consider the following:

- High-resolution CT with three-dimensional airway reconstruction
- Flow-volume loops
- Direct visualization with bronchoscopy (standard)

4. How about pressure-volume loops?

If there is a fixed obstruction, you see flattening of the volume curves with inspiration and expiration. A variable extrathoracic obstruction would cause flattening of volume loops on inspiration only, whereas a variable intrathoracic obstruction would cause flattening of the volume loops on expiration. If there is a plan for a bronchoscopy, then no.

5. What else can be done to rule out dynamic obstruction?

Echocardiography can rule out external compression of the heart by the mass. The patient also has bilateral effusions and ascites, and echocardiography may help to rule out the heart as the cause, and it can evaluate for a possible tamponade or significant pericardial effusion, because the patient complains of dyspnea.

6. Echocardiography shows some external compression of the right atrium, but there is no significant obstruction to the filling and flow, and the patient has normal systolic function. Bronchoscopy shows no dynamic obstruction or distortion of the lumen. Do you want any additional consultations?

- Pulmonary consultation to discuss obstruction and to discuss the need for pressure-volume loops versus bronchoscopy
- Cardiology consultation to see if there is a need for any further optimization of the patient's cardiovascular status, depending on the echocardiography results
- Ear, nose, and throat consultation for a possible rigid bronchoscopy if there is an airway collapse after induction
- Cardiovascular surgery consultation for a possible CPB
- Neurology consultation to rule out recurrence of myasthenia gravis

7. What do you do about bilateral pleural effusion?

Depending on the size of the effusions and whether the patient is symptomatic, I would consider draining them. This particular patient has orthopnea, and I would likely drain the effusions.

Intraoperative Questions

1. How would you proceed with the anesthesia?
From a cardiovascular point of view, I would make sure that the patient receives an intravenous bolus before induction to ensure the patient has adequate preload and to keep right filling pressures high to prevent cardiovascular collapse due to external compression of the right ventricle.

From an intubation point of view, because there was no dynamic obstruction or distortion of the lumen, I would proceed with normal induction, pre-oxygenate the patient well, and keep the patient in a sitting position (less obstruction). I would have an ears, nose, and throat specialist with a rigid bronchoscope on standby. I could also consider awake intubation.

2. Which things will you keep in the room?

- A good luck charm
- Ear, nose, and throat specialist with a rigid bronchoscope
- CPB pump

3. How do you position this patient for induction?
The patient should be sitting, so that gravity's pull on the mass would work with you, not against you, after the patient is under general anesthesia and paralyzed.

4. Considering the massive ascites, do you want to do an RSI?
Yes, the ascites will increase pressure on the gastroesophageal junction, increasing the likelihood of aspiration.

5. Would you use muscle relaxants?
If using an RSI, yes. If the patient has recurrence of myasthenia gravis, the response to succinylcholine could be unpredictable. Patients with myasthenia gravis are very sensitive to neuromuscular blocking agents (NMBAs). Because the patient is going for exploratory laparotomy, the use of an NMBA will likely be necessary. In this case, I would closely monitor neuromuscular blockade.

6. After induction, you place the patient in the supine position, and you notice that the pulse oximeter is showing a value of 92% and the end-tidal value dropped to 25 mm Hg CO_2. What do you do?
The differential diagnosis includes partial disconnect, decreased cardiac output, decreased ventilation, and pulmonary embolism.

Make sure the patient is hemodynamically stable, and then hand bag the patient with 100% F_{IO_2} to make sure that there is no obstruction. Check for a partial disconnect, and listen to the patient's lungs to make sure the ETT is in the appropriate position.

Assuming that ETT placement was confirmed, the possible cause of decreased saturation and end-tidal CO_2 is hypoventilation due to atelectasis caused by the increased intra-abdominal pressure related to ascites. I would manually bag the patient and apply recruitment maneuvers until the saturation improves. I would make sure that the patient has PEEP throughout the case, adjust O_2 flow as needed, and try to keep the peak inspiratory pressure between 30 and 35.

How It Actually Happened

Many consultations were needed. We discussed the case with the surgeon, emphasized the importance of ruling out airway obstruction, and bargained for 24 hours more. We obtained a CT scan, echocardiogram, and pulmonary consultation. The pulmonologist performed bronchoscopy and ruled out dynamic obstruction. We did not think that pressure-volume loops would be beneficial because the patient could not lie down and bronchoscopy provided all the relevant information. We drained the pleural effusion. We discussed the case with CT specialist and ear, nose, and throat surgeons. Arrangements were made for a pump team to standby for possible femoral-femoral and for ear, nose, and throat surgeons for possible rigid bronchoscopy.

However, because there was no true dynamic obstruction, we decided to do an RSI with the patient in a sitting position, and there was no airway disaster. Although in the literature there are case reports about serous airway obstruction after institution of muscle relaxation, they have occurred in the pediatric age group.

CASE 31: NOTHING TRIVIAL IN THE OUTPATIENT CENTER

Preoperative Questions

1. What are the anesthetic concerns for this patient?

Morbid obesity is a concern, with the associated cardiovascular, respiratory, difficult airway, and gastrointestinal complications. Stroke volume and cardiac output increase, often leading to systemic hypertension, increased mean pulmonary artery pressure, and an elevation in right and left ventricular stroke work. Eventually, this may lead to right and left ventricular failure. Cardiac dysrhythmias may result from hypoxia or ischemic heart disease, or both. These patients are at risk for venous stasis and emboli. Pulmonary concerns arise from the deposition of fatty tissue on the chest and abdominal walls. There is an impairment of lung volumes and gas exchange. Expiratory reserve volume, FRC, and therefore total lung capacity are reduced. Airway closure occurs during normal ventilation, leading to lower PaO_2 values than in nonobese patients. The supine position and the induction of general anesthesia further reduce FRC. Endotracheal intubation and mask ventilation may be difficult because of the deposition of fatty tissue in the pharyngeal tissue. Obesity is a very important independent risk factor for obstructive sleep apnea; 60% to 90% of patients with obstructive sleep apnea are obese. These patients may be at risk for adverse perioperative outcomes. Obese patients have increased volume and acidity of gastric juices preoperatively, leading to an increased risk for pulmonary aspiration.

COPD may result from long-standing tobacco use, and a bronchospastic component may respond to bronchodilators. It is characterized by increased airway resistance or increased airway responsiveness, or both. It constitutes a spectrum of diseases, including asthma with increased bronchial reactivity in response to various respiratory irritants that is reversible with bronchodilators and chronic bronchitis characterized by excessive mucus production, atelectasis, intrapulmonary shunting, and hypoxemia, leading eventually to emphysema with its associated alveolar destruction and airway collapse. Airway hyperreactivity can be ascribed to reduced airway caliber and an autonomic imbalance with increased parasympathetic activity in the lung. Forced exhalation during spirometry, such as forced expired volume in 1 second (FEV_1), reflects airway resistance. Perioperative complications range from bronchospasm to ventilator dependence as a result of retained secretions, atelectasis, pneumonia, pneumothorax, and respiratory failure.

2. What other information would you like in the patient's history?
Attention is directed to the airway and cardiopulmonary systems. The following information would be helpful:

- Anesthetic history (e.g., severe sore throat postoperatively, any discussion of difficult intubation with a previous anesthesiologist)
- History of hypertension
- History of cardiac disease or symptoms (e.g., angina, MI, chest pains, palpitations, exercise tolerance)
- History of pulmonary symptoms (e.g., sputum production, recent upper respiratory infection [URI], shortness of breath at rest, dyspnea on exertion, exercise tolerance, use of steroids in the past, ER visits and hospitalizations for pulmonary complaints, snoring, nocturnal awakening or gasping, daytime sleepiness)
- History of gastroesophageal reflux or hiatal hernia
- Medications and allergies

This patient denies a history of hypertension, chest pains, or palpitations, and she has fair exercise tolerance. She carries groceries into the house and can climb a flight of stairs without shortness of breath. She has not had any ER visits for pulmonary symptoms, nor has she been treated with systemic steroids. She does have sputum production in the morning but denied any recent URIs. Her only medications are the inhalers (PRN), and she has no allergies.

On further questioning, it is revealed (by her husband who is seated beside her) that she snores excessively at night, waking him up. He also reports that she turns often and sometimes vocalizes. She denies daytime sleepiness. You ask whether she has had a sleep study. The answer is no, but you make a presumptive diagnosis of obstructive sleep apnea.

3. Define obstructive sleep apnea and obstructive sleep hypopnea.
Obstructive sleep apnea is a syndrome characterized by recurrent episodes of partial or complete obstruction of the upper airway during sleep. Obstructive sleep apnea is strictly defined as cessation of airflow for more than 10 seconds despite ventilatory effort, occurring five or more times per hour, and it is usually associated with a decrease in arterial oxygen saturation of more than 4%. Obstructive sleep hypopnea is defined as a reduction in airflow of more than 50% for more than 10 seconds, occurring 15 or more times per hour of sleep, and it may be associated with a decrease in oxygen saturation of more than 4%. Both disrupt sleep, alter cardiopulmonary function, and may cause daytime sleepiness.

According to the ASA practice guidelines, predisposing physical characteristics include a BMI greater than 35, neck circumference of 17 inches in men and 16 inches in women, craniofacial abnormalities, anatomical nasal obstruction, and tonsils nearly touching in the midline. Symptoms associated with obstructive sleep apnea include snoring, observed pauses in breathing during sleep, awakening from sleep or frequent arousals, and daytime somnolence or fatigue. The estimated prevalence of obstructive sleep apnea is 2% among women and 4% among men. However, 60% to 80% of patients at risk for obstructive sleep apnea remain undiagnosed. These patients are at increased risk for adverse outcomes when they receive sedation, analgesia, or anesthesia, and their risk increases as the severity of obstructive sleep apnea increases.

4. Discuss the pathophysiology of obstructive sleep apnea.
Obstructive sleep apnea occurs because of the relationship of the anatomy and muscle function in the upper airway during sleep. In adults, a night of sleep typically consists of four to six cycles of non–rapid eye movement (NREM) sleep, followed by REM sleep. There are four stages of NREM and one stage of REM sleep. Stage 3 and 4 NREM sleep and REM sleep are deep, restorative periods of sleep that are characterized by slowing of EEG waves. These stages of sleep result in loss of muscle tone, causing pharyngeal narrowing. The most compliant sites are the lateral pharyngeal walls, which are a predominant site of adipose deposition in obese patients. Increased deposition of fat increases the likelihood that loss of muscle tone will cause collapse of the pharynx. As upper airway resistance increases, the negative pressure generated by a diaphragmatic contraction increases, and pharyngeal collapse increases. PaO_2 decreases, $PaCO_2$ increases, and ventilatory effort increases, thereby increasing neural transmission in the reticular activating system and causing arousal of the individual.

5. Discuss the systemic effects of obstructive sleep apnea.
Decreased oxygenation may cause cardiac dysrhythmias, especially bradycardia. However, one half of the patients with apneic events have long sinus pauses, second-degree heart block, or ventricular arrhythmias. There is a higher incidence of nocturnal angina and MI among these patients. Increased sympathetic tone with each repetitive event produces pulmonary and systemic hypertension, which can lead to right and left ventricular hypertrophy.

6. Discuss the parameters measured in a sleep study and how the severity of obstructive sleep apnea is graded.
A presumptive diagnosis of obstructive sleep apnea may be made on the basis of symptoms, but a definitive diagnosis is determined by the results of a sleep study. It consists of monitoring the EEG, electro-oculogram (EOG), oral and nasal sensors for movement of air, electromyogram (EMG), end-tidal CO_2, pulse oximetry, noninvasive blood pressure, and ECG. Pulse oximetry desaturation data, ECG results, and changes in vital signs are reported. The total number of apnea and hypopnea episodes per hour is called the *apnea-hypopnea index* (AHI). The AHI is used quantitatively to classify the severity of obstructive sleep apnea. Mild obstructive sleep apnea has an AHI value of 6 to 20, the moderate form has a value of 21 to 40, and the severe form has a value higher than 40. The total number of arousals per hour is reported as a total *arousal index* (AI). According to the ASA practice guidelines, the literature supports the efficacy of CPAP in improving AHI and oxygen saturation levels in the nonperioperative setting. There are insufficient data to evaluate the impact of the preoperative use of CPAP on perioperative outcomes, but the consultants agreed that preoperative use of CPAP or nasal intermittent positive-pressure ventilation (NIPPV) may improve the preoperative condition.

7. How is the perioperative risk of obstructive sleep apnea determined?

Obstructive sleep apnea has a scoring system similar to that for cardiac risk. The following is adapted from the ASA Task Force guidelines:

A. Severity of sleep apnea based on sleep study or clinical indicators: 0 to 3 points are assigned for degrees of severity from none to severe.

B. Invasiveness of surgery: 0 to 3 points are assigned for degrees of invasiveness from superficial, minor procedures to major surgery.

C. Requirement for postoperative opioids: 0 to 3 points are assigned for degrees of opioid use from none to high-dose or neuraxial.

D. Estimation of perioperative risk

The scoring system may be used to determine the preoperative risk of obstructive sleep apnea. It takes into account the severity of obstructive sleep apnea with the invasiveness of anesthesia or surgery or the requirement for postoperative opioids (whichever is greater). A score of 4 may signify increased perioperative risk from obstructive sleep apnea, and a score of 5 or 6 may signify significantly increased risk. One point may be deducted if CPAP or NIPPV has been used preoperatively and the patient will be using it postoperatively.

Author's Note: The ASA website has all our guidelines. Check them out and make sure you know THE LATEST. Remember, any book is "stuck in time," whereas websites are updated. THAT DOESN'T MEAN YOU SHOULD STOP BUYING MY BOOKS THOUGH. You can always use my book for a footrest. What website can do that?

8. What is this patient's perioperative risk of obstructive sleep apnea?

This patient would be classified as having mild to moderate obstructive sleep apnea based on symptoms because we do not have a sleep study. She snores, occasionally vocalizes, but does not complain of daytime sleepiness. She requires general anesthesia and therefore would have a score of 4 or 5. She is at increased perioperative risk from obstructive sleep apnea.

9. What are you going to pay particular attention to during your physical examination?

Attention should be focused on the airway and the cardiopulmonary examination. Vital signs, including blood pressure, heart rate, and oxygen saturation, are important.

10. On examination, her blood pressure is 140/90 mm Hg, her heart rate is 88 beats/min, and her airway has a Mallampati score of 1 to 2. Her cardiac examination reveals regular heart rate and rhythm without any murmurs, gallops, or rubs. Examination of her lungs reveals decreased breath sounds bilaterally, but they are clear. What laboratory data and tests would you want?

• Complete blood cell count (polycythemia)
• Electrolytes (acidosis)
• ECG (rhythm disturbances or signs of infarction or ischemia)
• Chest radiograph (cardiomegaly, atelectasis)

PFTs are impractical preoperatively, and a careful history should identify factors that place the patient at increased pulmonary risk. A sleep study would be helpful to classify the severity of obstructive sleep apnea and perhaps determine whether to begin CPAP or NIPPV preoperatively. However, because the diagnosis of obstructive sleep apnea is presumptive based on history and there is some concern about this patient's ovarian pathology, you proceed with the case.

Cessation of smoking is desirable. Airway reactivity decreases, and mucociliary transport improves, but these benefits of smoking cessation take several weeks. If smoking can be stopped for even 48 to 72 hours, the carboxyhemoglobin content decreases, improving oxygen delivery to the tissues.

11. Is this case appropriate for an ambulatory surgery center? If this patient were scheduled to have a laparoscopic cholecystectomy instead, would this center be appropriate?

There are insufficient data in the literature to guide the decision about inpatient or outpatient management or about the appropriate time for discharge. However, the consultants involved in the ASA practice guidelines agree that procedures normally performed on an outpatient basis on patients without obstructive sleep apnea may be performed on an outpatient basis on patients with obstructive sleep apnea when local or regional anesthesia is administered. The consultants are equivocal about performing superficial surgery or gynecologic laparoscopy under general anesthesia on an outpatient basis on these patients. They do agree that for these patients at increased risk, the outpatient facility should have the availability of equipment for addressing a difficult airway, respiratory equipment, radiology and laboratory facilities, and a plan in place for transfer to an inpatient facility. Upper abdominal laparoscopy, airway surgery, and tonsillectomy in patients with obstructive sleep apnea who are younger than 3 years should not be performed in an outpatient setting. Similarly, obstructive sleep apnea patients with a severity score of 5 or greater should not have surgery in an outpatient center.

12. Would you consider any premedications for her?

Because of the increased volume and acidity of gastric juices, you would premedicate her with cimetidine, ranitidine, or metoclopramide and a nonparticulate antacid such as Bicitra. An inhaled bronchodilator used just before induction can be useful. Sedatives should be avoided because airway obstruction is the concern. A discussion regarding the risk of perioperative venous thrombosis should take place with the surgeon, and a decision should be made concerning the perioperative use of low-dose anticoagulants.

The patient is induced in a rapid-sequence fashion, intubated by direct laryngoscopy without incident, and maintained on a combination of a propofol infusion and sevoflurane.

Operative Questions

1. The patient is induced in a rapid-sequence fashion, intubated by direct laryngoscopy without incident, and maintained on a combination of a propofol infusion and sevoflurane. What are your concerns intraoperatively?

The major concern for this patient is her respiratory status. A deep plane of anesthesia should be maintained to avoid airway hyperreactivity. She may require suctioning and inhaled bronchodilators. Close attention must be paid to the insufflation of the abdomen and compression of the diaphragm, because this may further decrease an already reduced FRC due to obesity and the induction of general anesthesia. Similarly, requests for any Trendelenburg position must be considered carefully because it will further decrease the FRC.

Although opioids are probably necessary in this procedure to supplement the general anesthetic and may inhibit mucus secretion and bronchoconstriction, their use should be minimized as much as possible because of the respiratory depressant effects in the recovery period. The surgeon should be encouraged to use a long-acting local anesthetic at the laparoscopy sites.

2. The case proceeds relatively uneventfully, except for a constant debate between you and the surgeon about how much Trendelenburg positioning the patient can tolerate. Her lungs remain clear, with occasional rhonchi. Her oxygen saturation levels are 95% to 96% on 50% F_{IO_2} throughout. How will you extubate this patient?

This patient should be extubated awake after full reversal of any neuromuscular blockade in the semi-upright position.

3. The patient is awake and extubated. You start to disconnect the monitors, leaving the pulse oximeter on while you turn to jot down a few last notes on your anesthesia record. You suddenly hear those terrifying low tones of the pulse oximeter, look up, and find the patient has dozed off and the saturation level is 79%. You spring into action and stimulate the patient. The oxygen saturation rises to between 93% and 94%. You proceed to transfer the patient to the PACU. How long should you monitor the patient in the PACU?

Supplemental oxygen should be administered until the patient can maintain her baseline oxygen saturation level on room air. If the patient had been treated with CPAP or NIPPV preoperatively, oxygen should be administered in the recovery period. She should be maintained in the semi-upright position. The goal is to have no episodes of desaturation or obstruction when left undisturbed. The consultants of the ASA Task Force recommend that patients with obstructive sleep apnea be monitored for a median of 3 hours longer than those without obstructive sleep apnea and 7 hours longer than the last episode of hypoxemia or obstruction on room air. This patient was monitored in the PACU for 7 hours. She was eventually discharged from the ambulatory surgery center. The subsequent postoperative course was uneventful.

4. How will you manage postoperative pain?

This patient should be treated with nonsteroidal anti-inflammatory agents and perhaps with low-dose oral opiates to minimize the sedative effects and the risk of airway obstruction. If her pain remained uncontrolled, she should be transferred to the inpatient facility to manage her pain in a monitored setting.

American Society of Anesthesiologists (ASA) Task Force on Perioperative Management of Patients with Obstructive Sleep Apnea: Practice guidelines for the perioperative management of patients with obstructive sleep apnea. Anesthesiology 2006;104:1081-1093.

Benumof JL: Obesity, sleep apnea, the airway, and anesthesia. ASA refresher course lectures. Anesthesiology 2002;30:27-40.

Brodsky JB: Anesthesia for bariatric surgery. ASA refresher course lectures. Anesthesiology 2005;33:49-63.

Gal TJ: Reactive airway disease: Anesthetic perspectives. IARS review course lectures. Anesth Analg 2002;March(Suppl):45-53.

Roizen MF, Fleisher LA: Anesthetic implications of concurrent diseases. In Miller RD (ed): Miller's Anesthesia. Philadelphia, Elsevier/Churchill Livingstone, 2005, pp 1028-1034.

Sladen RN: Preoperative evaluation of the compromised patient. IARS review course lectures. Anesth Analg 2004;(Suppl):108-115.

Stierer TL: Postoperative obstructive sleep apnea. Paper presented at the Society for Ambulatory Anesthesia 21st Annual Meeting, May 2006, Washington, DC.

References included here because OSA is a tough issue and it's a rich "source" of oral board questions.

CASE 32: THE BIG HIT

1. What is HIT? Explain the differences between type 1 and type 2 HIT.

Heparin-induced thrombocytopenia (HIT) is a transient but recurring IgG-mediated antibody response against the platelet factor 4 (PF4) and heparin complex. It can occur with any exposure to heparin, but it is more common with high-dose unfractionated heparin. Thrombocytopenia is the most common event in HIT, and it occurs in at least 90% of patients. A high proportion of patients with HIT can develop thrombosis.

Although it is mainly associated with unfractionated heparin (UFH), it can also occur with exposure to low-molecular weight heparin (LMWH), but at significantly lower rates. Despite the low platelet count, it is a thrombotic disorder, with very high rates of thrombosis, in the arteries with or without venous complications. HIT typically develops 4 to 14 days after the administration of heparin.

There are two forms of HIT: type I and type II. Patients with type I HIT have a transient decrease in platelet count without any further symptoms. There is recovery even if heparin continues to be administered. Platelet counts rarely fall below 100,000/µL. This form of HIT occurs in 10% to 20% of all patients on heparin. It is not an immune reaction, and antibodies are not demonstrated.

Type II HIT is an autoimmune reaction, with antibodies formed against PF4 and heparin complex. It appears that heparin binding to PF4 causes a conformational change in the protein, rendering it antigenic. The antibodies found are most commonly of the IgG class, with or without IgM and IgA class antibodies. IgM and IgA antibodies are rarely found without IgG antibodies. Type II HIT develops in about 3% of all patients on UFH and in 0.1% of patients on LMWH, and it causes thrombosis in 30% to 40% of these patients. Clot formation is mainly arterial and rich in platelets (i.e., white clot syndrome), in contrast with fibrin-rich clots, which are red because of trapped red blood cells. Most thrombotic events occur in the lower limbs, and skin lesions and necrosis may also occur at the site of the heparin infusion. The most important enzyme in type II HIT is thrombin, the generation of which is increased after platelet activation. The risk for HIT is higher among women than men, and HIT occurs more commonly in surgical than in nonsurgical settings.

2. How is HIT diagnosed?

The diagnosis of HIT should be entertained in any patient with a significant fall in the platelet count while on heparin therapy ($<150 \times 10^3$/µL or a 50% or greater decrease in platelet count after 5 days of therapy). The definitive diagnosis requires the following steps:

- Thrombocytopenia while on heparin
- Exclusion of other causes of thrombocytopenia
- Improvement in the platelet count after cessation of heparin therapy
- Presence of heparin-dependent platelet antibody determined by an in vitro test

In most cases, the diagnosis is made on the basis of clinical findings. The most common serologic test is the PF4/heparin polyanion enzyme immunoassay.

3. What are the preoperative considerations from an anesthesiologist's point of view?

Besides the usual preoperative issues, these patients face morbidity derived principally from venous and arterial thrombosis in the face of thrombocytopenia. Thrombosis, not bleeding, constitutes the principal risk for these patients, and fatal thrombosis or embolism is not uncommon.

If the patient is facing surgery, especially cardiac surgery, consider an alternative to heparin as an anticoagulant. Your setup should be completely heparin free. If planning to use a Swan-Ganz catheter, use a heparin-free catheter. Bleeding is a major issue after surgery because there are no reversal agents for the alternative anticoagulation.

4. What are your options regarding anticoagulants?

The three alternative anticoagulants available are bivalirudin, argatroban, and lepirudin.

5. What is the mechanism of action of the alternative agents?

All three agents are thrombin inhibitors. Bivalirudin (Angiomax) is a synthetic, 20–amino acid peptide. It has a short half-life of about 25 minutes. The half-life is prolonged in patients with renal failure. Bivalirudin is considered to be a safe alternative to heparin based on its pharmacologic and pharmacokinetic profile.

Lepirudin (Refludan) has a longer half-life (80 minutes), and it cannot be used repeatedly because it has immunogenic properties. Argatroban is used as an alternative to heparin mostly in noncardiac surgery.

6. What is the dosing regimen?

The dosing regimen for bivalirudin for on-pump cases includes the following recommendations:

Bolus: 1 mg/kg bolus
Maintenance: 2.5 mg/kg/hr infusion
Pump: 50 mg are added to prime the pump
Subsequent dosing: Repeat doses of 0.1 to 0.5 mg/kg are administered to maintain a target activated clotting time (ACT) greater than or equal to 2.5 times baseline. The infusion continues until 15 minutes before CPB separation.
Special cases: Lower doses are employed for renal impairment.

The dosing regimen for lepirudin includes the following recommendations:

Bolus: 0.4 mg/kg body weight (up to 110 kg)
Maintenance: 0.15 mg/kg body weight (up to 110 kg)/hr as a continuous intravenous infusion

The dosing regimen for argatroban includes the following recommendations:

Bolus: 350 μg/kg
Cardiopulmonary bypass pump: Add 150 μg/kg
Maintenance: 25 μg/kg/min

7. What are the advantages and disadvantages of the available alternative drugs?

Bivalirudin has a short half-life (25 minutes) but relies on renal clearance. Argatroban is metabolized by the hepatobiliary system. Lepirudin has a long half-life (80 minutes), and it is immunogenic, making repeat dosing a problem.

8. How will you monitor the level of anticoagulation?

The level of anticoagulation is measured using the activated clotting time (ACT) in the OR setting. Generally, an ACT greater than 420 seconds or 2.5 baseline is an acceptable level of anticoagulation for on-pump procedures. A slightly lower level of ACT is accepted for off-pump procedures. Infusion is usually continued up to 15 minutes before weaning from CPB. The ACT should be frequently monitored.

9. How will you reverse the anticoagulation?

There is no direct reversal for the direct thrombin inhibitors. However, a combination of modified ultrafiltration, hemodialysis, and the administration of recombinant factor VIIa, FFP, and cryoprecipitate may reverse the anticoagulant effects.

10. When the cell saver technician wonders what he should use for anticoagulation, what will you tell him?

Citrate phosphate dextrose (CPD) should be used as the reservoir anticoagulant in a 1:12 ratio of CPD to blood.

How It Actually Happened

We had to look up stuff, too. I ran home and started looking up HIT. Fortunately, there is extensive recent literature on HIT. It appears that bivalirudin (Angiomax) has the best safety profile, and it has been used successfully. We opted for Angiomax and loaded the patient with a 1-mg/kg dose 10 minutes before cannulation of the aorta. At the same time, the infusion was started at 2.5 mg/kg. We checked the ACT, and it was below 403 seconds. Everybody in the room was thrilled. The operation began, and I finally had my coffee break. I stopped the infusion, weaned the patient off bypass, and waited for the bleeding to stop and the ACT to come down. It took approximately 60 to 70 minutes for the ACT to come down, and the surgeon started seeing clots. This was the second hardest part of the case. The first was finding a heparin-free Swan-Ganz catheter, because nobody knew what we were taking about! We waited for bleeding to stop and clots to appear, and we kept the patient warm. When the ACT was nearing normal, we transferred the patient to the cardiovascular ICU. The remainder of the hospital course was uneventful.

Spiess BD, DeAnda A, McCarthy HL et al: Off -pump coronary artery bypass graft surgery with anticoagulation with bivalirudin: A patient with heparin-induced thrombocytopenia syndrome type II and renal failure. J Cardiothorac Vasc Anesth 2006;20:106-111.

CASE 33: HOME IS WHERE THE OXYGEN IS

Preoperative Questions

1. What is the life span for a patient with ovarian cancer? What would you tell the patient about the operation preoperatively?

The prognosis for ovarian cancer is probably less than 6 months. For this patient to have this type of surgery, there is a very high possibility that the patient would need a prolonged intubation and ICU stay and perhaps would never wake up again. These issues need to be explained to the patient and her family during the preoperative visit, so the family will not be surprised when this happens.

2. Do you need any further workup on this patient? What tests would you order?

Based on the information provided, this patient needs a more extensive workup in several areas, including her cardiovascular system, pulmonary function status, liver function, renal function, coagulation study, and metastatic status.

3. Does the patient need any workup for cardiac function? Does the patient need cardiac catheterization?

Based on the patient's history, she has shortness of breath, requires supplemental oxygen at night, and has very low exercise tolerance. The patient needs further cardiac workup, such as an ECG and pharmacologic stress echocardiography. Because of her inability to walk, we need to evaluate whether the patient has any myocardium at risk and determine her left ventricular function. The patient may or may not need cardiac catheterization based on the results of the ECG and the stress test.

4. Does the patient need any pulmonary function tests? If so, what tests do you order?

The patient has significant smoking history, has COPD, and has moderate-sized ascites, which may have a restrictive effect on respiration. A chest radiograph and spirometry test with a flow-volume curve could provide much information. The chest radiograph will show if the patient has lung infection, pulmonary edema, pleural effusion, a metastatic nodule, and cardiomegaly. Both tests will show a respiratory pattern with obstructive and restrictive features (mostly an obstructive pattern). Spirometry can determine whether the airway obstruction has any reversible component.

5. Would you drain the ascites before surgery? Why or why not?

Draining ascites before the operation would not benefit the surgery and anesthesia, and if the patient is not adequately resuscitated, she may develop hypovolemia and hepatorenal syndrome, causing acute renal failure.

6. Do you think the patient needs oxygen 24 hours each day? How much oxygen would you give the patient: 2 L/min, 4 L/min, or 6 L/min? Why?

The patient has COPD and possibly has pulmonary metastasis and left ventricular dysfunction. She can benefit from around-the-clock supplemental oxygen. Low-flow oxygen, such as 2 L/min of O_2, would be a better choice than a higher flow. Because she is a chronic CO_2 retainer, her respiratory center is not sensitive to hypercapnia, and the only effective stimulus is her hypoxic drive. High-flow O_2 would take away this hypoxic drive and cause respiratory depression.

7. How do you interpret the ABG results?

The ABG determination shows hypoxemia with a P_{O_2} of 56 mm Hg and hypercapnia with a P_{CO_2} of 45 mm Hg. There are many causes for this, including a long history of COPD, pulmonary edema, pulmonary infection, and pulmonary metastasis.

8. Would you transfuse the patient preoperatively? Why or why not?

The patient has several reasons for her anemia, including nutrient deficiency and malignancy. Considering the patient's long history of COPD, she should have a higher than normal hematocrit, and this low hematocrit may mean that the bone marrow has metastases. Because she is in late stage cancer and has very low cardiac reserve, transfusion would be beneficial for keeping the hematocrit above 30%.

9. Would you premedicate this patient?

It may not be helpful to premedicate this patient, who is a chronic CO_2 retainer, because sedation would suppress the hypoxic drive and further compromise her respiratory function. This is dangerous, especially in an environment in which intensive monitoring is not available.

Intraoperative Questions

1. What monitors do you choose for this patient? Would you put arterial line and central line in this patient? What about using a Swan-Ganz catheter?

Besides the basic ASA monitors of ECG, noninvasive blood pressure (NIBP), pulse oximetry, and temperature, an arterial line and central line are necessary to monitor blood pressure and the patient's fluid status. The arterial line should be placed before induction because the patient's left ventricular function is decreased. If the patient is very nervous, mild sedation in small increments titrated to effect would be helpful, because close monitoring and emergency treatment are immediately available in the operating room.

2. You decide to place an arterial line before induction, but the patient is very anxious. Would you give sedation?

Placing a pulmonary artery catheter is controversial. Studies have shown that placement does not improve outcome and may even increase mortality. I would not place a pulmonary artery catheter.

3. How would you induce this patient? What agents would you use? Would you use ketamine? What muscle relaxant would you choose? What is the Hoffman reaction?

This patient should be treated as if she had a full stomach. An RSI is warranted. Etomidate or thiopental are good choices. Ketamine is a good choice because of its ability to provide analgesia, amnesia, and stimulation of catecholamine release to maintain cardiovascular stability. She has probably been bedridden for a relatively long time, and muscular atrophy is a concern if succinylcholine is to be used. Her hepatic and renal functions may not be optimal based on her condition. Cisatracurium or atracuronium is a good choice because these drugs are metabolized by the Hoffman reaction.

4. What factors can affect the Hoffman reaction?

A Hoffmann reaction is nonenzymatic degradation at body temperature and pH that occurs independent of hepatic or renal clearance. It is important to keep the patient normothermic and at a neutral pH.

5. What agent would you use for anesthesia maintenance? What are your concerns?

Maintenance of anesthesia can be achieved with any intravenous or inhalant anesthetics. A rapid offset would be advantageous if early extubation is a goal.

Inhalant anesthetics, especially desflurane, are better choices considering their low blood gas coefficient, rapid onset and offset time, and low level of metabolism by the body.

6. After opening the abdomen, the patient's blood pressure suddenly drops. What is your differential diagnosis?

When hypotension happens, it is always good to think in a systematic way to approach the cause: preload, contractility, afterload, heart rate, and rhythm. In this manner, you are less likely to miss some important issues. In this situation, it is mostly caused by decreased venous return because of a sudden decrease of the intra-abdominal pressure causing dilation of abdominal venous beds. A fluid challenge would likely correct the problem.

7. During surgery, peak airway pressure suddenly increases. What is your differential diagnosis? Can capnography allow early detection of an endobronchial intubation?

You should develop a systematic approach to treat high peak aspiratory pressure. One way is to think from the outside to the inside: ventilator, breathing circuit, ETT, trachea, lungs, pleural cavity, diaphragm, chest wall, and abdomen. The most likely causes in this situation are secretion or a mucous plug of the ETT, ETT kinking, endobronchial intubation, pneumothorax, light anesthesia, and inadequate muscle relaxation. You can hand ventilate the lungs to check the compliance, suction the ETT, check bilateral breath sounds, check neuromuscular blockade, and check other vital signs to rule out light anesthesia. If the breath sound is unilateral, after endobronchial intubation is ruled out, pneumothorax is highly likely; a chest tube should be placed before proceeding further after the diagnosis of pneumothorax is confirmed. Capnography cannot tell an endobronchial intubation.

8. How do you diagnose pneumothorax? Would you place a chest tube?

Suspicion is the key to the prompt and accurate diagnosis of pneumothorax intraoperatively. You should auscultate the chest to check for bilateral breath sounds, check the patency of the circuit and the valves, suction the ETT to rule out a mucous plug, and use fiberoptic scope and obtain a chest radiograph to confirm the diagnosis. A chest tube should be placed after the pneumothorax has occurred.

9. What intravenous fluid would you use: crystalloid or colloid?

The choices of intravenous fluid for administration during major surgery are controversial. The choice of fluid matters in major surgery because different fluids have different effects on different body systems. Because no single type of fluid is superior in all ways to others, the best practice is to administer combinations of crystalloid and colloid fluid to maximize the benefits and minimize the side effects.

10. The patient's O_2 saturation slowly drops into the low 90s. What would you do? How does PEEP work?

Low O_2 saturation indicates hypoxemia until proved otherwise. Causes include low F_{IO_2}, inadequate alveolar ventilation, $\dot{V}/\dot{Q}$ mismatch, anatomic shunt, and low cardiac output. Other vital signs should be checked. Increase F_{IO_2} to 100%; check the integrity and patency of the whole circuit from the ventilator to the ETT; make sure that ventilation is adequate; assess pulmonary compliance by hand ventilation; verify the correct position of the ETT; listen to both lungs; rule out aspiration and bronchospasm; add PEEP to the circuit; check the blood pressure, heart rate, and ECG to rule out cardiac causes; and give fluids and transfuse to maintain cardiac output and hemoglobin level. PEEP improves oxygenation by increasing functional residual volume.

How It Actually Happened

There are no surprises here. The case was a struggle, and saturation was a headache. The postoperative course was a struggle, and saturation was a headache. It is hard to look good in a case like this!

14

Answers to Grab Bags

CASE 1: EAR TUBES

As you are calling for all help within three counties, you put the patient's head down, turn her head to the side, suction like mad, reach in and scoop out the big stuff, give succinylcholine (barring contraindications such as spinal cord injury, neuromuscular disease, burns), and intubate. After the patient is intubated, you suction like mad, going all the way to putting a fiberoptic scope down and getting stuff out that way or calling a chest surgeon and doing rigid bronchoscopy and pulling out chunks. You then arrange intensive care unit (ICU) care and ventilation, using supportive care (e.g., ventilation, positive end-expiratory pressure [PEEP]) but avoiding the unproven techniques of antibiotics and steroids.

Misery of miseries, this happened to me. Curiously, I later found out the patient binged and purged every morning and had binged that morning on Mexican food, which explained the voluminous emesis and poor gastro-esophageal junction function (that rhymes; I like that). It sort of shattered my faith in no oral intake (NPO) forever. Who knows what other weird "eating things" patients do and never tell us about?

Oy vay! I still get nightmares about this case. My salvation was calling for help early and getting people in the room to help me!

CASE 2: RADIATION THERAPY FOR A MENTALLY RETARDED MAN

This is a toughie, but it is the kind of thing you see in special procedures. Because you hate to intubate each and every time, you attempt sedation with propofol. The radiologists need only about 30 seconds of holding still, and there is no pain involved. The propofol bolus should keep him calm, while you are watching the pulse oximeter like a hawk. He then is rolled into the room while a propofol infusion is running. The key is to know what worked the last time. If, by chance, you stumble into this case on the fifth or sixth try, read the earlier notes, and see what others used. If you are a pioneer doing this for the first time, make a note of what worked and what did not, and leave a nice note telling how much the patient needed. Be kind to those who follow.

This case is an excerpt from real life, as is the whole book. Dexmedetomidine was a possibility but a little time consuming. With lots of help from his caregivers' talking, reassuring, and hand-holding (all good medicine that is very low on side effects!), we gave a small bolus of propofol, watched the pulse oximeter, ran a low-level infusion, and got through it.

CASE 3: KNIFE IN THE BACK

You cannot lay him on his back, but you have to secure his airway. You could induce with the mask on his side and intubate on his side, but that is iffy. I would do an awake intubation with sedation, and after the airway was secured, I would induce as usual. Because the injury is fresh, you could use suxamethonium (within 24 hours), but the awake intubation makes that question moot.

This was among the freakiest things I ever saw. The patient was stuck by his girlfriend (what else is new?) and he could move one side but did not know it was moving, and he could sense the other side but could not move it—just like the textbook. I cannot imagine what kind of life this poor guy had afterward. Pulling the knife out was a beast, because it was not possible to "wiggle it a little" to work it loose. That would cut what was left of his spinal cord. We eventually had to get an enormous orthopedic surgeon to yank it out.

CASE 4: FEVER IN THE INTENSIVE CARE UNIT

The whole picture says sepsis, with a high temperature, low blood pressure, tachycardia, and a large A-a gradient (on 60% oxygen, the patient's saturation level should be 100% with a PO_2 of about 250 to 300 mm Hg). Because the patient had recent exploratory surgery, the concern is an infectious process (e.g., dead gut, abscess). Proceed by supporting the airway, breathing, and circulation (ABCs), giving ventilatory and circulatory support (e.g., volume resuscitation, vasoconstrictor to get blood pressure up), and obtaining a consult to find and cure the cause of the infection.

CASE 5: SMOKING CESSATION

I would recommend that the patient continue smoking up to the night before surgery. There is some evidence that states the lungs can become hyperreactive for up to 2 weeks after quitting smoking. Twelve hours without smoking is enough to decrease plasma levels of carboxyhemoglobin substantially. Smoking perioperatively causes mucous hypersecretion, narrowed small airways, and impaired ciliary transport, making it difficult for the patient to clear secretions.

CASE 6: TACHYCARDIA AFTER KNEE ARTHROSCOPY

Assess the patient for hypoxia, pain, and hypovolemia, which are the three most common causes of postoperative cardiac dysrhythmias. The patient is on a pulse oximeter, and the blood pressure cuff is on, so that helps with hypovolemia. Pain assessment amounts to asking, "Are you having pain?"

If the patient has supraventricular tachyarrhythmia (SVT), I would follow the advanced cardiac life support (ACLS) algorithm for SVT. Vagal maneuvers include the use of adenosine or verapamil, a β-blocker, and digoxin. If it is a wide complex, use the lidocaine. If all else fails, administer cardioversion.

CASE 7: BONE PAIN AND SARCOMA

Ewing sarcoma can be a very painful disease because it involves the bone. This patient will probably require some type of controlled-release opioid such as oxycodone or a fentanyl patch with an opioid for breakthrough pain. These patients also can be put on methadone for neuropathic pain. As for any acute or chronic pain management, treatment needs to be titrated to effect. A nerve block can be considered, depending on the location and extent of the tumor.

CASE 8: INTRAVENOUS FLUIDS

Decades of cases have failed to prove the benefit of colloid over crystalloid. You can hang your hat on a few things:

- Free water in the face of brain injury is not advisable (D_5W for a subdural evacuation is not a good idea).
- Glucose-containing solutions, unless they are absolutely needed, are not a good idea, because hyperglycemia can exacerbate neural and renal injury.
- Giving fresh-frozen plasma (FFP) or other potentially infectious agents for pure volume expansion rather than to fulfill a need (e.g., factor deficiency) is bad judgment.

Other than those guidelines, the mantra is the same as for any recipe: give just enough and not too much, and evaluate the patient for response. That is the word of fluids in the operating room (OR).

CASE 9: SEDATION IN A HALO

The halo makes routine intubation nearly impossible and mask ventilation difficult—you could do it with the mask turned around, but it would be a pain. This sedation starts with assessing the patient, talking things over, reassuring him that you will be there the whole time, and explaining what is going on. The more talking *ahead* of time, the fewer drugs *at* the time. Institute sedation with dexmedetomidine (keeps respirations going, provides sedation and some analgesia, and maintains the patient's ability to interact) with a small dose (e.g., 1 mg) of midazolam. Alternatives are midazolam/fentanyl and propofol/midazolam/fentanyl, but each of those combinations constitute "dancing with apnea wolves," so I would avoid them.

CASE 10: SWAN-GANZ CATHETER

Swan-Ganz catheters have a checkered past and a dubious future, but we are stuck with them, just as we are stuck with receding hairlines, polyps, and erectile dysfunction, so we have to find a way to cope. The mushy recommendations for Swan-Ganz catheters boil down to this: Although of no proven benefit regarding outcome, a Swan-Ganz catheter should be used if you need it. How is that for a circular argument? One option for this situation is to place a Swan-Ganz introducer in everyone having a heart operation so you can always "float one if you need it," but put one in only if you really feel you will need it for postoperative management.

- There is no need for a Swan-Ganz catheter in a guy with an ejection fraction (EF) of 50% who is undergoing coronary artery bypass grafting (CABG).
- You may need the additional information for a patient undergoing repeat CABG and mitral valve replacement who has an EF of 20%.

Make sure everyone is up to snuff on transesophageal echocardiography (TEE), because it can guide you intraoperatively, and if in trouble in the ICU, you can always drop a TEE probe and have a look postoperatively. Most importantly, do not place a Swan-Ganz catheter for its currently number one indication: the presence of a telephone. Most Swan-Ganz catheters (personal prejudice) are placed because people do not want to do bedside evaluation (i.e., look at the blood gas, consider what the TEE probe showed intraoperatively, see what happens when you turn on the various inotropes, follow urine output, and get the patient extubated as soon as feasible). Most people want to phone in, get some numbers, give an order, and go back to sleep.

CASE 11: POSTOPERATIVE RIGIDITY

The evaluation process always begins with the physical examination and review of the vital signs, being careful to notice trends and changes. The patient's current vital signs should guide further immediate therapy. As always, begin with ABCs. Consider ordering a chest radiograph and arterial blood gas (ABG) determination because this is an acute change in status. Inadequate or obstructive ventilation can cause tachypnea. Relieve airway obstruction and support oxygenation and ventilation. Proceed to mechanical ventilation as needed.

Tachypnea alone may be the patient's reaction to pain or fever. Treat the pain and the cause of fever. Rigidity increases oxygen consumption. Because the thermoregulatory threshold is lowered during general anesthesia, this could be an exaggerated form of postoperative shivering. It would cause increased oxygen consumption and increased production of carbon dioxide, with the subsequent increase in minute ventilation. Treatment goals in this case are to restore normothermia, so do not forget to rewarm the patient. The shivering can be treated with meperidine or other opioids.

Rigidity in the postoperative period is uncommon and should prompt you to rule out life-threatening causes such as malignant hyperthermia and neuroleptic malignant syndrome. We often see shivering in the postanesthesia care unit (PACU), and it should be differentiated from rigidity. Malignant hyperthermia can manifest at various times in the operative and postoperative period.

Neuroleptic malignant syndrome should be considered. Testicular torsion can result in a necrotic testis, and the surgical manipulation of these tissues can release potential bacterial loads into the systemic circulation. This can precipitate rapid onset of systemic inflammatory response syndrome (SIRS), which can lead to sepsis. This could explain the patient's state.

CASE 12: PERIPHERALLY INSERTED CENTRAL CATHETER AND DESATURATION

The visitors are likely helping him continue his drug abuse. His vital signs need to be monitored very closely for a drop in oxygen saturation, respiratory rate, and blood pressure. We certainly do not want this patient to overdose while in the hospital. The respiratory depression indicates opioid abuse. The patient may be using his peripherally inserted central catheter (PICC) to get high. Confronting the patient may or may not reveal what is happening. If we are not giving the patient pain medicine, urinalysis may show opioids. A contract of care should be made with the patient and documented in the chart regarding the use of illegal drugs and medications not ordered by his physician. To continue treating the patient in the hospital, we may need to treat his withdrawal symptoms and provide psychological support while in the hospital. Limiting the patient's access to his visitors is a good idea.

CASE 13: AORTIC VALVE REPLACEMENT IN A PREGNANT PATIENT

Ideally, we would like to preserve fetal perfusion and oxygenation and reduce the risk of fetal harm. None of this can happen if an unstable patient is stuck on cardiopulmonary bypass (CPB). The goal is to come off CPB with adequate perfusion, oxygenation, and ventilation. This is the best-case scenario for the patient and the fetus.

Correct ventilation and oxygenation, and then optimize volume status, oxygen delivery, and coagulation status. Provide hemodynamic support with inotropes and vasoactive medications as needed. I would use norepinephrine if it improves blood pressure and allows separation from CPB. α-Agonists (i.e., vasopressors) can increase uterine tone by increasing systemic vascular resistance and thereby place the fetus at increased risk. I would argue that hypotension and low perfusion states would be a worse case scenario.

Epinephrine can provide inotropic support along with increased systemic vascular resistance. Physiologic doses of vasopressin can help maintain blood pressure. We often place intra-aortic balloon pumps (IABPs) to augment perfusion so the patient can be separated from CPB. I would consider epinephrine and vasopressin before the use of an IABP.

CASE 14: SUBCUTANEOUS EMPHYSEMA

Most likely, a perforation of the trachea or bronchi has occurred while placing a double-lumen tube. This can occur because of trauma while placing the double-lumen tube or overinflation of one of the cuffs. Proper positioning should be confirmed immediately with fiberoptic examination. If this does not improve or resolve the subcutaneous emphysema or the ventilator alarms, it increases the odds that there is trauma to the airway below the tracheal cuff. This trauma may be temporarily dealt with by lung separation techniques. A high tracheal injury may be allowed to heal by placing a tracheostomy. Airway injury below the level of the tracheal cuff would likely require a thoracic surgeon.

CASE 15: PATIENT IN THE TRIPOD POSITION

This looks like epiglottitis. With her psychiatric history, it could be some bizarre reaction to her psychotropic drugs (e.g., neuroleptic malignant syndrome), but the tripod position and drooling point toward epiglottitis. Get her to the OR without delay, and perform an inhalation induction with the ear, nose, and throat (ENT) specialist standing by to do a tracheostomy. When intubating, do not touch or manipulate the fiery red epiglottis, because it is huge, and could bleed or fall apart.

CASE 16: ATTENTION DEFICIT DISORDER AND ELECTROPHYSIOLOGIC STUDY

The preoperative visit with patient and caretaker is important. Various people with these diseases react in different ways. This patient may be cooperative if you explain what is going on and keep in touch during the case. Very light sedation with constant reassurance may be all that is needed. Other patients may react entirely differently and require a general anesthetic. Talk to the care-taker because they know the patient best and are a gold mine of information.

CASE 17: FIRE ALARMS

You cannot abandon the patient. Tell the surgeon to put on a bandage; grab an oxygen tank, Ambu-bag, and a ton of propofol; and roll out to safety. Do the rest of the case with a finger on the pulse (if that is all you have) under jury-rigged total intravenous anesthesia (TIVA) out in the parking lot if you have to. Hard times require hard decisions.

CASE 18: ETOMIDATE FOR SEDATION

Because etomidate induces general anesthesia, anyone giving it must be able to manage a general anesthetic. The karma for conscious sedation is this: Make sure the patient is conscious and still responsive. Running propofol or other "general anesthetics in a bottle" is not a good idea and will lead to airway trouble. Give a little, and see what happens. That is how you sedate.

CASE 19: EPIDURAL PLANNED BUT THE PROTHROMBIN TIME IS HIGH

Do your best to correct the prothrombin time (PT) with fresh frozen plasma (FFP), and then recheck the PT to make sure you did correct it. If so, place the epidural. This case is worth "taking the risk," because the patient is in such terrible pain and this may be an end-of-life situation (talk with the oncologist), so do what you can to make the suffering patient feel better. Systemically, you can try combination therapy, and you can be pretty aggressive about dosing. Consulting a pain expert is a plus in this situation.

CASE 20: MEDIASTINAL MASS

Ay caramba! Unfortunately, the radiology manufacturers have not yet come up with a "slanted approach" to their beds going into the magnetic resonance imaging (MRI) and computed tomography (CT) chambers. Often, if we could just "sit them up a little," we would be okay. I would intubate her while awake, keep her breathing spontaneously, use no muscle relaxant, and then have her anesthetized in the CT machine. It is a little clunky, but the safest bet.

CASE 21: ANKLE PAIN

Evaluate the patient by obtaining a history and performing a physical examination. This patient turned out to have a classic story of an injury to an extremity that never really got better. The achy pain that was relieved by ibuprofen for the first couple of weeks after her tennis injury is gone, but in its place is this constant burning pain that keeps her from wearing her sock and shoe. When you gently brush the skin over the ankle joint, she winces, and you notice that the pain does not follow a dermatomal pattern. The diagnosis is complex regional pain syndrome (CRPS) type I, the artist formerly known as reflex sympathetic dystrophy (RSD). Does she need an MRI scan? No, unless you suspect there is a soft tissue injury. Plain x-ray films can be obtained if you suspect a bone injury; the same is true for a CT scan. A bone scan may be justified, because it may show the beginnings of the characteristic bone loss associated with CRPS. Treatment starts with neuropathic pain medicines, such as tricyclic antidepressants and anticonvulsants. You could also do a lumbar sympathetic block and prescribe physical therapy. The key to treatment is to restore function and keep the patient from losing hope.

CASE 22: BLOOD PATCH IN A JEHOVAH'S WITNESS

Fortunately, this nice woman had an uncomplicated cesarean section by spinal anesthesia, and as I was riding in the elevator to go see her, thoughts of cell saver machines and hetastarch raced through my head. How can I get blood to not leave her body but get it into her epidural space? Should I give her Lovenox and then start poking around in her back? I think a Jehovah's Witness can take Lovenox. Then, I saw it. I will take a butterfly and attach it to an extension tube. I will connect a stopcock, a 20-mL syringe, and another extension tube, and when I get the loss of resistance, I will connect it to the Touhy. I get to her room, and there she is walking around and getting ready to see her baby in the nursery. I introduce myself, and she asks whether I have something for her migraine because her husband left her medicine at home.

CASE 23: PATIENT CANNOT MOVE LEGS

I went to see the patient and reviewed the anesthesia record. He could not move his legs, but it was not surprising considering that he had been bolused with 10 mL of 0.5% bupivacaine just before the end of the procedure. The patient was very comfortable, and about 1 hour later, he started moving his legs. However, occasionally, I am called to see these patients, and they were not recently bolused. You should think about reasons other than the anesthesia to have postoperative neurologic deficits. I reviewed the patient's medical history to see whether anticoagulants were part of the picture. You must perform a focused neurologic examination to get an appreciation of what you are dealing with. Most cases of nerve injury after orthopedic surgery are caused by surgical traction resulting in nerve stretching, not by the anesthesia. In the perioperative period, the most important thing to do is keep a close watch on the situation. Let the surgeons know what is going on. An MRI or a CT scan can be considered if spinal hematoma is suspected. They occur more frequently in older women with bad backs after many larger needle sticks while on anticoagulants. They do not usually occur in the PACU, but instead form on postoperative day 1 or 2. A neurology consult should be considered after residual anesthetic is ruled out.

CASE 24: PAIN CONTROL IN THE POSTANESTHESIA CARE UNIT

Determine the nature of the pain. Is it located where expected after an operation? This patient had total knee arthroplasty under general anesthesia and had a femoral nerve catheter placed. On further investigation, it turned out that the catheter was bolused with 30 mL of 0.5% ropivacaine preoperatively, so I checked to see if the distribution of the operative leg was numb, and it was. It turned out that all of the pain was in the posterior aspect of the knee, and the patient was quite tolerant to opioids. He normally took extended-release oxycodone (80 mg) twice daily and then a bunch of short-release oxycodone and acetaminophen each day. The little voice in the back of my head said, "Give more fentanyl." I did. I am not a big fan of mixing opioids in the PACU, so I gave another 900 μg of fentanyl, and he started to feel a little better. I consider 50 μg of fentanyl equivalent to 5 mg of morphine and 1 mg of hydromorphone in the opioid-naïve patient, but that fentanyl number starts to approach double as patients develop more tolerance.

CASE 25: NEPHRECTOMY AND HEPARIN

Subcutaneous heparin is okay with neuraxial stuff. Intravenous heparin needs more attention. The American Society of Regional Anesthesia (ASRA) guidelines recommend waiting 2 hours to give intravenous heparin. If the surgeon asked you to give clopidogrel or any low-molecular-weight heparin, just say no. These drugs are the bane of epidurologists.

CASE 26: CELIAC PLEXUS BLOCK

This case happened when I was the pain medicine fellow and was doing the celiac plexus block. I thought we could do this under local anesthesia and sedation, but the much-smarter-than-I anesthesiologist pointed out that this patient was at very high risk for aspiration and definitely needed to be intubated. The patient was an easy intubation and was maintained with controlled ventilation on sevoflurane and fentanyl. With the celiac plexus block, there are several organ systems to be wary of as you pass a long needle to the anterior portion of the L1 vertebral body right in front of the aorta. You first have to avoid the lungs as you guide the needle forward, and when the patient is being ventilated, you should hold his or her breath as the needle approaches or risk another procedure for the day—a chest tube. Luckily, we missed the lung, edged close to the kidney, and twisted past the vertebral disk, inferior vena cava, and renal and splenic veins to land right in front of the aorta and inject our radiopaque dye, hoping for that crescent-moon shape in front. Then we moved onto the ethanol. Things to look for postoperatively are hypotension (e.g., with a sympathectomy), lung collapse, hematuria, catastrophic nerve damage, or paralysis from the ethanol, and pain relief.

CASE 27: EPIDURAL STEROIDS

I went to see the patient, and she was not pleasant. She was perhaps the most miserable pregnant lady I ever met. She sneezed a few days earlier and felt a sharp, stabbing pain in her low back that shot down the back of her leg all the way to the foot. MRI showed a very large, herniated nucleus pulposus impinging on both S1 nerve roots. Fortunately, she only felt one of them. I told her I was willing to try giving her an epidural steroid injection, but she had to understand the risks involved. I also explained that continuing on opioids for the rest of her pregnancy would likely result in her baby having to be detoxed after birth. I discussed with her obstetrician the use of the usual adjuvants, and nonsteroidal anti-inflammatory drugs (NSAIDs) were frowned on. The obstetrician approved of giving gabapentin, but I was a little trepidacious. After all the risks, benefits, and alternatives were explained, I decided to try to find a surgeon to make a little incision under local anesthesia and suck that disk out of there. I could not find one and ended up giving her 80 mg of Depo-Medrol with a few milliliters of bupivacaine at the L5-S1 interspace (I think). Her VAS pain score of 9/10 went to 7/10. I prayed that the baby would be okay, and she was. The mother was converted to oral hydrocodone and discharged home. She saw my colleague in our outpatient clinic, and they bonded well. My kind and gentle Russian-American colleague taught her some deep-breathing exercises, and 9 weeks later, she had a scheduled cesarean section done without incident under spinal anesthesia. She had stopped her opioid well in advance, the baby had normal Apgar scores, and everyone was happy.

CASE 28: LASER FOR POLYPS

You are worried that you can adequately control the airway without exacerbating the disease process. A generic intubation can "knock polyps down into the trachea," and you could end up with polyps down there later. No good!

You also have concerns about an airway fire, because the laser, high oxygen levels, and vaporized material add up to an airway fire. You are concerned about eye safety for the patient and the OR staff. You have concerns about infection, because the vaporized material could be inhaled by the people in the OR, and they could get polyps. All this in one case! What to do?

- Use jet ventilation with a low inspired oxygen and no nitrous oxide.
- Use tight-fitting masks for everyone in the OR, and use eye protection appropriate for the laser's wavelength for the staff.

CASE 29: OPEN REDUCTION AND INTERNAL FIXATION OF A WRIST

After a complete history and physical examination and after ruling out additional injuries, you can do the case with an axillary block. Regional purists would say you should block each of the nerves individually, but you also can perform the block with a through-and-through perivascular injection of local anesthetic.

CASE 30: MASSETER SPASM

Masseter muscle spasm raises the suspicion level enough to assume susceptibility to malignant hyperthermia. Even if he has had two subsequent operations with suxamethonium (who the hell did that?), he could manifest malignant hyperthermia this time, so why take the risk? The preoperative CPK level does not help. It is easy enough, in this era of infusion pumps and propofol, to do a trigger-free anesthetic, so just do it!

CASE 31: PREECLAMPSIA

Magnesium antagonizes release of acetylcholine at the neuromuscular junction. Clinically, you see lethargy, drowsiness, flushing, and diminished tendon reflexes (a good thing to follow clinically!), and it can progress to hypotension, coma, paralysis, and death. Follow the patient clinically with the tendon reflexes, her level of consciousness, and her vital signs.

In the OR, with blood pressure this high, I would follow closely with an arterial line and would titrate nicardipine to decrease the blood pressure. If she needs a cesarean section, I would use succinylcholine for intubation. If she needed further relaxation in the case, I would use reduced doses of vecuronium and follow the twitch monitor closely, because magnesium potentiates nondepolarizing muscle relaxants.

CASE 32: PANCREATECTOMY

Use a low thoracic insertion site, such as T7-8, aiming at a band of anesthesia that covers the surgical area. You can infuse 0.125% bupivacaine plus fentanyl, titrating to patient comfort. To minimize respiratory depression, I would follow the patient's comfort levels (i.e., pain scale of 1 to 10) and respiratory rate. If hypotension occurred, I would stop the local anesthetic component of the infusion, resuscitate with fluids, and run in a narcotic infusion until the blood pressure normalizes and the patient can again tolerate the sympathectomy from the local anesthetic.

CASE 33: CEREBRAL ANEURYSM

At the moment of truth, I would drop the blood pressure with nicardipine. I would keep the patient eucarbic because hyperventilation can cause cerebral ischemia. Hypothermia has not been shown to be protective, nor has a "pentathol coma," so I would not use pentathol. That much pentathol can cost in terms of blood pressure and time to emergence.

Etomidate, like barbiturates, reduces cerebral blood flow and the cerebral metabolic rate, and it does not depress the cardiovascular system. I would still not use it, because I am most comfortable with this as an induction agent and would not want to be using it at an "unfamiliar time," such as during aneurysm clipping.

CASE 34: VIDEO-ASSISTED THORACOSCOPIC SURGERY

The tube is in the right place, but air is sneaking across the occluding balloon and getting to the other side. I would inflate the balloon a little more. If that did not work, I would change the ventilation to pressure control, making sure I did not go past 22 cm H_2O. Aha! Less pressure means less sneaking past the balloon, and the lung will stay down!

CASE 35: ASTHMA

Use ketamine as an induction agent, hoping that its sympathomimetic properties prevent an exacerbation of the asthma. I would also add narcotics and lidocaine in this rapid-sequence induction to further blunt the airway response to intubation.

CASE 36: ASTHMA AND APPENDECTOMY

Resecure the airway, and then go with inhaled β-adrenergic agents, turn potent inhaled agents on if the bronchospasm continues, and give steroids. These measures will take hours to take effect, but you may be happy to have that help in a few hours! Sedate the patient, and keep the endotracheal tube (ETT) in until the bronchospasm has improved and it is safe to retry extubation.

CASE 37: TRIGGER POINTS

The complications of trigger point injections include skin infection, postinjection soreness, hematoma, intravascular injection, nerve damage, vasovagal reactions, and pneumothorax from chest wall injection.[1,2]

CASE 38: HEAD INJURY

There are several recommendations for treating hyperventilation in the setting of severe traumatic brain injury (TBI):

- In the absence of increased intracranial pressure (ICP), chronic and prolonged hyperventilation therapy ($PaCO_2$ of 25 mm Hg) should be avoided after TBI.
- The use of prophylactic hyperventilation ($PaCO_2$ of 35 mm Hg) during the first 24 hours should be avoided because it can compromise cerebral perfusion during a time of reduced cerebral blood flow.
- Hyperventilation may be necessary during brief periods for increased ICP refractory to sedation, paralysis, cerebrospinal fluid (CSF) drainage, and osmotic diuretics.
- There is a risk of causing cerebral ischemia with aggressive hyperventilation. Additional parameters to identify ischemia include jugular venous oxygen saturation, arterial-jugular venous oxygen content differences, brain tissue oxygen monitoring, and cerebral blood flow monitoring.

Recommendations for steroids include the following:

- Steroids are not recommended for improving outcome or reducing ICP.
- Most evidence indicates that steroids do not improve outcome or lower ICP.

Recommendations for anticonvulsants include the following:

- Most studies show prophylactic anticonvulsants reduce *early* post-traumatic seizures but do not reduce the incidence of *late* post-traumatic seizures.
- Routine seizure prophylaxis later than 1 week after head injury is not recommended.
- Phenytoin and carbamazepine have been shown to reduce the incidence of early post-traumatic seizures.
- Phenytoin or carbamazepine can be used in high-risk patients during the first week after head injury.

CASE 39: UNSTABLE NECK

In airway management of the "uncleared" neck, intubation options include oral intubation using a Macintosh blade after intravenous induction, Bullard laryngoscope, flexible fiberoptic scope, and flexible fiberoptic bronchoscope. Many favor flexible fiberoptic bronchoscope because of the neutral position of the head and neck, little spinal movement, awake intubation, and protective reflexes that may be left intact. However, no data suggest better neurologic outcomes with its use. Direct laryngoscopy after induction with manual in-line stabilization is deemed acceptable practice by American College of Surgeons. No data suggest definitively better outcomes with any particular technique.

Manual in-line stabilization (MILS) reduces total spinal movement during laryngoscopy to a greater degree than use of collars. MILS may reduce overall spinal movements during airway maneuvers but may not guarantee immobility at the point of injury. Spinal movements may be restricted at the caudal end by the weight of the torso and MILS at the cervical (occiput) end, but the cervical midpoint may remain unrestricted. Traction forces may result in distraction at the site of injury. Studies using cadaver models have failed to demonstrate reduction of movement with MILS with posterior column injury.

Stabilization maneuvers make visualization more difficult, but they offer a better view than leaving the collar on. In one study, a grade 3 or 4 laryngoscopic view was obtained in 64% of patients with a collar, tape, and sandbags, compared with 22% stabilized with MILS. The main factor was reduced mouth opening. Another study of 157 normal patients compared a standing sniffing position view with a MILS view plus cricoid pressure. In 55%, the view remained the same; in 36%, the view worsened by one grade; and in 9.5%, the view worsened by two grades. MILS has less impact on airway maneuvers than other forms of immobilization. Removal of the anterior portion of collars (with the neck maintained by MILS) improves the mouth opening and aids airway maneuvers. Cricoid pressure may counter the worsened laryngoscopic view during MILS.[3,4]

CASE 40: PULMONARY ARTERY CATHETER KNOT

Several methods that have been described:

- Simple manipulation and traction (knot may become lodged or cause damage) may be used.
- Under fluoroscopy and using a large introducer, pull the knot to include the knot within the introducer and then withdraw both.
- Percutaneously, with a balloon angioplasty catheter passed through right femoral vein, direct the catheter through the loop of the knot and inflate the balloon to partially open the knot. An Amplatz gooseneck snare introduced through the right basilic vein is guided through the knot by a Terumo wire. The end of the Swan-Ganz catheter is snared and pulled back through the loop, untying the knot.
- Snare the knot with a Dotter basket.
- Use a tip-deflecting guidewire to untie the knot.
- Pull the catheter down to the femoral vein and access by cut-down.
- Perform a cardiotomy.[5-7]

CASE 41: AIRWAY FIRE

Follow airway fire protocol:

1. Stop ventilation, and remove the ETT.
2. Turn off the oxygen, and disconnect the circuit from the machine.
3. Submerge the tube in water.
4. Ventilate with a face mask and reintubate the patient.
5. Assess the airway damage with bronchoscopy, serial chest radiographs, and ABG determinations.
6. Consider bronchial lavage and steroids.

Articles have questioned whether categorically removing the ETT is prudent in all cases, such as if the risk of losing a difficult airway was greater than the potential damage caused by leaving the tube in after the fire is extinguished. Individualized case-based judgment may be appropriate.[8-10]

CASE 42: STEROIDS IN A MUSCULAR MAN

Anabolic steroid use can cause cardiomyopathy, atherosclerosis, hypercoagulability, hepatic dysfunction, and psychotic behavior (roid rage). The heavy musculature can make the patient's airway difficult to manage, and a stormy emergence can endanger the patient and staff. A heavily muscled chest pulling against a closed glottis is a setup for negative-pressure pulmonary edema if you extubate with less-than-perfect timing.

You need a good history, a physical examination, and laboratory tests looking specifically at hepatic disorders. To avoid a stormy emergence and negative-pressure pulmonary edema, I would tailor the anesthetic accordingly (heavy narcotics and I would be willing to wait around a while before he emerges).

Ephedra is like taking ephedrine in high doses for a long time, so look for signs of cardiovascular damage in the history and physical examination results. During the case, I would be aware that he may develop hypotension; his sympathetic nervous system is "wrung dry" requiring direct-acting vasopressors, such as epinephrine.

Garlique can cause easy bleeding. In case reports, delayed emergence has been linked to St. John's wort. An ingredient in this herb, hypericin, is thought to have activity with the γ-aminobutyric acid (GABA) receptor. It functions like a sedative with a long half-life.

Complicating all this herbal medicine is a lack of regulation or standardization in the food supplement industry. One batch of St. John's wort may have a high level of hypericin, and the next batch may not, so determining dosage is difficult.

CASE 43: LEFT BUNDLE BRANCH BLOCK

Damned hard is the quick answer. You could be a techno-weenie and say, "I would put in a TEE probe and look for new regional wall motion abnormalities," but that is just plain not practical. You would have to put in the probe and be constantly scanning for something new—and try that when he has a spinal!

The best you can do is look for "something else" telling you the heart is in trouble (e.g., ectopy, hemodynamic change), because it is tough to draw conclusions about the ST segments themselves. If the patient is awake, you can go with the old standby—chest pain—but if he has diabetes, you may not be able to draw from that well. If you have a high index of suspicion, sample troponins after an "event" (e.g., hypotensive, hypoxic intubation), and look for chemical markers of ischemia. In short, you are screwed.

CASE 44: CARBON MONOXIDE

High flows over a long time can dry out the carbon dioxide absorbent. Exposure of dry absorbent to an anesthetic agent (which can happen if a machine is left on all weekend with 2 L/min of O_2 flow going) can produce carbon monoxide.

Change the absorbent, stay on 100% oxygen, and follow serial blood gas samples. If the carbon monoxide level remains high, send the patient for hyperbaric oxygen therapy. To prevent this, make sure no machines are kept on overnight, and change the CO_2 absorbent on a regular basis.

CASE 45: AIRWAY IN A PREECLAMPTIC PATIENT

Have a smaller tube ready, as well as extra hands and equipment (e.g., bougie, fiberoptic scope) in case the airway is not easy. To blunt the sympathetic response to intubation (and avoid an intracranial hemorrhage), have an arterial line in and a vasodilator (e.g., nicardipine, nitroglycerin) ready to inject if the blood pressure spikes.

CASE 46: MONOAMINE OXIDASE INHIBITORS

The bad boys in terms of MAO interactions are ephedrine (i.e., produces an exaggerated response) and meperidine (i.e., hypertension, convulsions, and coma). As long as you avoid those medications, you can do a safe anesthetic.

CASE 47: TRACHEOSTOMY AND LUNG ISOLATION

Obtain the patient's history, and perform a physical examination, focusing on the need for a tracheostomy and how big the tracheostomy stoma is. A good approach is to place a Univent tube in the stoma and use the blocker to block the lung you want blocked (duh). Putting a big-hogger double-lumen tube through a tracheostomy may be pushing it. An important thing to remember is that you can (absent a tracheal resection) intubate from above in a patient with a tracheostomy stoma.

CASE 48: PARENTAL PRESENCE

Explain to the mother that children can get disoriented as the midazolam takes effect and that only reassurance and careful watching are needed. If she looks like she will be an obstruction, do not bring her back with you. If she is cool, back you go.

CASE 49: HYPOTHERMIA FOR HEAD INJURY

Studies have shown no improvement in outcome with mild hypothermia and cerebral protection. Patients for aneurysm clipping were put in a hypothermic group (33° C) or a normothermic group (36.5° C), and there was no difference in outcomes.

Hypothermia is hard to achieve because the body is pretty good about defending its core temperature. Then you have to worry about getting the patient too cold, producing coagulation problems and rhythm disturbances. Although in theory it may help to "cool the patient to protect the brain," I would not do it for absence of proof.

NOTE: As you take the boards, should you quote a study? Yes, you can quote the gist of it if that is what guides your choices. Word comes through the grapevine of people advising "Never quote a study, because they will take you to task on it." That is bogus advice. You are a physician, a consultant. Quote what you feel is worth quoting!

CASE 50: CARBON DIOXIDE INSUFFLATION IN VIDEO-ASSISTED THORACOSCOPIC SURGERY

The best response is "Something is happening, and I do not like it, so stop doing that something." A small amount of insufflation should not cause a tension pneumothorax or severely impede venous return, but it may not be a small amount (i.e., the gauge could be wrong), or the patient might not have read the book on how he is supposed to respond; maybe he is a lot drier than you think, and this small amount of insufflation is too much for him. Pull out, stop insufflating, make sure there is no pneumothorax, regroup, and start over.

CASE 51: CONSTRUCTION IN THE OBSTETRICS DEPARTMENT

In the obstetrics department, you never want to use up your last room on an elective case. What if a patient requiring an immediate cesarean section comes along? Wait at least until everything is cool in one of the extra rooms before you go back with this elective case.

CASE 52: FLOW VOLUME AND ANTERIOR MEDIASTINAL MASSES

You do not need to take any special precautions. In an asymptomatic adult, it is not likely that you induce and, all of a sudden, cannot ventilate or do anything else. If the patient is symptomatic, it is a different story.

- Femoral-femoral bypass is at least a possibility (with perfusionists sticking around).
- Rigid bronchoscopy should be available.
- Everyone in the room should be informed that you may have to put the patient on the side or even prone if things go haywire.

In a child, you have to be ready for the worst, just as you do for a symptomatic adult. Children are more cartilaginous and more prone to a mediastinal mass squishing down and flattening everything than are adults. Adults are more calcified and stiff, and we are less likely to get squished by our own mediastinal mass. At least there's one good thing about being old.

CASE 53: APROTININ (Historical question only!)

No, no, a thousand times no! Aprotinin has been tarred and feathered with accusations of serious end-organ damage, particularly renal failure, and graft occlusion.[11] I therefore would not use aprotinin in this case. We already have a pair of kidneys on the ropes, and we have old grafts and, soon, new grafts to worry about.

CASE 54: BOTOX

Obtain the patient's history, and perform a physical examination, focusing on where you can place lines (sometimes very challenging in this population) and how accessible and intubatable the airway is. Use inhalation induction (no succinylcholine), secure the airway, and place an intravenous line.

Although botulinum toxin is a long-acting muscle relaxant, its use in the muscles of cerebral palsy patients has not caused adverse effects. Of course, the first complication is always waiting to happen, so I would watch neuromuscular function closely throughout the case.

CASE 55: TRANSJUGULAR INTRAHEPATIC PORTOSYSTEMIC SHUNT PROCEDURE

This case can go just wonderfully and usually does. The radiologist uses the intrajugular approach, puts his spike through the liver (scary as hell, but there it is), and all is well. Then again, a big spike, big organ with a big blood supply, and a poor coagulation system are the makings of a cardiovascular wipeout from bleeding. You have to be ready with large-access lines and blood that has been typed and crossmatched. Because all these patients have poor coagulation, I would not give prophylactic fresh frozen plasma (FFP). No matter the numbers, if there is not an indication to give it now (e.g., bleeding in a field), I would not give it. The risks are volume overload and transfusion-related lung injury.

CASE 56: VAGINAL BIRTH AFTER CESAREAN SECTION

She will need to be informed about the risk of uterine rupture. She probably should deliver in an OR with a team ready to put her to sleep and perform a laparotomy in the event her uterus ruptures. The risks of this procedure should be explained and consent obtained early in case this emergency is encountered. The patient must understand that she risks requiring a hysterectomy or ligation of the hypogastric arteries, or both, to control bleeding. In the face of a well-functioning epidural, uterine rupture is still accompanied by continuous abdominal pain and hypotension. In an attempt to make these changes easier to detect, the anesthesiologist can use dilute concentrations of local anesthetics in the epidural.

CASE 57: MULTI-ACCESS CATHETER INSERTION GONE BAD

I would listen to the patient's chest fields for signs of a pneumothorax or hemothorax. If this is likely and the patient is hemodynamically stable, I would call a surgeon to put in a chest tube. The patient may need a more emergent needle decompression. If the patient is truly in respiratory distress, he may have to be intubated. Knowing that achondroplastic dwarfs are likely to have small airways and foramen magnum stenosis, I would avoid direct laryngoscopy and instead opt for a fiberoptic intubation through the laryngeal mask airway (LMA) already in place. The size of the tube is based on the patient's weight, not age. I would want a chest radiograph and arterial blood gas (ABG) determination, and I would like to know if he has equal pulses in his radial arteries.

CASE 58: DELIRIUM IN AN ELDERLY PATIENT

Postoperative delirium is a transient, potentially reversible disorder of cognition and attention according to Stoelting and Dierdorf. We first seek potential causes such as pneumonia, electrolyte abnormalities, hypoxemia, and medication interactions. Otherwise, it is a good idea to promote normal awake-sleep cycles with use of correct lighting and decreased noise. Absolutely avoid the use of restraints.

CASE 59: NERVE BLOCK AND COUGHING

The diagnosis is anxiety, pneumothorax, hemothorax, and ipsilateral phrenic nerve block. Management should provide 100% oxygen, regardless of saturation and make sure the patient is ventilating and is hemodynamically stable. An electrocardiogram (ECG), blood pressure measurement, and pulse oximetry should be instituted if not already ongoing. Preparation for endotracheal intubation and hemodynamic support must be made. Mental status must be followed. Small doses of midazolam can alleviate anxiety while avoiding excessive sedation. Get an immediate chest radiograph. Anxiety is always a diagnosis of exclusion.

CASE 60: HEADACHE

I would ask her if the headache is worse when she stands up and if it is better when lying flat. Did these symptoms come on suddenly or have they been slowly progressing. Does she have a fever or photophobia? I would tell her it is most likely a postdural puncture headache, which usually resolves after 12 to 72 hours. Conservative treatment includes lying flat, analgesics such as Tylenol or NSAIDs, oral or intravenous fluid, caffeine, stool softeners, and a soft diet. If these do not help or the pain is unbearable, I would tell her to come in because she may need an epidural blood patch. A more sinister problem is the possible onset of meningitis or arachnoiditis, which could result from contamination of the equipment used during the epidural. An indwelling epidural catheter also can become colonized.

CASE 61: CEREBROSPINAL FLUID DRAINAGE

CSF drainage can reduce brain tension, but you must drain only when the dura is open to prevent brain herniation. Draining about 10 to 20 mL of CSF is the recommended amount. If you suck out 100 mL, you really are looking at a possible herniation! Tell the surgeon about your booboo, and watch for signs of herniation. You may consider reinfusing some of the CSF (keeping strict aseptic technique, of course) to prevent herniation.

CASE 62: PHEOCHROMOCYTOMA

No, you do not proceed. A patient with a pheochromocytoma is one case you really want optimized, even if that means admission and in-house monitoring of blood pressure. Pushing ahead for economic reasons is penny-wise and pound-foolish. The complications of wild blood pressure swings in an un-optimized pheochromocytoma patient could result in myocardial ischemia, stroke, renal damage, or death—quite a price to pay for being in a rush!

CASE 63: CERVICAL EPIDURAL

This is a formula for disaster for several reasons:

- The patient is prone, and you cannot get at the airway.
- The patient is morbidly obese, in the prone position, and quick to desaturate.
- With inadequate sedation, the patient could jump at the wrong time, risking neurologic damage.
- To get the cervical epidural in, you must flex the neck, which is the wrong way for airway maintenance.
- She is demanding, so "hold still" will not work.

My plan? Not to sound like a broken record (no, the drug company people do not pay me to say this), take the time to do a dexmedetomidine load, and run an infusion. It is the only sedative that will lessen the risk of all the bad things mentioned in the preceding list. She will be sedated, keep breathing, and have some pain relief. It is just what you need.

CASE 64: PAIN RELIEF AFTER KNEE SURGERY

You want to make sure the patient is in the care of a responsible adult who can watch for the bad things:

- Catheter fell out (inadequate pain relief)
- Infected catheter
- Leak at any connection site

The infusion apparatus should protect against an overdose, but the patient should still be advised of signs of toxicity and be provided with an emergency number to contact.

CASE 65: EQUIPMENT CHECK

A positive-pressure test can ascertain problems only as far back as a check valve in the system, so you would miss the area from beyond the check valve. This includes the vaporizers themselves and the oxygen/nitrous/air manifold. That is the area checked by the negative-pressure test. The bulb that you use to push in opens and keeps open the check valve, and you then have to open each vaporizer individually to see if there is a leak. The negative-pressure test also works if your system does not have a check valve.

CASE 66: PACEMAKER

Thank God and our lucky stars that Marc Rozner, PhD, MD, is around to clear the fog on "all things that go pace in the night." I would be lying if I failed to admit I stole this from his 2006 American Society of Anesthesiologists (ASA) refresher talk (number 239 if you are thumbing through it).

Magnet-activated switches were put in pacers "to produce pacing behavior that demonstrates remaining battery life, and sometimes, pacing threshold factors." We have forever kidded ourselves into thinking that magnets automatically put the patient into a continuous asynchronous mode. **BUT NO, SAYS ROZNER** (using capitalized, boldface letters). You cannot say for sure what will happen when you put a magnet on, so "calling the manufacturer remains the most reliable method for determining magnet response."

So there. But what about a magnet in the case of an automatic implantable cardioverter defibrillator (AICD)? (After all, what self-respecting vice-president does not have an AICD?) We again go to the Book of Rozner for a reading to show us the way and the light: "Antitachycardia therapy in some Guidant and CPI devices can be permanently disabled by magnet placement for 30 seconds." So get those magnets away from those AICDs, or I'll sic Rozner on you!

CASE 67: CONSENT

You do not need separate consent for anesthesia (look around you; lots of hospitals do not), but a lot of places do get separate anesthesia consent, because there are risks inherent to the anesthetic state alone (e.g., awareness) that are separate from surgical risks, and it is reasonable for the anesthesiologist to address these concerns with the patient. You want to balance the information, tailoring it to the "reasonable person" (which, you hope, your patient is). For example, you can mention awareness as a possible risk and then detail how you will watch closely and augment that with bispectral (BIS) index monitoring to minimize (you can never completely eliminate) that risk. If a patient asked for an ad hoc consent form, I would write one up on a progress note and make sure everyone signed it, including witnesses.

CASE 68: GASTROSCHISIS

You will need to be in constant communication with the surgeon because there are two major concerns: volume management (i.e., large amounts of fluids are lost through the exposed viscera) and ventilation (i.e., as the contents are returned to the abdomen, you create a restrictive defect). As the contents are replaced, let the surgeon know if the pressure drops (because pushing in large amounts of viscera can cut off venous return of blood—a kind of abdominal compartment syndrome that can impair circulation to the bowel, kidneys, and legs), and let the surgeon know if ventilation becomes difficult. Often, the surgeon has to do a staged repair, not returning all the contents to the abdomen at once.

One way to measure "how much is too much" is to measure intragastric pressure. You place a nasogastric tube in the stomach and measure a column of saline. Keep the pressure lower than 20 mm Hg.

CASE 69: PYLORIC STENOSIS

Pain control in the neonate is tempered by concern about apnea with narcotics. Infants at highest risk are premature, those with multiple congenital anomalies, those with chronic lung disease (which is related to prematurity), and those with a history of bradycardia and apnea. An adequately volume-resuscitated patient with pyloric stenosis is not at any increased risk for apnea, but I would follow the guidelines for all neonates: Use a conservative approach, and monitor all infants younger than 60 weeks' postconceptual age for 24 hours after surgery.

For pain relief, I would avoid narcotics (i.e., respiratory depression) and would place an epidural and give 1.25 mL/kg of 0.25% ropivacaine. For additional pain relief, I would administer acetaminophen rectally, being aware of its side effect of hepatotoxicity.

CASE 70: COCAINE USER

Long-term propofol can lead to a number of problems, including fat embo-lus syndrome and acidosis. I would use propofol for short-term sedation (i.e., overnight).

Dexmedetomidine is a good choice for long-term sedation, because it allows the patient to be cooperative and to breathe but keep sedated, and it is hemodynamically smoother due to dexmedetomidine's ability to decrease central sympathetic outflow. Fentanyl and midazolam are also reasonable options, although they are more likely to cause respiratory depression.

Much of the choice depends on the ICU staff. For example, a staff familiar with dexmedetomidine and knowledgeable about its shortcomings (e.g., drop in blood pressure, bradycardia) would constitute a good setting for its use. If the staff members are unfamiliar with the drug, its dosing, and its side effects, you are safer going with, for example, the old standby of a narcotic plus benzodiazepine infusion.

CASE 71: SEIZURE DISORDER

Resign yourself to the fact that there may be a seizure in the perioperative period, and make sure the preoperative and postoperative staff are aware of the risk. This is an emergency, so you will do a standard rapid-sequence induction. The only special thing you might do is avoid things that would increase cerebral metabolic rate (e.g., ketamine) or that could cause epileptiform movement (e.g., etomidate). Pentathol is an attractive choice. At least the patient will not have a seizure when that drug is on board!

All those agents probably have jacked the patient's ability to metabolize drugs, so the patient may "go through" narcotics and muscle relaxants quickly. Use these methods to follow the patient:

- Twitch monitor for the muscle relaxation
- Respiratory rate for the narcotics

CASE 72: CRANIAL MAPPING

This is a preoperative visit worth stretching out longer than usual. Go into detail about how you will be there, how you will keep the drapes off the face as much as possible, and how you will keep talking to him. The more trust you build up, the fewer drugs the patient will need.

How should you sedate him? Well, damn, here we go with dexmedetomidine again. It keeps them breathing and calm, and it provides some pain relief. To play the devil's advocate, a low-dose propofol infusion, with meticulous attention to "keeping the patient talking, ergo breathing," could do just as well.

CASE 73: DIASTOLIC DYSFUNCTION

Moderate diastolic dysfunction means the heart is stiff; the heart is not good at relaxing during diastole to allow complete filling of the ventricle. This translates clinically into the following alterations in your plan:

- You need higher filling pressures to fill the ventricle.
- You may find yourself infusing more fluid than you normally would to keep the same blood pressure.

In a practical sense, there is no "diastolic dysfunction pill" or "diastolic dysfunction procedure" that will magically make this patient better. Go on the usual clinical grounds—the history and physical examination results—and see how much the patient can do, such as being able to lie flat or walk up a few flights of stairs. If he seems good to go otherwise, proceed. Damn the diastolic dysfunction; full speed ahead!

CASE 74: SLEEP APNEA

Respiratory, respiratory, respiratory! The concern is respiratory misadventure during airway management. A thick tongue and neck and rapidity of desaturation add up to airway trouble if you do a general anesthetic. Postoperatively, there is concern about respiratory depression, including delayed respiratory depression after the patient has gone home.

"The next morning, the patient was found dead in his bed." What a nightmare!

The ASA has practice guidelines (just guidelines, mind you) about obstructive sleep apnea. If the patient scores greater than or equal to 5 on the scale, he or she is not considered a good candidate for outpatient surgery. This is the basis of the obstructive sleep apnea grading system:

A. Severity of sleep apnea based on sleep study or clinical indicators
B. Invasiveness of surgery and anesthesia
C. Requirements for postoperative opioids
D. Add them up to get an estimation of perioperative risks

So with all this information, what do you do? There is no problem with something done under regional or local anesthesia. If patients require general anesthesia or narcotics, they must be watched overnight.

CASE 75: RENAL FAILURE

You are supposed to wait 4 to 6 weeks after placement of a stent to have elective surgery. The concern is that clot formation in a new stent has not had time to endothelialize. Is an arteriovenous graft truly elective? I say no, because the patient needs effective dialysis, and keeping a big central line in for another 4 weeks (doing dialysis through a central line) runs the risk of the line getting infected, clotting, or needing replacement. I would proceed with the graft.

CASE 76: NERVE GAS

God help us if this happens. Most nerve agents are basically insecticides, causing a monster cholinergic response in us. (It is creepy to think about us being eliminated like so many cockroaches.) You must be prepared with heroic doses of atropine to counter the cholinergic thunderbolt from the weapon. Key in this maneuver is protecting the hospital personnel themselves, because nerve gas can be re-aerosolized as the patients' clothes are removed. You need protective gear, and you must be ready to give yourself atropine if you are affected.

Respiratory insufficiency is one of the many problems caused by these weapons, so you will be involved in a lot of airway management. This is no mean feat in protective gear and with patients with profuse secretions.

CASE 77: CENTRAL LINE STERILITY

Put on a gown like the Anesthesia Patient Safety Foundation says! The wire is contaminated, so pull out and go again. And wear that gown from now on.

CASE 78: KIDNEY PROTECTION DURING ABDOMINAL AORTIC ANEURYSM

No pharmacologic kidney protection is required during abdominal aortic aneurysm (AAA) procedure. The surgeon is behind the times. Dopamine and mannitol do nothing for the kidneys; do not use them. The best management for protecting the kidneys is a short clamp time (yell at the surgeon to hurry up!) and adequate volume resuscitation. Nothing else matters.

CASE 79: MYASTHENIA GRAVIS

No succinylcholine; no suxamethonium drip. You do not know what kind of a response the patient will have, so do not risk it. If some fool did do it, follow the twitch, but more importantly, follow the clinical signs to make sure the patient is able to be extubated: hand grip, head lift, adequate tidal volumes, normal respiratory rate, and an ability to handle secretions.

CASE 80: UREMIA AND PLATELET FUNCTION

Uremia affects platelet function, and how the hell did a 44-year-old woman with renal failure get pregnant and carry to term? Those amazing humans!

There are platelet function studies, but the best assessment is based on the patient's history and physical examination. Look for signs of easy bleeding and bruising. In particular, look for venipuncture sites, and see if there are big hematomas there.

If the history and physical examination results indicate it is okay to proceed, I would use regional anesthesia, but be aware that a bleeding problem is more likely in her than in the nonuremic patient.

CASE 81: MANDIBLE FRACTURE

Aha! You thought we would provide answers for all of these grab bags! Guess again! Figure this one out for yourself.

CASE 82: PREGNANT NURSE

No one is sure what the story is on working in the OR during pregnancy. In particular, no one has ever controlled for stress as a contributing factor, and saying that she should not work in the OR because we do not know the risks may result in even *more* stress. For example, the nurse may be supporting a family, and leaving the OR job may put a financial burden on her.

I would tell her to get out of cases in which they do radiology studies or radioactive implants (e.g., prostate seeding). I would let the other anesthesiologists know so they could avoid nitrous oxide in those rooms, and I would not alter this advice based on which trimester she is in. The same suggestions apply to working in the recovery room.

CASE 83: GENERAL ANESTHESIA IN A PREGNANT PATIENT

The risks are minimal, and the best way to take care of baby is to take care of mom. I would tell her not to worry. At 20 weeks, it is too early to change horses in midstream and do a cesarean section if you saw anything, so I would do an examination only before and after the operation.

At 37 weeks, it is a different story. I would have the fetal heart rate monitor on the entire time and would have a labor and delivery nurse watching it throughout the case. If you really got in trouble (which you will avoid by taking good care of the mother), you could do a cesarean section.

CASE 84: KID WITH A BAD AIRWAY

This one is good enough to be an entire stem question! Because of concerns about the loss of the airway and possible need for an emergent tracheostomy with airway collapse, the baby was brought to the OR for induction of anesthesia. Because the child became stridorous when supine, induction was done with the baby supported at a 60-degree upright position. The existing intravenous access was adequate. The attending pediatric surgeon was scrubbed and ready to do an emergent tracheostomy if needed. The equipment for the tracheostomy and an appropriately sized rigid bronchoscope was available. Induction with sevoflurane, oxygen, and nitrous oxide was successful, and although not great, ventilation by means of the mask was adequate. Airway visualization was complicated by the large tongue being forced into the oral cavity by the mass below in the sub-mental space and by involvement of the mass in the posterior pharynx. Despite attempts with an appropriate tube size (4.0), it would not pass, and a 3.5-French, uncuffed endotracheal tube (ETT) was successfully placed. The leak with the child upright was 10 cm H_2O. With the child supine, the leak increased to 18 cm H_2O because of compression of the trachea by the mass and showed the degree of tracheal malacia because of the chronic tracheal compression by the cystic hygroma mass. The child was taken to MRI anesthetized with a propofol infu-sion running to maintain anesthesia and rocuronium for neuromuscular block-ing. The MRI/MRA scan took approximately 1.5 hours. The child was transferred back to the OR with the same setup as before. Neuromuscular blocking was reversed, anesthesia was discontinued, and the patient's leaks were reassessed. With the same leaks upright and supine as were seen after intubation, the deci-sion was made for trial extubation. With the baby fully awake, she was extubated in a 60-degree upright position. There were no differences in her ventilation between preoperative values and after 15 minutes in the OR, and she was taken to the PACU. She was scheduled for removal of the mass 6 days after the scan.

CASE 85: EPIDURAL AND COMPLEX REGIONAL PAIN SYNDROME

This one little grab bag could be your entire oral board examination! Complex regional pain syndrome (CRPS) is a group of sympathetically maintained neuropathic pain disorders.

Type I (i.e., RSD) typically develops as a consequence of trauma (e.g., con-tusions, lacerations, and fractures) affecting the limbs, with or without an obvious peripheral nerve injury. The pain has a burning quality and often is accompanied by diffuse tenderness and pain in response to light touch. Autonomic nervous system dysfunctions manifest as changes in skin tempera-ture, cyanosis, edema, and hyperhidrosis.

Type II (i.e., causalgia) typically follows high-velocity injuries (e.g., gun-shot) to large nerves. The pain usually has an immediate onset and is associ-ated with allodynia, hyperpathia, and vasomotor and sudomotor dysfunction. Anything that increases sympathetic tones, such as fear, anxiety, light, noise, or touch, exacerbates the pain. It most commonly affects the brachial plexus, especially the median nerve, and the tibial nerve.

The mechanism of decreasing pain by a spinal cord stimulator is based on the gate-control theory of pain. Reception of large nerve fiber information, such as touch, a sense of cold, or vibration, turns off or closes the gate to reception of painful small nerve fiber information. The expected end result is pain relief. By electrically stimulating large fibers of the spinal cord with a spinal cord stimulator, painful small fiber information is shut down at that spinal segment, and all other information downstream from that segment is shut down as well.

Because of the location of the spinal cord stimulator electrodes, I believe lumbar epidural for labor analgesia would be a reasonable option for this patient. However, I would first confirm the specific anatomy of the lead place-ment and the path of the extension wire with radiographic studies (so that I would not damage the wire on insertion of the epidural needle). I would also use meticulous sterile technique for the epidural procedure because there is a potential for increased risk of infection in a patient with a pre-existing foreign body. I would also inform the patient that there is always a possibility of disrupting the function of the spinal cord stimulator.

What Actually Happened

We placed a labor epidural at L3-4 with no problems. Not all of the pain specialists at our institution agreed about whether the patient could use the stimulator during the epidural analgesia, so we kept it off. The patient had excellent analgesia for her labor and had an uneventful, spontaneous, vaginal delivery. She started to use her stimulator again approximately 6 hours after the epidural infusion was discontinued.

CASE 86: PREMATURE INFANT AND PATENT DUCTUS ARTERIOSUS

Although a lethargic, 3-day-old preemie and a "generic adult" seem miles apart, you want to take a similar approach to understanding any change in the mental state (lethargy in this case). Look at the big three reasons, which encompass damned near everything: pharmacologic, metabolic, and neurologic, and then take into consideration the characteristics specific to a preemie.

Pharmacologic reasons: Did the child get any medications in the ICU? It is unlikely, given the prematurity and a cardiac problem, but you want to consider it. An immature system is extremely sensitive to any sedatives.

Metabolic reasons: Almost anything could tip this kid into trouble, including hypoglycemia (a premature infant has little in the way of metabolic reserve), hypoxemia, hypothermia, or acidosis. Another thing to consider is a baby's normal sleep pattern. The kid may be sleeping.

Neurologic reasons: Consider the child's prematurity. Realize that an intracranial lesion is a possibility.

CASE 87: PERICARDIAL WINDOW

Lack of a pulse means you are not perfusing, the same as pulseless electrical activity (PEA). However, it is not PEA *all* the time, only *some* of the time. Hmmm. Aha! This patient's tamponade is so bad he is almost in complete PEA, but it is occurring only part time, happening during part of his respiratory cycle. He has respiratory variation to the point of losing his pulse completely. This condition can give pause to even the most experienced anesthesiologist.

Suffice it to say we did this case under local anesthesia and in a big hurry. After the patient's cardiac output returned and he could perfuse his brain, he went to his baseline mental status, which was combative and disoriented. We could tell he was getting better as he tried to reach in the field with one hand and tried to strangle me with the other. Careful—the life you save may *take* your own!

CASE 88: TRANSESOPHAGEAL ECHOCARDIOGRAPHY PROBE PLACEMENT

Cardiologists need no help when it comes to dressing (they all dress better than we do), but placing that transesophageal echocardiography (TEE) probe can tax them. If they are encountering problems, ask whether there is any contraindication (e.g., esophageal operation, diverticulum, injury) and then use a laryngoscope to get a good view and avoid forcing the probe and getting an esophageal tear (frowned on in medical circles, but much admired in plaintiff's attorneys' circles). If the patient is awake, he or she is probably inadequately sedated. Try dexmedetomidine; it sedates well, controls sympathetic outflow, and keeps the patient breathing.

A thoracic gunshot could have injured the esophagus, if not by direct missile injury, then by the blast effect. Make sure the esophagus is "safe" before you proceed.

CASE 89: BURNS

Betadine does not cause burns by itself (think of how many cases we do with Betadine), so something else must have acted in concert. Have the room gone over with a fine-tooth comb for any electrical leaks. Then check with the hospital administration, and see if there is some new chemical in the cleaning process of the sheets, blankets, or drapes.

In the meantime, make a complete report, document everything. Disclose what happened to the family and patient, and get appropriate consultation (dermatology or the burn service) to ensure the patient gets the appropriate care.

CASE 90: CORNEAL ABRASIONS

At the end of a case, before transporting the patient to the ICU, it is common to take the tape off the eyes. An unconscious and often paralyzed patient goes into the ICU, where the first thing that happens is massive rearranging of lines. It is easy to see an arterial line or a stopcock dragging across the eye, pulling up the lid a little, and producing a corneal abrasion. The best thing to do is keep the eye protected until everything is nice and neat and educate the staff on the proper ways to protect the eyes.

CASE 91: OBESE PREGNANT PATIENT

This is a difficult situation for the obstetrician and anesthesiologist. For the obstetrician, the worries are a possibility of uterine rupture and not being able to monitor the baby's well-being. For the anesthesiologist, the issues are morbid obesity, recent ingestion of solid food, and possible increased length of surgery.

If you cannot pick up a heartbeat, you cannot assess fetal well-being. The overall incidence of uterine rupture is less than 1%. However, trauma and scar tissue increase the risk. The problem is that the clinical presentation varies, and diagnosis can be difficult. Fetal distress is an early and reliable sign. Abdominal pain is not always present. In a retrospective study, abdominal pain occurred in less than 10% of uterine rupture cases.

To get ready, you prepare for possible blood loss with a blood type and screen a large-bore, peripheral intravenous line. For aspiration prophylaxis, you use intravenous metoclopramide and oral Bicitra.

Your anesthetic options include regional and general anesthesia. Irrespective of the technique chosen, you should always be prepared for general anesthesia as backup. An LMA, a variety of blades, a bougie, fiberoptic devices (e.g., Bullard laryngoscope), and a video-assisted laryngoscope transtracheal jet ventilator should be immediately available. Make sure adequate help is available.

An epidural can be time consuming because of technical difficulties in locating the space and can be unreliable because of suboptimal blocks (unilateral or patchy), especially in morbidly obese patients. A single-shot spinal may not last long enough for the procedure, which may be lengthy due to technical problems. Moreover, spinal needles are much more flexible and may contribute to technical problems in locating the intrathecal space.

Continuous spinal anesthesia is achieved by deliberate placement of a catheter in the intrathecal space. Although there are dedicated continuous spinal kits available in Europe, they are not available in the United States. However, it can be performed using the Touhy needle and the catheter in the epidural kits. The advantages are the ability to titrate to the desired level and the duration of the blockade. Plain 0.5% bupivacaine is a good choice because it is not hyperbaric, and the level can be titrated easily. The risk of postdural puncture headache appears to be less when the catheter is placed for a short period and more so when it is left in place for a longer time. The original reports of neuropathy described a maldistribution leading to exposure of some of the nerves to higher concentrations of hyperbaric local anesthetic. You also must make sure that the catheter is not mistakenly giving epidural dosing.

What Actually Happened

We discussed our concerns with the obstetrics team. Although monitoring the baby is important, we wanted to make sure that we were prepared for blood loss and had an anesthetic plan that was safe and reliable.

We gave metoclopramide (10 mg IV) and sent a blood specimen for type and screen. We gave Bicitra (30 mL PO) just before anesthesia. We prepared all the necessary equipment for a difficult intubation. We did continuous spinal anesthesia with the patient in the sitting position. The placement was easy, and the remainder of the course was uneventful.

CASE 92: WHIPPLE IN A DIABETIC PATIENT

Pain in cancer patients may be caused by a multitude of factors, such as complications of treatment, postoperative surgical pain, neuropathy caused by chemotherapy and radiation fibrosis, or effects of the tumor (e.g., recurrence in surrounding tissues, distant metastases, nerve compression). The patient may have somatic, visceral, or neuropathic pain or a combination thereof, which is not uncommon in cancer patients. The patient may have coexisting problems that are causing pain, which may be overlooked in light of the extensive history of pancreatic cancer. Thorough evaluation of the patient's pain complaint is necessary. Quality, frequency, duration, radiation, and aggravating and alleviating factors must be thoroughly assessed. The patient's medical history should be carefully studied to see what cancer treatment he has had. Close attention must be paid to any coexisting diseases for which medication is being taken. The physical examination should be conducted to see if the pain is referred from the back, if it is of neuropathic origin, if it is related to an acute abdomen, or if it is has a noncancer origin. All necessary laboratory tests (especially liver and kidney tests) and diagnostic procedures (e.g., radiography, MRI, CT scan, bone scan) should be performed if indicated. In this case, pain may be caused by surgical complications, adhesion, obstruction, tumor recurrence and metastases, radiation enteritis, mucositis, fibrosis of the retroperitoneal space, mesenteric ischemia, or colitis after chemotherapy. The case should be discussed in detail with the oncologist, who can give you information about the patient's condition and life expectancy.

The finding of decreased sensation in the hands and feet leads me to believe that the patient is experiencing neuropathic pain, probably caused by chemotherapy and his diabetes. However, you must rule out pathology of the spinal cord, radiation plexopathy, vitamin insufficiency, and cachexia due to cancer.

After thorough evaluation of the patient's pain, he should be treated according to the World Health Organization stepladder approach:

Step 1: Manage the pain by nonopioid medications, with or without adjuvants.

Step 2: If pain persists or is increasing, add weak opioids to nonopioid analgesics and adjuvants.

Step 3: Strong opioids are used with nonopioid analgesics and adjuvants until the patient achieves complete analgesia.

Because of the severity of this patient's condition, treatment would be initiated at Step 3. Interventional procedures (e.g., celiac plexus block) may be employed at any step in the ladder. To determine the patient's effective dose for analgesia, the patient would be started on intravenous patient-controlled analgesia (PCA) and then transferred to long-acting, oral opioids with breakthrough medication in equipotency doses. Adjuvants such as tricyclic antidepressants or antiseizure medication such as gabapentin would be added for his neuropathic pain. Clonidine would also help. Treatment of the patient's pain should be a multidisciplinary task and should include physical therapy, psychotherapy, and alternative treatments such as acupuncture. If oral medication does not achieve analgesia, intrathecal delivery of opioids, clonidine, and local anesthetic should be considered. It is imperative to constantly re-evaluate the patient and adjust treatment accordingly by changing medication or performing more invasive (surgical) procedures.

Many care providers are reluctant to treat cancer patients with the high doses of opioids that are necessary for pain relief because of the belief that the patient will become addicted to the drugs. In reality, addiction is rare among cancer patients. Studies have shown that undertreatment of pain may cause pseudo-addiction. As soon as the pain control is adequate, drug-seeking behavior disappears.

References

1. Alvarez DJ, Rockwell PG: Trigger points: Diagnosis and management. Am Fam Physician 2002;65:653-660.
2. Frontera WF, Silver JK: Essentials of Physical Medicine and Rehabilitation. Philadelphia, Hanley & Belfus, 2002.
3. Crosby ET: Airway management in adults after cervical spine trauma. Anesthesiology 2006;104:1293-1318.
4. Ghafoor AU, Martin TW: Caring for patients with cervical spine injuries: What have we learned? J Clin Anesth 2005;17:640-649.

5. Bhatti WA Sinha S, Rowlands P: Percutaneous untying of a knot in a retained Swanz-Ganz catheter. Cardiovasc Intervent Radiol 2000;23:224-234.

6. Kao MC, Lin SM: Knotted continuous cardiac output thermodilution catheter diagnosed by intraoperative transoesophageal echocardiography [correspondence]. Br J Anaesth 2003;91:451-452.

7. Tremblay N, Taillefer J, Hardy J: Successful non-surgical extraction of a knotted pulmonary artery catheter trapped in the right ventricle. Can J Anesth 1992;39:293-295.

8. Chee WK, Benumof JL: Airway fire during tracheostomy: Extubation may be contra-indicated. Anesthesiology 1998;89:1576-1578.

9. Morgan GE, Mikhail MS: Clinical Anesthesiology, 4th ed. New York, Lange Medical Books, 2006: 840.

10. Ng JM, Hartigan PM: Airway fire during tracheostomy: Should we extubate? Anesthesiology 2003;98:1303.

11. Fergusson DA, Hébert PC, Mazer CD, er al: A clinical trial comparing aprotinin with lysine analogues in high-risk cardiac surgery. N Engl J Med 2008;358:2319-2331.

Part III

Oldies but Goodies

15

Stem Questions and Grab Bags without Answers

This chapter contains an assortment of stem questions and grab bags. Most do not have answers, but some provide hints. A few updates are thrown in here and there.

CASE 1: TOTAL ABDOMINAL HYSTERECTOMY IN A PATIENT WITH HEPATITIS

A 42-year-old, 60-kg woman is scheduled for a total abdominal hysterectomy because of heavy bleeding from large fibroids. She has a history of chronic hepatitis, for which she is on prednisone (15 mg each day). Attempts at weaning from steroids have failed over the years. Her blood pressure is 150/85 mm Hg, pulse is 90 beats/min, respiratory rate is 14 breaths/min, hematocrit is 27%, and serum aspartate aminotransferase (AST) level is 100 U/L (normal is 40 U/L). The total bilirubin level is normal. She started taking "that purple pill they're always advertising on TV" for heartburn that she gets after eating gyros at her local Greek restaurant.

Preoperative Questions

1. You evaluate the patient's hepatic status. The AST level was formerly called the serum glutamic-oxalo-acetic transaminase (SGOT) level. What does an elevated AST (SGOT) level mean? Do you want any more specific tests? What is the effect of liver disease on anesthesia care? Does presence or absence of ascites matter? How? Do you drain the ascites first?
2. For anemia, do you transfuse preoperatively? Why or why not? What is lowest hematocrit you will accept for an elective case? What if the case is emergent? Do you recommend iron or erythropoietin preoperatively? Are there problems with either? How long can you wait? What if her insurance runs out this month? How do you determine volume status preoperatively?

Intraoperative Questions

1. For anesthesia care, is an epidural a good idea? Will you use a continuous or single-shot form? What changes will you make in light of liver disease, anemia, or hypovolemia? Does her height make a difference? If it did, why not use a spinal? Does it depend on the surgeon? Which local anesthetic will you use for a spinal or for general anesthesia? What is transient ischemic radiculopathy? Can you use lidocaine in that case? Does general anesthesia offer any advantages over regional?
2. The patient prefers general anesthesia to regional anesthesia. Do you try to talk the patient into regional anesthesia? What if the patient "always wakes

up wild" after a general? Which induction agent will you use? Is there any advantage of etomidate or propofol over pentathol? How about a midazolam induction? What about inhalation? Will you use ketamine? Which agent gives most stable induction? What are the hepatic impacts of these drugs?

3. For muscle relaxation, is cisatracurium a good idea? Would you use Pavulon (pancuronium) if the surgeon is slow? Would you consider using rocuronium? Defend your choice. Will you start with suxamethonium? Why or why not? What does 2/4 twitches mean? What does 0/4 mean? If you are at 0/4 at the end of the case, how do you reverse? How do you reverse if you are at 4/4 and have no fade? What is most sensitive clinical indicator of muscle relaxant reversal?

4. Fibroid removal turns into the St. Valentine's Day Massacre. Blood loss is 750 mL. The patient has been bleeding excessively from the start. When do you transfuse? How do you monitor blood loss? How accurate is it? How do you evaluate the patient's coagulation profile? Do you use a thromboelastogram (TEG)? What do the various patterns mean? Should you just "give everything"? How do you scientifically treat a coagulopathy?

Postoperative Questions

1. The patient is experiencing emergence delirium. Thirty minutes after arrival in the postanesthesia care unit (PACU), the nurse tells you the patient is going out of his mind and thrashing violently. What is the differential diagnosis, and what is the treatment? You determine that pain is the culprit. Do you use intravenous or intramuscular morphine? Do you use patient-controlled analgesia (PCA)? Do you use epidural or intrathecal narcotics? If epidural, is it better to go with morphine, fentanyl, or sufentanil?

2. The patient has oliguria. The patient's urine output has been 15 mL/hr for 2 hours postoperatively. What are the possible causes, and what is the treatment? Do you need a Swan-Ganz catheter to determine the Svo_2? Should you use transesophageal echocardiography (TEE)? What if she develops acute tubular necrosis in the face of liver disease? How long do you wait before you dialyze?

Grab Bag

1. How do you perform anesthesia in a 6-week-old child who needs a hernia repair? Is your approach different in the outpatient setting? What if the infant was a preemie? Describe the risks to the patient's eyes. What intravenous fluids and what amount of glucose would you administer?

2. Should you use Nubain (nalbuphine hydrochloride) to reverse a case in which you gave too much fentanyl? Detail the risks of Narcan (naloxone). Discuss the use of nalbuphine in the outpatient setting.

3. What safety devices are common to all anesthesia machines? What is the fail-safe device? Do you need an O_2 analyzer? Where do you place it? What electrical safety devices do you need in the operating room (OR)?

CASE 2: CHORIOAMNIONITIS AND PREECLAMPSIA

A 17-year-old, 61-kg girl, who is 33 weeks' pregnant and toxemic, is admitted with ruptured membranes. She develops chorioamnionitis and worsening preeclampsia and is scheduled for emergent cesarean section. She has been given Demerol for pain, along with magnesium and hydralazine. The blood pressure is 180/115 mm Hg, pulse is 105 beats/min (increasing to 120 beats/min with contractions), respiratory rate is 30 breaths/min, temperature is 40°C, and hematocrit is 34%.

Preoperative Questions

1. The patient has toxemia. What is preeclampsia? What are the signs? How is preeclampsia different from eclampsia? How do hydralazine, Nipride (nitro-prusside), and magnesium work? What are the side effects of each? How does each interact with anesthetic agents? What are the major complications of preeclampsia in the mother and baby? How do we assess fetal well-being? What are the various concerning patterns, and what do we do about them?
2. Should you treat the fever before starting the anesthetic? Why or why not? How? Will you use Tylenol or antibiotics? What are the effects on the baby?

Intraoperative Questions

1. Should you use regional or general anesthesia? What are the advantages and disadvantages of each? In the face of fever, do you worry about epidural abscess? Is it likely to happen? If so, how do you diagnose and treat it?
2. It appears to be a difficult intubation. What if the patient is mentally challenged and will not hold still for regional? Will you do a rapid-sequence induction (RSI)? You get an unexpected grade III view and cannot pass an endotracheal tube (ETT). What now? You make two more attempts but cannot pass the ETT. Now what do you do? If she did not cooperate before, how will she cooperate now? Will you do it while she is still "drunk" from the first induction?
3. After you got the tube in, what would you use for maintenance before delivery? Why? Is propofol okay for induction? Which muscle relaxant would you use? What crosses the placenta? After delivery, do you change anything? Why?
4. The baby arrives small, floppy, cyanotic, and apneic and has a heart rate of 60 beats/min. What do you do about the fetal distress? What if meconium is present? Do you use naloxone to reverse your anesthetic drugs? Do you institute muscle relaxant reversal? How do you give drugs if you cannot get an intravenous line placed and are not good enough to get the umbilical lines?
5. There are coagulation headaches. The obstetrician tells you to give oxytocin. What is oxytocin, and how can it hurt or help? Bleeding from the uterus is audible across the room. What is the differential diagnosis, and what is the treatment? What laboratory tests do you order? Should you get the pro-thrombin time (PT), a TEG, or the level of fibrin splits? Does treatment include fresh-frozen plasma (FFP), platelets, cryoprecipitate, or Amicar? Why or why not for each agent?

Postoperative Questions

1. In the PACU, the patient has a full-blown grand mal seizure. What is the treatment? What is a seizure, and how does it damage the brain? Do you need to intubate? What is the effect of the patient being a "full stomach"? When is a mother no longer a full stomach—a week or a month?
2. The patient has postoperative tachycardia. Three hours postoperatively, the heart rate shoots to 170 beats/min. What are the most likely causes and the

less likely causes? How would you proceed? What is the danger of a heart rate of 170 beats/min in a young woman with preeclampsia? Is there any difference after the infant is delivered?

Grab Bag

1. A newborn has coronary heart disease (CHD) and a ventricular septal defect (VSD). Discuss the mechanism of cyanosis.
2. A class I patient just had a laparoscopic cholecystectomy and developed apnea in the PACU. What is the differential diagnosis?
3. Discuss hypoxic pulmonary vasoconstriction during a one-lung case.
4. You reverse a patient, but then he poops out, and you have to quickly give suxamethonium and reintubate him. What kind of a block do you now have, and what is your response?

Update: Central Lines

1. Name the complications of central lines: wire or catheter embolus, cardiac tamponade, carotid puncture, hemothorax, pneumothorax, and pulmonary artery rupture.
2. Name the complications that had the highest death rate: hemothorax, cardiac tamponade, and pulmonary artery rupture.
3. Name a few more complications: hydrothorax or pleural effusion, fluid extravasation in the neck, air embolus, and other vessel injuries.
4. Describe how these complications could have been prevented: ultrasound guidance, pressure monitoring, and getting a chest radiograph.

CASE 3: SMALL BOWEL OBSTRUCTION AND RENAL FAILURE

A 65-year-old man is scheduled for an exploratory laparotomy because of small bowel obstruction. He has chronic renal failure (CRF) and has undergone 5 years of hemodialysis. He is taking clonidine and metoprolol for hypertension. He feels sick all the time because of his CRF and does not do much. His blood pressure is 180/100 mm Hg, pulse is 90 beats/min, respiratory rate is 24 breaths/min, temperature is 38°C, hemoglobin level is 8 g/dL ("that is what I always run"). The patient is in obvious pain, vomiting, and grimacing.

Preoperative Questions

1. How do you decide whether he needs dialysis before surgery? What if this case were elective? Can you still do a "quickie dialysis" if it is urgent? Are there any problems immediately after dialysis? What tests of renal function do you want? What other organ systems are involved, and how will you evaluate them? How do you evaluate fluid status?
2. Is the blood pressure adequately controlled? If the case were elective, would you cancel until the blood pressure is optimized? How long does the blood pressure have to be controlled—an hour, a day, a week, a month? How does poorly controlled blood pressure increase the risk of anesthesia, even in light of our newer, shorter-acting drugs? The patient says he has been too sick to take his clonidine and metoprolol for 2 days. What are the dangers of this? Should you give something intravenously now?

Intraoperative Questions

1. What monitors do you need for fluid status? If patient is not anuric, do you bother with a Foley catheter? Do you need to place an arterial line for blood pressure measurement? How about a blood pressure cuff? How does a blood pressure cuff work, and what are its limitations? What about newer noninvasive blood pressure devices? What are the advantages of this new modality? How about just keeping a finger on the pulse?

2. What are major considerations, starting with the most important, for this patient? Do you use preoperative antacids, Reglan, a nasogastric tube? If a tube is in, do you keep it in or take it out? What are the problems with masking in case of missed intubation? How does the nasogastric tube act as a wick? Which induction agent and which relaxant do you use for induction? Are there special considerations because of the patient's renal failure, full stomach, or recent vomiting? What is the priming principle? How will you decrease fasciculations, or does that not make a difference? Is nitrous narcotic or "garbage bag" anesthetic better? Which is best for the heart, for the kidneys, or for the gastrointestinal tract? What can you do to get him on his feet faster?

3. Twenty minutes after induction, the blood pressure drops to 55/30 mm Hg. What is the differential diagnosis, and what is the treatment? After the blood pressure is okay, you notice that you do not feel a thrill over his arteriovenous fistula. Is there anything you can do?

4. The patient has hypoxia. The arterial blood gas (ABG) determination after an hour shows a P_{O_2} of 65 mm Hg on F_{IO_2} of 0.5. What is the A-a gradient? Your certified registered nurse anesthetist (CRNA) says to go with 10 cm H_2O of positive end-expiratory pressure (PEEP). Do you agree or disagree? Are other steps needed? How does a pulse oximeter work? What are problems with PEEP and with a high F_{IO_2} value? What if that same ABG determination showed a P_{CO_2} of 70 mm Hg?

Postoperative Questions

1. Do you plan to keep the patient on a ventilator postoperatively? Why? What is the advantage of continued ventilation? What is the disadvantage? Which ventilator setting and which modality do you use? How can you be sure the ventilator is working right? What are the potential problems with any ventilator? How can you determine if there is a pipeline crossover? How do you decide when to extubate? What if the patient were an extremely difficult intubation? Would you use any special precautions or techniques?

2. In the intensive care unit (ICU), the patient is thrashing and fighting the ventilator. High-pressure alarms are going off. The ICU nurse says you should sedate the patient. What is your response? What are the options? What other things may be going on? If the patient has pain, should you go with an epidural in an intubated patient? Should you sedate with dexmedetomidine? What is this drug?

Grab Bag

1. The first twin is out okay, but the second needs a version, and the obstetrician requests relaxation. How? Do you use nitroglycerin or go to general anesthesia? Do you use high-dose halothane, or is sevoflurane just as good?

2. The patient is petrified of acquired immunodeficiency syndrome (AIDS) but is about to undergo repeat coronary artery bypass grafting (CABG). He asks, "Doc, is donor directed better? Can I donate myself ahead of time? Are blood extenders okay? How low can you let my blood count go?"
3. The patient comes to you with hemophilia. What are mechanism and genetics of this disease? Do you give Amicar, cryoprecipitate, FFP, factor VIII, or factor VII? What if she is scheduled for a laminectomy for symptomatic footdrop?

Update: Ambulatory Care

1. Does preoperative clinic visit really make a difference? Yes, it reduces cancellations eightfold and drops testing costs by 60%.
2. What are the biggest problems?—Pain and postoperative nausea and vomiting are the most serious problems.
3. What if the surgeon gives inadequate local anesthesia? The anesthesiologist oversedates, and the patient stays longer.
4. Is there a need to take orally or void? No.
5. What is the most common complication of thyroidectomy? Hypocalcemia is the common complication.
6. Among tonsillectomy and adenoidectomy patients, who is more likely to bleed? Older patients are more likely to bleed.
7. Who is more likely to have respiratory problems? Younger patients more often have respiratory difficulties.
8. Does mild intraoperative hypothermia prolong the PACU stay? Yes.

CASE 4: RENAL TRANSPLANTATION AND ALCOHOL ABUSE

A 50-year-old, 70-kg woman with CRF scheduled for renal transplantation. She had dialysis 12 hours earlier. Her hemoglobin level is 6 g/dL, potassium level is 5.1 mEq/L, and creatinine level is 4 mg/dL. She had hepatitis at age 30 and has history of alcohol and Vicodin abuse after a back injury. Her blood pressure is 160/100 mm Hg, heart rate is 65 beats/min, respiratory rate is 18 breaths/min, and temperature is 37°C.

Preoperative Questions

1. Do you need further laboratory workup? Why or why not? Which liver function tests will tell you the most? What is the significance of these laboratory test results for your anesthetic?
2. What is cause of anemia in renal failure patients? Should you treat preoperatively? Why or why not? What compensatory mechanisms are there for anemia? If treatment is necessary, what do you give—whole blood, donor directed, or products along with packed cells? Should you skip all this and give erythropoietin? How do you explain the risk of being infected with human immunodeficiency virus (HIV) from treatment?
3. You fret about hyperkalemia and get a repeat potassium test. It is 5.8 mEq/L. Do you proceed, dialyze first, or use Kayexalate? Do you give medical treatment? What is the medical treatment? Explain how insulin, glucose, and bicarbonate work? How does hyperkalemia short circuit the heart?

Intraoperative Questions

1. Which lead of the electrocardiogram (ECG) will you monitor, and why? Does lead placement really make a difference? What is Eindhoven's triangle? What is the best method of detecting ischemia? What would the ECG show if patient were hyperkalemic, hypokalemic, hypercalcemic, or severely anemic?
2. Is regional anesthesia an option? Where exactly do the surgeons sew in the new kidney? Can you do this with an epidural or spinal? What if the surgeons want you to give heparin intraoperatively to avoid clotting in the vessels? If you use a regional, which kind and which anesthetic? If you use a general, which induction agent and which maintenance agent? Does it make a difference? What about factor A and sevoflurane? Is a nitrous narcotic better? If the patient has a spinal cord injury, can you use suxamethonium? Why or why not?
3. Intraoperative anuria develops. Thirty minutes after new kidney is in, there is still no urine. Do you give a diuretic or more fluid? Do you get cardiac output up with dobutamine? Is it better to give renal dopamine or colloid? Is it time to get invasive and put in a central venous pressure (CVP) or Swan-Ganz catheter? Should you use TEE? If you hit the carotid with the sheath, what do you tell the surgeons?
4. Do you reverse the muscle relaxants at the end of the case? Even if you used cisatracurium and you have 4/4? How about 4/4 and no fade? How do you evaluate clinically? What will acidosis tell you, and will that make you keep the patient intubated? What else can throw off a neuromuscular situation—antibiotics, liver status, or the length of the case? Which anticholinesterase would you use? Does it make a difference? Do you use atropine or glycopyrrolate? What would happen if you forgot to include that?

Postoperative Questions

1. How would you treat postoperative pain? How do epidural or intravenous opioids work, and which is more effective? What if the patient is a VIP? What are the side effects of the epidural compared with the intravenous approach? What are the respiratory effects? Is there a difference given that the patient is "tolerant" from years of Vicodin abuse? Do you use intercostal blocks? What are the advantages and dangers? How do you conduct an intercostal block?
2. The patient has postoperative hypertension. In the PACU, the blood pressure is 220/110 mm Hg. What is the differential diagnosis? What are the special dangers of this operation? What is a Goldblatt kidney? Could that be the cause? Which drug will you use to get blood pressure down? How will that affect renal and hepatic blood flow? Does it make a difference? What if you give labetalol and the patient develops wheezing? What is the differential diagnosis, and what is the treatment?

Grab Bag

1. Discuss the anatomy of the epidural space and the structures encountered during placement of a catheter.
2. What is the train of 4? What is post-tetanic facilitation? What is tetanus? How do we evaluate muscle paralysis?

3. What would you do if a patient says he is "allergic" to Novocaince, but you were planning on doing a lidocaine spinal for transurethral resection of his bladder tumor (TURBT)?

CASE 5: TRANSURETHRAL RESECTION OF THE PROSTATE, DIGOXIN, AND LEFT BUNDLE BRANCH BLOCK

An 85-year-old man is scheduled to have cystoscopy for possible transurethral resection of the prostate (TURP) because of benign prostatic hypertrophy (BPH). He takes digoxin (0.25 mg/day) and sublingual nitroglycerin "every now and then." He has a 4/6 systolic murmur. His blood pressure is 140/100 mm Hg, heart rate is 65 beats/min, respiratory rate is 12 breaths/min, temperature is 37°C, and potassium level is 3.0 mEq/L. The ECG shows a left bundle branch block (LBBB).

Preoperative Questions

1. Are you concerned about his cardiac status, especially the murmur? What could it be, and why is it a problem? How will you tell if it is innocent or sinister? Do you insist on an echocardiogram? The echocardiogram shows significant aortic stenosis, and catheterization shows a gradient of 80 mm Hg. What are the risks of anesthesia and surgery? How do you answer when the patient asks whether he should get his heart fixed first?
2. Catheterization also shows significant coronary artery disease (CAD). Should he have his cardiac surgery first? What if his symptoms are minimal? What if he refuses cardiac surgery? What is significance of an LBBB? What about a new LBBB?
3. What is angina? What is angina at rest and what about the diabetic? What is the difference between stable and unstable angina? Should your preoperative clinic or the surgeon be starting this man on β-blockers? Why? What are the implications of the POISE study?
4. Does a potassium value of 3.0 mEq/L worry you? What is the difference between chronic and acute potassium depletion. Should you replace the potassium before you proceed? What are the dangers of this approach?

Intraoperative Questions

1. If the patient has an "eggshell aorta" and inoperable CAD, how will you do the anesthetic for his TURP? Will you use a spinal, an epidural with slow dosing, or a local? What are the special risks of aortic stenosis?
2. If the patient has a PT of 15 seconds, do you still use regional anesthesia (assume there was no stenosis)? How about if clotting studies were normal, but he took aspirin or Plavix?
3. If you go with a general anesthetic, is it better to have spontaneous ventilation or to put on ventilator? What are the advantages and disadvantages of spontaneous ventilation? Which induction agent is best? Should you use esmolol at induction or an esmolol infusion? Why or why not?
4. Can you do this without an arterial line? Why or why not? Do you need a CVP or Swan-Ganz catheter? Defend your choice. If you use a central line, where should you place it? Give the pros and cons of each choice.
5. You use a CVP line. After an hour and a half of dissection, the CVP rises from 4 to 22 mm Hg. What is the differential diagnosis, and what is the treatment?

Do you tell the surgeon to stop? Is there an artifact? How will you tell? How about the sodium level? How often do you monitor it? How can you treat a sodium of 122 mEq/L, 112 mEq/L, or 102 mEq/L?

6. The patient oozes from venous sinuses. Why? Which tests do you use? How do you diagnose disseminated intravascular coagulation (DIC) or fibrinolysis? Does the information from a TEG help? What is the treatment??

Postoperative Questions

1. Thirty minutes after touchdown in the PACU, the patient goes into bigeminy. Which tests do you order? What is the treatment?? Do you start lidocaine or amiodarone? Is there a drop in the sodium level? What is the danger of rapid sodium replacement?

2. You used general anesthesia, and at the end, the patient fails to awaken. Is the cause pharmacologic, metabolic, or neurologic? What steps do you take while you figure it out? What is the treatment of each cause? What do you tell the anxious wife and the indifferent children?

3. The patient is in agony from the Foley catheter, and he keeps threatening to pull it out. How can you help the patient out? Is there anything else it might be? What is the differential diagnosis, and what is the treatment?

Grab Bag

1. In the management of abruptio placentae, what is considered urgent? Are there special problems such as DIC? Do you use a spinal, epidural, or general? Why? What if there is a language barrier? What if the father wants to be there when the patient is unstable?

2. The technician finds high levels of N_2O in the room, and the Occupational Safety and Health Administration (OSHA) is miffed. How can you fix this, especially with the laryngeal mask airways (LMAs)? Can you tell OSHA that this is not a problem? How do you do high and low pressure checks of the machine?

3. A man says he is "allergic to suxamethonium." What does this mean? How do you tell malignant hyperthermia (MH) from pseudocholinesterase deficiency on the basis of the history or laboratory test results? Does the creatine phosphokinase level help? Does the dibucaine number help? What does that mean anyway?

Update: Pediatrics

1. What is the state of the art for no oral intake (NPO)? Clear liquids up to 2 hours preoperatively, breast milk for 4 hours, formula for 6 hours, and solids for 8 hours.

2. What is the scoop on upper respiratory infections (URIs)? If there is purulence below the cords, cancel the operation.

3. What is the effect of second hand smoke? It causes a 10-fold increase in laryngospasm.

4. What sedation should you use? Use oral midazolam in a dose of 0.5 mg/kg.

CASE 6: CESAREAN SECTION AFTER LUMBAR LAMINECTOMY

A 39-year-old primigravida is scheduled for a cesarean section because she has active herpetic lesions. At age 23, she fell off a horse, hurt her back, and had a lumbar laminectomy and fusion for disk problems. She takes aspirin. She has 3+ edema, has clonic ankle reflexes, and is taking magnesium. Her blood pressure is 175/115 mm Hg, pulse is 80 beats/min, respiratory rate is 16 breaths/min, and temperature is 36.8°C.

Preoperative Questions

1. Is this eclampsia or preeclampsia? What is the difference, and what is the significance? What is the pathophysiology of preeclampsia and the involved organs? What are the complications and treatment? How much magnesium do you give? Does magnesium cross the placenta? What is the effect on the fetus? What is the interaction with anesthetic agents?
2. The fetal heart rate is 120 beats/min. Is this good or bad? What else do you look for? Which patterns are normal, and which are concerning? What happens to variability when a mother goes under anesthesia? If variability is lost, do you perform a cesarean section right away (assume a mother who is 26 weeks' pregnant was having an appendectomy, went under general anesthesia, and the fetal variability went away)?

Intraoperative Questions

1. Laminectomy was performed at the L5-S1 level. Would you use general anesthesia, a spinal, or an epidural? What are the pros and cons of each? The patient demands an epidural because she is an "empowered health care consumer." What is your explanation of the risks and benefits? What if her back pain worsens later and she blames "the needle in my back"? How does a laminectomy alter your landmarks?
2. Five minutes after placing an epidural, the patient seizes. What is the priority of treatment? What is the differential diagnosis? Do you go to a cesarean section right away? Now she is intubated, but she is waking up from the seizure and wants the tube out. Do you sedate? What is the effect on the fetus? Do you use dexmedetomidine? What do you tell the pediatrician?
3. The epidural is spotty, and the patient is howling bloody murder. Do you change to general anesthesia? What are the risks of general anesthesia, particularly for a patient with preeclampsia? What special airway measures (e.g., LMA, bougie, fiberoptic scope, smaller tube) at hand do you use?
4. The blood pressure jumps to 220/130 mm Hg with her crummy epidural. What is the differential diagnosis, and what is the treatment? Can you use Nipride or glycerin? What are the risks to fetus? Are other drugs, such as labetalol or hydralazine, better? What is uteroplacental insufficiency? What is an abruption? What is placenta previa?

Postoperative Questions

1. After delivery, the mother complains of chest pain while the surgeons are externalizing the uterus. What is the differential diagnosis, and what is the treatment? How likely is cardiac ischemia, and how do you rule that out? The mother becomes nauseated. What do you do to relieve her nausea?
2. Twelve hours postoperatively, the mother complains about severe headache. What is the differential diagnosis, and what is the treatment? How can you tell whether this is something terrible (e.g., bleed in head) or a typical spinal headache? What if you got a wet tap earlier? Does the patient need a blood patch right away, or should you wait?

Grab Bag

1. What kinds of vaporizers do we use? Why is the desflurane vaporizer so weird looking? Why do we not want the vaporizer to tip over ever?
2. A 15-year-old boy shot himself in the hand. He has been drinking and is rowdy but somewhat cooperative. Will you do an axial block, Bier block, or interscalene block? What are the pros and cons of each and compared with general anesthesia? What are the pros and cons? What if the local anesthetic goes intravascular?
3. After excision of a laryngeal papilloma, the kiddie develops severe stridor. The surgeon wants to avoid further trauma with an intubation. What are the options, and what do you do? When would you reintubate?
4. Discuss use of a celiac plexus block and a stellate ganglion block. When would you use a neurolytic block?

Update: Spinal Lidocaine

1. What is transient neurologic syndrome? Pain or dysesthesia develops within 24 hours of spinal anesthesia but resolves within 72 hours. Symptoms occur when the patient returns home.
2. Is motor block ever a part of this? No, never; look for something more sinister.
3. What is the treatment? Nonsteroidal anti-inflammatory drugs (NSAIDs) and time constitute the only treatment. At least it tends to resolve in 3 to 4 days.

CASE 7: BLEEDING TONSIL

A 4-year-old, 20-kg boy comes back with a bleeding tonsil. The operation completed 10 hours earlier. His hemoglobin level was not determined preoperatively, because he was perfectly healthy. Estimated blood loss during operation was 50 mL. The patient is restless and anxious. His blood pressure is 80/50 mm Hg, pulse is 130 beats/min, and respiratory rate is 24 breaths/min.

Preoperative Questions

1. What was this patient's starting blood volume? What is it now? How do you estimate blood loss in a bleeding tonsil? How much blood does the kid swallow? Does a repeat hematocrit help, or should you even bother to get one? If it is 25%, do you transfuse? When would you transfuse? If the child had a history of heart surgery as an infant, would it influence your decision?
2. What laboratory tests do you order in the emergency room (ER)? What if there is only typed and screened blood available? What is the chance of a reaction compared with typed and crossed blood? Mother says she will donate right now because she does not want kid to get AIDS. What do you say?
3. What vital signs are appropriate for age and situation? How does a child's heart differ from an adult's? Is the tachycardia caused by emotion or hypovolemia? How will you tell?
4. The kid is restless. Do you sedate? What are the dangers of sedation compared with the dangers of a kid becoming wild and out of control? He keeps pulling pulse oximeter off. How do you determine oxygenation?

Intraoperative Questions

1. Should you give a fluid bolus in the ER or the OR? What do you use for the bolus and why? Do you transfuse blood? In your rush, you gave a bag of heparinized saline; do you now give protamine or something else?
2. Do you premedicate with atropine or glycopyrrolate to dry up the patient? Do you use anti-aspiration medications such as citrate, Reglan, or ranitidine? Why or why not? Is there any evidence-based medicine for these decisions?
3. Do you use a nasogastric tube? What are the pros and cons? Does it help or hurt? How does it act as a wick?
4. The blood bank is cleaned out. The surgeon wants to get going. Do you delay while blood comes from another hospital or just forge ahead?
5. The intravenous fluid infiltrates, and the kid is a tough stick. Now what? Do you use intramuscular ketamine, inhalation induction, a tibial intraosseous line, or central line? If you use a central line, where do you place it?
6. Assume an intravenous line is in. Do you do an RSI, modified RSI, or cricotracheotomy? What size tube and blade should you use? Which stylet should you use?
7. You did not give atropine. You intubate, the child's heart rate slows, and he arrests. What is the remedy?
8. For maintenance, do you use intravenous propofol or inhaled agents? Make a case for and against each.
9. The patient desaturates and becomes bradycardic. What is the differential diagnosis, and what is the treatment? The heart goes into ventricular fibrillation. Take me through a Pediatric Advanced Life Support (PALS) scenario to resuscitate this child.
10. Should you extubate deeply? If not, how do you extubate smoothly?

Postoperative Questions

1. The patient's axillary temperature in the PACU is 34°C. Is this a concern? Why? How do you warm the patient? Going back in time, how could you have prevented this?
2. The kid's eyes get yellow 2 weeks later. Is this hepatitis or halothane hepatitis? The surgeon is blaming you. How do you do a workup?

Grab Bag

1. The child presents with epiglottitis. An experienced hand says you should breathe down with halothane rather than sevoflurane. Do you agree? What is the reasoning? Walk through an entire case of epiglottitis, from the diagnosis to securing the airway safely.
2. A hernia operation is scheduled, and the patient is healthy. The PT and PTT results come back high, and no one knows why. What now? The surgeon says, "Come on. It is a hernia, and I'll do it under local." Is this a good idea? How would you do a block for this?
3. A symptomatic patient with a large mediastinal mass has scary flow-volume loops. You suggest an awake fiberoptic intubation, but he refuses. Now what? If you induce and lose the airway, what do you do next?

Update: Blood Therapy

1. What are the risks? The risks of blood therapy are 1 in 900,000 for HIV, 1 in 1.6 million for hepatitis C, and 1 in 180,000 for hepatitis B. The most common risk is still a reaction caused by clerical error.
2. What is transfusion-related acute lung injury? Between 4 and 6 hours after receiving blood, the patient becomes hypoxemic and has respiratory distress, hypotension, and fever.
3. How low can you go? The patient can tolerate a hemoglobin level of 5 g/dL but no lower.

CASE 8: COLECTOMY IN A PATIENT WITH CIRRHOSIS

A 60-year-old, 60-kg, cirrhotic man is scheduled for a right colectomy because of cancer. He has ascites, jaundice, and spider angiomas. The blood pressure is 100/80 mm Hg, pulse is 100 beats/min, temperature is 36.8°C, and hematocrit is 27%.

Preoperative Questions

1. Are tests for PT, albumin, enzymes, and bilirubin important? Why is there so much focus on the albumin level? If malnutrition seems to be a factor, does it pay to get the albumin level up before operating? Should you use nasogastric feeds or hyperalimentation? What are the implications of hyperalimentation treatment on the CVP?
2. Does ascites influence the anesthetic? What is the effect on volume of distribution? What is volume of distribution, and how can it be greater than the patient's actual volume?
3. Should you do paracentesis? If not, under what circumstances would you? Should you give vitamin K, FFP, or platelets? How far do you go to optimize his coagulation status?

Intraoperative Questions

1. How does the volume of distribution in the cirrhotic patient affect your dosing? Do you induce with pentathol, propofol, or etomidate? Is one better than another? What about cost?
2. For maintenance, are sevoflurane, N_2O, and O_2 okay? Is a nitrous narcotic better? What is the prime concern about this anesthetic? How do we ensure adequate flow to the kidney, the heart, the brain, and the liver?
3. Should you use bispectral (BIS) index monitoring? How much does it cost? Does it make a difference in patient safety? How can we make sure there is no recall?
4. Is suxamethonium okay or desirable for intubation? Why not rocuronium? Do you avoid long-lasting anesthetics? Is there a difference between rocuronium and cisatracurium? What if you give suxamethonium, and 1 hour later, there are 0/4 twitches? What is a dibucaine number?
5. On 50% O_2, the saturation level is only 91%. Do you need to get an ABG determination? If the ABG result confirms a low oxygen level, what is the differential diagnosis, and what is the treatment for this hypoxemia?

6. What are the special fluid needs of the cirrhotic? Does the patient require albumin, plasma, or Hespan? What is Hespan? It may be cheaper, but are there problems with it? How will you manage glucose, or is there a concern? If the sodium level starts out at 122 mEq/L, do you correct it? What is the sodium concentration of normal saline or lactated Ringer's solution? Do you give hypertonic saline? What is the risk of central pontine demyelinolysis?

7. If urine output drops, how will you manage? Can it be an indication for transfusion? How do you document this?

Postoperative Questions

1. At extubation, the patient vomits and aspirates. He wheezes and becomes cyanotic. What is the treatment?? Do you use antibiotics or steroids? Explain the concept of best PEEP. Do you need an oximetric Swan-Ganz catheter to manage the best PEEP?

2. You extubate, and the patient obstructs, makes a big respiratory effort, and develops pink frothy fluid in the trachea. What is the mechanism of this complication, and how do you treat it?

3. The patient fails to awaken at the end of the case. Is there anything specific to a liver patient that you should consider? What else is in the differential diagnosis? Will the BIS help? Should you get an electroencephalogram (EEG)?

Grab Bag

1. The power goes out at the hospital. You have just started a heart. What are your priorities, and do you proceed with the case?

2. A genitourinary specialist asks you to use high-frequency jet ventilation (HFJV) during extracorporeal shock wave lithotripsy (ESWL) to keep the stone from moving. Do you agree? Does HFJV have any other place in clinical medicine? What are specific risks of HFJV and of ESWL?

3. A 6-year-old boy with Down syndrome presents for tonsillectomy and adenoidectomy. He had a recent URI and has history of heart murmur. What are your concerns, and how do you manage this case?

Update: Cerebral Protection during Hypothermic Circulatory Arrest

1. What agents are generally used? Pentathol, propofol, and steroids are used for cerebral protection during hypothermic circulatory arrest.

2. Is there consensus on the best agent? There is no consensus, and there is no evidence-based medicine backing up one or another.

CASE 9: SICKLE CELL DISEASE, ASTHMA, AND EYE INJURY

A 15-year-old African-American boy with a history of asthma and sickle cell disease suffered an eye injury 1 hour earlier. He presents for repair of his globe. The hematocrit is 23%. The blood pressure, heart rate, and respiratory rate are normal. He was last transfused 2 years ago.

Preoperative Questions

1. How do you assess the severity of asthma on clinical grounds? Would any laboratory tests help? Do you need an eosinophil count, ABG determination, or chest radiograph?
2. How do you assess his sickle cell disease? Do you transfuse to make sure his hemoglobin S level is less than 50%? If this were an elective case and you had more time, would you do the same?
3. What if he had protein in his urine? What is the significance of that? What is the effect of silver sulfadiazine on renal function?

Intraoperative Questions

1. This patient has an open eye and full stomach. Describe how you would do induction to protect the eye. What if the airway looked difficult? Explain the pros and cons of using suxamethonium or long-acting agents. Is an LMA an option? How about LMA as a last resort option? What are the risks of aspiration compared with losing the eye?
2. How do you do an RSI in an asthmatic and not trigger bronchospasm? Would you use ketamine? Describe the problems with ketamine and methods to diminish those problems.
3. What are the special precautions given the sickle cell disease? What is a sickle cell crisis, and how do you prevent it? Will a Foley catheter ensure adequate fluid replacement? Do you need a central line?
4. In the middle of the case, the surgeon says the blood is dark, and indeed it is. How do you diagnose and treat?
5. Intravenous fluid infiltrates halfway into induction, and the patient vomits and aspirates. What is your next move? How do you get an "emergency intravenous line" placed in a big hurry when no other veins are present?
6. Postoperatively, the patient is restless and hypertensive, but he had not aspirated, and the case went normally. What is the differential diagnosis, and what is the treatment?
7. What is best option for preventing nausea and vomiting? How does ondansetron work? How does granisetron work? Why not give droperidol? What is long QT syndrome?

Grab Bag

1. A 19-year-old man wipes out on his all-terrain vehicle (ATV) and is admitted in a semicomatose state. A C5 fracture is seen on the radiograph. He moves all four extremities. He has a subdural hematoma but no other injuries. How do you manage the airway? What is the Glasgow Coma Scale? How do you allow a neurologic examination at end of case but keep the airway and neck safe?
2. Should you use an epidural for a patient with severe preeclampsia? What are the systemic effects of this disease, and how do we manage or cure them? How do you minimize hemodynamic swings in such a patient? Will a platelet count rule out bleeding problems? What are the risks of not putting in an epidural?
3. What are the safety features of your anesthesia machine? How do you know it is giving oxygen? What are the mechanical guarantees regarding O_2 besides the oxygen analyzer? How do you check calibration of your machine? Who is responsible for keeping the machines current? What is the concern if a vaporizer tips over? Does that apply to a desflurane vaporizer as well?

Update: Thoracic Aortic Aneurysm

1. What are some problems associated with somatosensory evoked potentials (SSEPs)? Because sensory monitoring detects posterior column ischemia better than anterior, paraplegia can happen even with normal SSEPs, hypothermia, and anesthetic agents, as can lower extremity ischemia, and all can interfere with the signal.

2. Discuss some methods for protecting the spinal cord. Methods include cross-clamp removal, cerebrospinal fluid (CSF) drainage, extracorporeal support, and providing perfusion to the lower part of the body.

3. How can you protect the kidneys? Volume management, mannitol, and mild hypothermia can be used. Dopamine has never been shown to provide renal protection against ischemia.

4. What percentage of thoracic aortic aneurysm patients has coexisting CAD? Eighty-seven percent have coexisting CAD.

5. What is a proven therapy to protect against adverse heart events? β-Blockade can be used, but proven? Again, refer to the POISE study.

CASE 10: CHOLECYSTECTOMY AND ASTHMA

A 45-year-old, 110-kg woman is scheduled to have an elective cholecystectomy. She takes aminophylline for her asthma. Her blood pressure is 150/100 mm Hg, pulse is 82 beats/min, respiratory rate is 16 breaths/min, and hematocrit is 51%.

Preoperative Questions

1. How does obesity affect the cardiovascular system, respiratory system, and airway? Can obesity affect liver function tests? How would you tell right heart failure from the effect of obesity alone? Do you need a preoperative ABG test to determine whether the patient is a CO_2 retainer?

2. Do you get pulmonary function tests (PFTs) to evaluate her asthma? If not, then under what circumstances do you order PFTs? Do you continue aminophylline? Do you get a level? Do you delay if the level is too low or too high? What if you feel premature ventricular contractions (PVCs) when you feel her pulse? Do you switch her to all inhaled drugs? Do you start her on steroids?

Intraoperative Questions

1. Do you need an arterial line for this case? What are dangers of an arterial line? What if the patient refuses or is too nervous? Do you use EMLA cream? Do you need it for induction? What about just feeling her pulse? Do you use newer, noninvasive means of continuous blood pressure measurement? What are drawbacks of the blood pressure cuff?

2. What are your special concerns about inducing anesthesia in this obese asthmatic? How will you avoid desaturation, aspiration, or a lost airway? Because of her asthma, should you avoid suxamethonium? If you use suxamethonium, should you defasciculate first? What if she gets weak after the defasciculating dose?

3. Does obesity affect the choice of anesthetic agent? Discuss the pros and cons of lots of narcotics (e.g., smooth wake-up process) versus the danger of obstructive sleep apnea. What is best anesthetic to prevent bronchospasm? Is halothane (if you can even find it anymore) better than the others?

4. The surgeon is ticked because the biliary tract is in spasm. He blames your fentanyl. What is your response? How can you help him get that cholangiogram? Should you use nitroglycerin, glucagons, or Narcan?
5. What special problems are associated with abdominal insufflation in a laparoscopic cholecystectomy ? What is a CO_2 embolus, and how do you treat it?
6. The patient wheezes, and inspiratory pressures climb. What is the differential diagnosis, and what is the treatment? What if you had put in a central line? If it is caused by insufflation, what can you tell the surgeon?
7. The patient jumps up off the table, and three people jump on her. She extubates herself, and you see the sevoflurane is bone dry. What do you do now?

Postoperative Questions

1. How does obesity affect airway management at the end of the case? Do you extubate deeply to help her asthma? What if you get in a cycle in which, no matter what, she always desaturates when you try to lighten her up?
2. Do you sit the patient up when you extubate? Discuss the pros and cons of this approach.
3. The surgeon wants help the next day with pain management. Discuss all the options (e.g., preoperative clonidine, intercostal blocks, intrapleural catheter, epidural, PCA). How would obstructive sleep apnea affect this decision? Do you need an ICU if she has obstructive sleep apnea?

Grab Bag

1. A 4-year-old child has epiglottitis. How do you manage this? How do you intubate, which blade should you use, and when is it okay to extubate?
2. A Jehovah's Witness thinks isovolemic hemodilution is the way to go with his repeat hip replacement. Discuss the pros and cons with him.
3. A cachectic 70-year-old man presents for colectomy with a shockingly low albumin level. Do you proceed or insist on nutritional support preoperatively? Why?

Update: Sedation during Regional Anesthesia

1. What advantages does dexmedetomidine have over propofol for infusion during regional cases? There is no need for airway support with dexmedetomidine compared with support needed for 40% of the propofol group.
2. What are potential problems with dexmedetomidine? Dexmedetomidine is associated with higher cost, slow onset of action, hypotension, and bradycardia.

CASE 11: SMALL BOWEL OBSTRUCTION WITH A PLATELET ISSUE

A 60-year-old, 75-kg woman has a small bowel obstruction. She had a splenectomy for idiopathic thrombocytopenic purpura (ITP) 4 months ago. She takes steroids in an attempt to raise her platelet count. She is on digitalis and hydrochlorothiazide. Her blood pressure is 180/105 mm Hg, pulse is 80 beats/min and irregular, respiratory rate is 20 breaths/min, hemoglobin level is 10 g/dL, temperature is 37.7°C, sodium level is 127 mEq/L, and potassium level is 3.0 mEq/L.

Preoperative Questions

1. What is patient's overnight fluid deficit? How is that altered by the presence of a small bowel obstruction? Does her diuretic alter things? How will this fluid state affect anesthesia? Should you "tune her up" before induction or put in a CVP and go for it?
2. What is ITP? Given her splenectomy, is she cured? If her platelet count was 30,000/mm^3, what would you do? Do you need other tests? Would you start platelets now, intraoperatively, or not at all? How will a TEG help? Will the bleeding time help? What are the results of the physical examination?
3. How does steroid use alter your anesthetic plan? How do steroids affect the sodium level? Does a sodium level of 127 mEq/L require therapy? Does it pose a danger? What happens if you correct too rapidly?

Intraoperative Questions

1. Awake intubation is forever touted as "the safest." What are the dangers of awake intubation? How can awake intubations go sour? What are the dangers associated with topicalization?
2. For induction, do you use ketamine, etomidate, or pentathol? What if you are in a developing country, and only pentathol is available? Is the lack of etomidate the kiss of death for the hypovolemic patient? Which muscle relaxant do you use for induction? What if there is a contraindication to suxamethonium (e.g., spinal cord injury)? How will you do a modified RSI?
3. For maintenance, is nitrous oxide contraindicated? What are the cardiac effects of nitrous oxide? Which maintenance drug is safest, or are they all the same? What if patient is a true cardiac cripple and absolutely cannot tolerate any potent agent at all? How will you do the anesthetic?
4. Atrial fibrillation now has a ventricular response of 140 beats/min. What is the treatment? What is the physiologic impact of atrial fibrillation? The systolic blood pressure is 70 mm Hg. Would you shock? What medications are needed? Now there is frothy fluid in the ETT associated with these hemodynamics. What is the differential diagnosis, and what is the treatment? Do you need a Swan-Ganz catheter, or would TEE be better?
5. Urine output drops. What is the treatment? Do you need a Swan-Ganz catheter now? How will you increase the urine output? Will you use a diuretic, dopamine, or epinephrine? Will you transfuse?
6. How does the BIS monitor work? What do you do if the BIS value drops to 0 or if it rises to 70?

Postoperative Questions

1. The patient has recall of the initial incision. What do you say to the patient? What is the mechanism of recall? Does the use of BIS prevent this?
2. How will you help with pain control? Will you go back in time and give a cyclooxygenase-2 (COX-2) inhibitor? Will you administer epidural bupivacaine or levobupivacaine?
3. The level of alanine aminotransferase (ALT), which was formerly called serum glutamate pyruvate transaminase (SGPT) is 400 U/L, and the lactate dehydrogenase (LDH) level is 250 U/L a week postoperatively. How will you evaluate this? What if you are asked to be an expert witness and the anesthesia record shows a long period of low blood pressure? Will you argue for the plaintiff?

Grab Bag

1. What special precautions apply to the birth of twins? What if the first one comes out and you need quick uterine relaxation for the second one?
2. What is a pressure-limited ventilator? What is a volume-limited ventilator? Which is better for acute respiratory distress syndrome (ARDS)? Is HFJV better for ARDS? What condition is better for ARDS? Does the patient receive the volume set on the ventilator? Why not?
3. Why does a small dose of pentathol go away so fast but a large dose last so long? Does propofol accumulate? Why or why not? Do potent inhaled agents "accumulate"? How does the volume of distribution differ in an alcoholic? What is the volume of distribution?

Update: Placenta Previa

1. What is a placenta previa? Placental implantation occurs over or near the cervical os, leading to third-trimester bleeding.
2. What do you do, and what do you avoid? Positive actions include large-volume access and type and cross of 2 to 4 units of blood. Avoid specular or manual examination.
3. What do you do if the patient is bleeding and 25 to 33 weeks' along? Use steroids to aid lung maturity.
4. How do you avoid supine hypotension syndrome? Use left uterine displacement by placing a wedge under the right hip.
5. What significant variable decreases in the pulmonary department? Functional residual capacity (FRC) decreases.
6. Is ketamine the agent of choice for the unstable patient? How about for the stable one? Use etomidate for unstable patients, and use propofol (less nausea and vomiting) for the stable patients.

CASE 12: CRANIOTOMY IN A CHILD

A 7-year-old, 28-kg girl is scheduled for a frontoparietal craniotomy for resection of a tumor. She had a seizure as a presenting symptom 2 weeks earlier, and she has had no appetite for a month and has lost 4 kg. She had bad asthma when she was 3 years old but has "outgrown" it. She uses a bronchodilator only when she plays outside on a cold day. She is on Dilantin to control seizures. Her blood pressure is 80/65 mm Hg, pulse is 110 beats/min, respiratory rate is 20 breaths/min, and temperature is 37°C.

Preoperative Questions

1. What is your primary concern regarding her neurologic status? Is it your responsibility to document all preexisting neurologic deficits? How will you tell her level of intracranial pressure (ICP)? Do you need an invasive reading of it before you start? How will her anticonvulsant therapy affect your anesthetic?
2. How will you evaluate her asthma? What further information do you need from her mother? Do you need PFTs? If you happened to have PFT results, what would you look for?
3. Does a 7-year-old child need premedication? What will you say to the child and to the mother? What are the risks of giving a premedication to a child with increased ICP? What will you give, when will you give it, and why?

Intraoperative Questions

1. Are air embolism monitors necessary? When, why, and which ones? Which is most sensitive? What is the latest sign? What is the pathophysiology of an air embolism? How should you measure blood pressure? Where should the transducer be? Does it matter where the monitor is when you zero it? Why? Do you need a CVP line in a kid? Do you need a multiport line to aspirate air?

2. How should you induce: by intravenous access, inhalation, or single-breath induction? Can you do this? Which agent should you use? Why not use halothane? What if the hospital administrator wants cheaper agents than sevoflurane?

3. Do you maintain by using an intravenous or potent anesthetic? What are the advantages and disadvantages of each? Describe the "pain needs" (e.g., brain, skull, meninges) during the case. How do you ensure a quick, smooth wake-up course so they can check for deficits?

4. Despite a CO_2 of 30 mm Hg, the brain is still bulging. What other methods do you have? Will you use Lasix or mannitol? Why not use Bumex?

5. The surgeon cuts an artery and wants deep hypotension. How will you accomplish this? What are risks? How low can you go? Do you use vasodilators or potent inhaled agents or labetalol? Why?

6. The patient's temperature drops to 32°C. What are the problems of hypothermia? What mechanisms do you have for warming the patient? Do you prefer to keep the patient a little cool for brain protection? Why or why not?

Postoperative Questions

1. Should you extubate early? What are the criteria for extubation? If you keep the patient intubated, which ventilator setting do you use? What is pressure support? What is the dead space in the circuit? How will you determine if this is a problem for this child?

2. The patient is unresponsive 20 minutes after turning off agents. How will you determine the problem? Do you need an EEG? Will BIS help? Why or why not? What metabolic problems may the patient have?

Grab Bag

1. Esophagectomy is planned. Should you use a Univent or bronchial blocker or a double-lumen tube for lung isolation? Is this an absolute indication for lung isolation? What is an absolute indication?

2. The pressure of the patient with a thoracic epidural in the PACU drops. Is it a volume problem or the epidural? Describe the special concerns with a thoracic or lumbar epidural. Should you discontinue the epidural or turn it off for a while? What if it is Friday, and you do not want to come in and check it over the weekend?

3. A new surgeon wants to do tonsils with an LMA. Is this a good idea? What are the advantages and disadvantages? What is the risk of aspiration? How do you avoid bucking at the end of the case? Can you do it with the patient on his side for a hip that is almost done, requiring only 10 minutes?

Update: Pediatric Trauma

1. What are leading causes of death among kids? They are trauma from motor vehicle accidents (MVAs), falls, bike accidents, drowning, burns, and abuse.

2. What is the most common form of fatal trauma? Head trauma is most often fatal.
3. Which organ is most frequently injured in the abdomen? The spleen is often injured.
4. Are spinal cord injuries as common in kids as adults? No.
5. Subdural hematomas in infants most often result from what? Shaken baby syndrome is responsible for most subdural hematomas in infants.
6. Which Glasgow number indicates severe brain injury? A score of 8 or less indicates brain injury.
7. Whom can you discharge from ER? Patients with a Glasgow Coma Score of 15 or higher and who have normal computed tomography (CT) findings can be discharged.
8. What are the pediatric mean arterial pressure guidelines to keep cerebral perfusion pressure (CPP) up? They are greater than 50 mm Hg for infants and 60 to 70 mm Hg for children.
9. What is the treatment for diabetes insipidus? Vasopressin is used.
10. How does a kid's thorax differ from an adult's? It is more compliant and has fewer fractures. Get an echocardiogram to look for cardiac contusion.
11. How is a child's abdomen different from that of an adult? It is more likely to get injured. It is less cushioned and protected.
12. What is the most sensitive indicator of intracranial injury? Scalp hematoma signals intracranial injury.

CASE 13: CATARACT AND A RECENT MYOCARDIAL INFARCTION

A 75-year-old woman with a pack-century of Marlboros under her alveoli presents for a cataract. She had a myocardial infarction (MI) 2 years ago, got two stents, and is now free of angina. She has swollen ankles, a barrel chest, and faint breath sounds. When lying flat, she gets short of breath and becomes anxious. Her blood pressure is 165/90 mm Hg, pulse is 100 beats/min, and respiratory rate is 24 breaths/min (breathing is rattly).

Preoperative Questions

1. What studies would the American College of Cardiology recommend? (Keep in mind the new recommendations.) Will the ECG alone be helpful? What do you expect to see on ECG given her poor respiratory status? Do you need a stress echocardiogram here? If you anticipate needing to go with general anesthesia, does it up the ante?
2. You perform the physical examination. What does edema mean? Explain the concept of Starling's forces in the lungs.
3. Do you need laboratory tests for electrolytes, even if this is just a cataract? How about an ABG determination, flow-volume loop test, or PFTs? Does any of this change when you add, " I will need to use general anesthesia"?

Intraoperative Questions

1. The surgeon always does these cases under a block. Do you agree? If you start this way, and she freaks out and sits bolt upright, will Precedex work better? Should you use a little ketamine in with a propofol drip? What are the dangers of a deep minimum alveolar concentration (MAC)?

2. To keep her airway from constricting, how will you induce? She is skinny; why not breathe her down or use intravenous lidocaine? What will the effect of positive-pressure ventilation be on her blood pressure? What are your concerns as you intubate? Will a smaller tube help? Will 5% lidocaine cream on the tube help, or will that be a problem?

3. The patient keeps bucking. When you try to deepen anesthesia, her pressure drops. This is an outpatient place; do you give her more narcotic? Do you paralyze and hope she does not remember? Will a BIS value help? How? What else could be causing the bucking? Is the ETT on carina? Why is that a problem?

4. The surgeon gives a too-concentrated drop of Neo-Synephrine in the eye. What will happen? What would happen if he injected 100 µg of epinephrine by mistake? What would you do?

Postoperative Questions

1. How will you time the extubation? Should it be deep? Suppose 20 minutes after extubation the PaO_2 is 52, $PaCO_2$ is 60, and the pH is 7.32 on 31% oxygen by nasal cannula? Should you reintubate, observe, or admit to the ICU? Should you take off the O_2? Explain the concern about the loss of the hypoxemic drive to breathe?

2. In the PACU, the patient is restless and moving all over the place. The PACU nurse suggests giving Romazicon. Do you agree? How about giving some physostigmine? What is the mechanism of a cholinergic crisis?

3. Despite two doses of ondansetron, the patient is still retching. What next? Explain the mechanism of the chosen drug. At what point would you admit the patient? The manager is very upset about this; what would you say?

Grab Bag

1. A 40-year-old woman is scheduled for a hysterectomy because of menorrhagia. She is on Coumadin for deep venous thrombosis (DVT). How do you manage her anticoagulation in view of her bleeding problem and her clotting problem?

2. An 8-year-old boy aspirated a safety pin. He has a family history of mental health.

3. How do you handle a massive CO_2 embolism introduced into the inferior vena cava during a laparoscopy?

Update: Rocuronium and Reintubation

1. Do more patients get reintubated with rocuronium than other agents? Yes.

2. Why is rocuronium so widely used? It has a large standard deviation in its recovery profile and a particularly long recovery profile in the elderly.

CASE 14: RETINAL REATTACHMENT IN AN ELDERLY PATIENT

A 90-year-old, 60-kg man is scheduled for retinal reattachment under general anesthesia. He takes Lasix and digoxin when he remembers to. The ECG shows a first-degree heart block and an old, inferior MI, but the man does not remember when he had that.

Preoperative Questions

1. Why does he have a first-degree heart block? Is this serious? Will you treat it? How? Why? What if he had a second-degree block (differentiate between Wenckebach and Mobitz type II) or a third-degree block? How do these differ? How about Wolf-Parkinson-White syndrome? Is his blood pressure normal? Will you cancel the case and optimize his blood pressure? Why and how? Does he need a stress test?

2. What are the mechanisms of action of digoxin and Lasix? What are the side effects and interactions with anesthesia? The potassium level is 5.5 mEq/L; will you proceed? How about 6 mEq/L? Does he need dialysis? Should you obtain a repeat potassium test? Why may a potassium level be erroneously high? Do you need a digoxin level? How is digoxin toxicity manifested?

3. What other tests do you want? Do you need a creatinine test, liver function tests, or PFTs? Explain in detail how 90 years take a toll on the heart, lungs, liver, kidney, and skin.

Intraoperative Questions

1. How will you maintain anesthesia? Are there any special considerations for the 90-year-old patient? How does age affect MAC, the solubility of agents, the volume of distribution, and the circulatory response to anesthetic agents?

2. This eye case does not require a lot of volume shifts. Do you need invasive lines because he had an MI? Do you need a central line? Would a hand on the pulse as you induce be enough? How about a noninvasive Tensys blood pressure monitoring system?

3. After you induce, the patient develops frequent PVCs and then a run of ventricular tachycardia. What is the differential diagnosis, and what is the treatment? When would you shock? What if he developed pulseless electrical activity (PEA)? What are the possible causes?

4. How do you set your ventilator? Do you need an ICU ventilator? Why or why not? What will the effect of ventilation be on intraocular pressure? What is the mechanism of blindness in a prone case? Can you use N_2O? Assume you did not know he had air in the eye and you turned on N_2O; what would happen?

5. If you set the ventilator too high and the pH goes to 7.6, what are the negative effects of this hyperventilation?

6. What special problems do you face as you extubate? How will you manage this safely?

Postoperative Questions

1. The nurse reports urine output of only 10 mL/hr in the PACU. Are you concerned? Will you get a urine specific gravity measurement? Why or why not? What is the syndrome of inappropriate antidiuretic hormone secretion (SIADH)? What is the normal response to surgery? What if the urine specific gravity is 1.010 or 1.030?

2. The patient complains bitterly about hoarseness and pharyngitis 24 hours postoperatively. How will you manage this? How will you help with the throat pain? Will you get a consultation with an ear, nose, and throat (ENT) specialist? How can you evaluate the vocal cords?

Grab Bag

1. Third-trimester painless bleeding occurs in a multipara. What is your diagnosis? What preparations do you make? Does a 14-gauge line run faster than a 16-gauge line? Why or why not? Where is most of the resistance in the intravenous line? Do you need to heat blood? Why? What if you overheat the blood and "fry" it?
2. How do you reverse muscle relaxants? What is happening on a molecular and receptor level? If a patient is flat and has only a little tetanus, do you reverse?
3. During a TURP, a patient starts to sing "Like A Virgin" and thinks he is the reincarnation of Madonna. What is going on, and what laboratory test do you get?

Update: Thienopyridine Drugs, Clopidogrel and Ticlopidine, and Other Bleeding Headaches

1. How do clopidogrel and ticlopidine work? They inhibit platelet aggregation by inhibiting the platelet ADP receptor.
2. What is your concern? Epidural hematoma may occur if you do a spinal or epidural anesthetic.
3. What are the American Society of Regional Anesthesia (ASRA) guidelines? Discontinue clopidogrel 7 days before a neuraxial injection. Discontinue ticlopidine 10 to 14 days before neuraxial anesthesia. Ticlopidine's half-life increases from 12 hours to 4 to 5 days after a steady-state level is reached.
4. How about aspirin? The ASRA says, in spite of the fact that aspirin irreversibly blocks the platelet cyclooxygenase, inhibiting the formation of thromboxane A_2 causes platelet aggregation. You can still do spinals and epidurals in the face of aspirin therapy. For example, you take someone off clopidogrel for 7 days, put him on aspirin, and then do the case 7 days later.
5. What is incidence of DVT in patients who have a hip operation and do not get prophylaxis? About 50% of these patients develop DVT.
6. What about a patient on Coumadin? You can do neuraxial work if the international normalized ratio (INR) is less than 1.4.
7. What about a patient on subcutaneous heparin? As long as the patient does not have heparin-induced thrombocytopenia (HIT) (check the platelet count of anyone on heparin), it is okay to do spinals and epidurals.
8. What about low-molecular-weight heparin (LMWH)? No neuraxial work should be done for at least 12 hours after the last dose. After the epidural is removed, wait at least 2 hours before starting the Lovenox (enoxaparin) again.

CASE 15: SMALL BOWEL OBSTRUCTION AND TIGHT MITRAL STENOSIS

A 70-year-old woman with known tight mitral stenosis (she refused surgery) presents with small bowel obstruction. She is on an angiotensin-converting enzyme (ACE) inhibitor and Lasix. She takes Coumadin because of her atrial fibrillation. Her belly is enlarged, and she is severely short of breath. The blood pressure is 110/60 mm Hg, heart rate is 110 beats/min, and the respiratory rate is 34 breaths/min. The ABG determination shows a PaO_2 of 55 mm Hg, $PaCO_2$ of 35 mm Hg, and pH of 7.19.

Preoperative Questions

1. How would you evaluate this patient's volume status? Do you need a Swan-Ganz catheter even before you start? How about an echocardiogram or TEE? What are the goals of preinduction volume management? If the potassium is 2.5 mEq/L, do you supplement? Why? How much? How fast? What are the dangers? If the nurse hangs it too fast and the T waves peak, what do you do?
2. How do you get a handle on her cardiac status? Will a chest radiograph help, or does this amount to re-arranging the deck chairs on the Titanic, and you should instead go to the OR? What are the goals of management in mitral stenosis? Contrast that with the goals in managing mitral regurgitation?
3. How do you interpret the ABG results? How can you attempt to optimize her respiratory status before you start the case? Why is she dyspneic? Will morphine help? How does morphine reduce dyspnea in the heart failure patient? What are the potential dangers?

Intraoperative Questions

1. What special monitors will you use? The surgeon asks that you keep a special eye on the V_5 lead. Is this appropriate? Why? Do automated machines keep track of the ST segment for us? When should you worry about ischemia? Contrast the significance of ST depression with ST elevation?
2. The surgeon says, "Her heart will not take a general; better do a high spinal." What is your response? What is the danger of regional anesthesia? Could you give a little FFP and then do an epidural? What are the dangers of giving FFP?
3. You induce, and feculent emesis goes down the trachea. What do you do? Should you have given antacids or histamine blockers? Would a nasogastric tube have helped? Do you give antibiotics or steroids now?
4. The induction went well. Two hours into the case, the patient develops supraventricular tachyarrhythmia (SVT) with rate up to 150 beats/min. What is the differential diagnosis, and what is the treatment? How does amiodarone work? Is this the best drug? When would you shock?

Postoperative Questions

1. How will you determine whether to extubate if she had aspirated? How will you titrate to the best PEEP? If she is on 40% oxygen, and she has a PaO_2 of 60 mm Hg, what is the A-a gradient? Explain the difference between shunt and dead space. What will you do to fix things? Do you need a mixed venous Swan-Ganz catheter? How does that work? What does an SvO_2 of 45% mean?
2. The nurse discovers a tooth in the gurney. What do you do?
3. The patient begins to shake after 45 minutes in the PACU. What does this mean? What is the mechanism? What is the danger? What is the treatment for shivering? What are the best rewarming methods? Explain the dangers of burns with Bair Huggers?

Grab Bag

1. Explain the mechanism of retinal ischemia in the prone patient. What are the best guidelines to help prevent this? Do goggles help or hurt? What do

you tell the patient who has gone blind from such a case? How do you explain this risk ahead of time?

2. What is ARDS, and what is the best treatment for it? Is HFJV a good option? Do you use extracorporeal membrane oxygenation (ECMO)? How does ECMO work?

3. After a VSD repair, a child is here for a central line placement. His baseline oxygen saturation is 91%. He is 4 weeks old. What special precautions do you take for this case?

Update: Nicardipine

1. What is nicardipine? It is a calcium channel blocker.

2. What is its proposed benefit? Especially in intracranial cases, this may be the way to drop blood pressure without increasing ICP or causing steal. A nonspecific dilator such as sodium nitroprusside can drop the blood pressure, but it also increases the ICP, which is a big no-no.

3. Compare nicardipine with labetalol. Because there is no β-blockade with nicardipine, there is no potential for triggering asthma.

4. What is the appropriate dosing? Each ampule has 10 mL of 2.5 mg/mL, or a total of 25 mg. For an acute bolus, dilute 1:10 so you get a syringe with 0.25 mg/mL. Give 1 mL at a time, and see what happens. You can also mix a drip. Add one ampule (25 mg) to a 250-mL bag, giving you a bag of concentration of 0.1 mg/mL. Start at 50 mL/hr (i.e., 5 mg/hr), and go up or down from there.

CASE 16: AORTIC VALVE REPLACEMENT AND A HIATAL HERNIA

A 60-year-old, 80-kg man with aortic stenosis is scheduled to have an aortic valve replacement (AVR). He has angina and occasional syncope. He has a hiatal hernia and takes "that purple pill" after eating Mexican food. He takes digoxin, metoprolol, and Lasix. The patient is afebrile and has a blood pressure of 130/100 mm Hg, heart rate of 60 beats/min, respiratory rate of 16 breaths/min, and potassium level of 3.1 mEq/L.

Preoperative Questions

1. What information do you request from the cardiologist? What else do you need to know? Do you need to know the gradient across the aortic valve? Suppose it is 100 mm Hg; is it significant? What does a low gradient mean? How can he have angina if his coronaries are "clean"? How clean is clean? Is a 50% reduction in the coronaries a problem? How about 20% or 70%? What is the natural history of aortic stenosis? Contrast that natural history with that of aortic regurgitation?

2. He will be the second case. Explain what your preoperative orders will be. He is NPO, but can he have a little water or black coffee in the morning? Which cardiac medications should he get and why? Do you add anything? Do you administer albuterol just in case he gets in trouble with his lungs? Can you give albuterol intravenously? What steps will you take regarding his hiatal hernia? Will you replace the potassium? What if he comes down to the holding area and a potassium-containing solution has infiltrated?

Intraoperative Questions

1. What information would a pulmonary artery catheter give you that a CVP line does not? If you use a Swan-Ganz catheter, what are the options open to you? What are the hazards of using a Swan-Ganz catheter? Is there any proven benefit? What does mixed venous oxygen represent? What is the significance of a low level? During cardiopulmonary bypass (CPB), how do you make sure flow is adequate? Does the BIS value or the EEG help? What do you do if urine output drops on bypass despite "adequate" flow?

2. Would TEE be of use? Is it mandatory given the valvular disease? What will you look for after bypass? What would make you repeat the valve operation?

3. Should you do an RSI given his hiatal hernia? Should you do a modified RSI, apply cricoid pressure, or do an awake intubation? What are the dangers of an awake intubation in a patient with aortic stenosis? What will you use to induce? What are hemodynamic goals? Which induction agent is best? Should you use esmolol? What should you do if the heart rate is 45 or 100 beats/min?

4. Given the aortic stenosis, how will you maintain anesthesia? If you use intravenous agents, how will you ensure no recall? How does a BIS monitor work? When is the biggest time for recall in a cardiac case?

5. You induce but do not see anything. The oxygen saturation is dropping, and the heart rate is rising. Do you give esmolol, or will that be a distraction as you work on the airway?

6. Coming off bypass, the heart rate is only 30 beats/min, and the patient has frequent escape beats. What is the differential diagnosis, and what is the treatment? How should you set up the pacemaker? What if it does not capture?

7. You give protamine, but there is no clot in the field. How do you create a better hematologic picture? Discuss blood alternatives in the case of a Jehovah's Witness. Will a mixed venous Swan-Ganz catheter help you decide when to transfuse?

Postoperative Questions

1. Three hours into the ICU, the urine output drops to 20 mL/hr. The surgeon says, "It is acute tubular necrosis. Restrict fluids from now on, or we'll overload!" What is your response? What is acute tubular necrosis, and how will you know if it is the problem?

2. Twelve hours later, the patient has not awakened, and the same surgeon is screaming bloody murder. The patient moves only the right side in response to pain. What is the diagnosis, and what is the treatment? Should you get a CT scan? Should you get a CT scan if the patient is hemodynamically unstable? Should you study the carotids and do a carotid endarterectomy (CEA)? Should you order an epiaortic echocardiogram to see if there was calcium in the aorta?

Grab Bag

1. How is fetal welfare monitored? Short-term and long-term variability are monitored. Why is bradycardia problematic?

2. What is your concern about the influence of local anesthetics on the fetal heart rate?

3. What is the treatment for a spinal headache after a "moist" tap?

4. You do a caudal with 0.5% bupivacaine for a vaginal hysterectomy. The patient gets tinnitus, bradycardia, and a seizure. What is the treatment? How could you have prevented this local anesthetic toxicity?

Update: Ultrasound Guidance for Brachial Plexus Block

1. Why do you need a high-resolution ultrasound for a brachial plexus block? Higher frequency gives better resolution.
2. What is the failure rate for blind technique in experienced hands? The failure rate is 10% to 15%.
3. What are the complications of blind techniques? Complications include direct nerve damage, pneumothorax, vascular injury, systemic toxicity, and spinal cord injury.
4. How does the brachial plexus appear on high resolution ultrasound? Hypoechoic nodules.

CASE 17: MANDIBULAR FRACTURE AND A SMELL NOT UNLIKE THAT OF ALCOHOL

A 49-year-old, 95-kg man is scheduled for exploratory laparotomy after an MVA. Has an open mandibular fracture, and he reeks of retsina (a Greek wine that has pine resin in it and takes some getting used to). He is wheezing but cannot answer questions, shouting only "OOPAH!" when you try to talk to him. The patient has a blood pressure of 90/60 mm Hg, heart rate of 110 beats/min, respiratory rate of 16 breaths/min, temperature of 36°C, and hemoglobin level of 9 g/dL.

Preoperative Questions

1. Why is he drowsy? What significance for anesthesia? How does the jaw fracture complicate things? What does acute intoxication due to the MAC? Contrast this with the chronic effects of alcohol. How do both effects of alcohol alter management?
2. Is he in shock? What is shock? How do you evaluate the cardiovascular status in this acute setting? How does a hematocrit value help? Do results of the ABG determination, ECG, echocardiogram, or physical examination help? Do you need to treat before inducing?
3. What does the wheezing mean? What is the differential diagnosis, and what is the treatment? How do you tell asthma from aspiration from pneumothorax? Do you need to place a chest tube "just in case"? For treatment, should you give an inhaler or aminophylline? Should you avoid N_2O?

Intraoperative Questions

1. What is the risk for aspiration at intubation? Given that, how would you induce? What is a Le Forte fracture, and how does it affect plans? Describe the pros and cons of an awake intubation, inhalation induction, RSI, and awake tracheostomy. What if he does not cooperate? What if you are fretting about an unstable neck fracture? How do you "clear" the neck, and can you do so in the current setting?
2. Immediately after intubation, the patient develops severe wheezing. What are the causes? What is the treatment? The end-tidal CO_2 is 28 mm Hg;

explain why it is low, or is it low? What are problems associated with hyperventilation? You have a terrible time and cannot move air at all. What is the differential diagnosis, and what is the treatment? If you are facing big-time aspiration, when would you extubate and try again? Do you convert to a tracheostomy? Do you place a chest tube?

3. How should you maintain anesthesia? Give the pros and cons of inhalation compared with total intravenous anesthesia (TIVA). Which is more likely to produce recall? Which muscle relaxant do you use, and how do you monitor the neuromuscular blocker? What is the train of 4? How do you monitor if the only twitch monitor is broken?

4. You take a break, and when you come back, the patient's blood pressure is 190/120 mm Hg. What is the differential diagnosis, and what is the treatment? What are the possible causes? What is Cushing's triad? What is the danger of correcting this blood pressure if the patient has an intracranial bleed? What is cerebral perfusion pressure?

Postoperative Questions

1. Urine output is 15 mL in the PACU after an hour. What are the possible causes? What is an adequate urine output? Is it different when a patient is on positive-pressure ventilation? Discuss the idea of the thoracic pump. Should you give Lasix? Why or why not? At what point do you decide that enough is enough as far as volume replacement goes?

2. The patient vomited on induction. How do you decide if this is significant? What would the signs be under anesthesia? Do you need to do fiberoptic observation, take a sample, or call a pulmonary specialist? How do you treat aspiration? What do you tell the family? Map out a plan for the next 2 days of respiratory therapy. What is the patient's prognosis?

3. Thirty minutes after arrival in the PACU, the patient's blood pressure is 80/40 mm Hg. What is the differential diagnosis, and what is the treatment? What are the most likely causes, and what are some unlikely but possible causes? Can you start a norepinephrine drip and hope that takes care of it? Can you use a dopamine drip? When would you go with an inotropic drip? How would you make a diagnosis of tamponade? How could this have happened? How would you diagnose an aortic dissection?

Grab Bag

1. Under what circumstances would you use HFJV? When would you use jet ventilation through a cricothyrotomy? How do you do that?

2. A new obstetrician suggests you do caudals every now and then, rather than using lumbar epidurals all the time. What is your response? How about caudals for kids undergoing hypospadias repair? How do you do such an anesthetic?

3. How do you induce a patient with porphyria? What is the mechanism of organ injury with porphyria?

4. A child has a tracheoesophageal fistula. How do you manage the airway?

Update: Cerebral Aneurysms

1. Describe the mechanisms of brain injury during neurosurgery. Mechanisms include brain retraction, direct vascular injury, and mechanical disruption

from the surgeon. Hypotension or hypertension, decreased O_2 content, hypo-osmolarity, and hyperglycemia may be caused by the anesthesia. These mechanisms can act synergistically.

2. How do you allow good head drainage? Allow at least 2 fingerbreadths per 70 kg of body weight between the mandible and the clavicle. Use CSF drainage and no cerebral vasodilators. Delay mannitol until removal of the bone flap or aural reflection so that the bridging veins do not tear. The peak effect of mannitol occurs in 45 minutes.

3. Do even mildly hypotonic fluids contribute to brain swelling? Yes. Never withhold fluid to the expense of stable hemodynamics.

4. Contrast arteriovenous malformations (AVMs) with aneurysms. Aneurysms bleed and cause subarachnoid hemorrhage. AVMs usually bleed into the parenchyma of the brain, and vasospasm is less likely.

5. What are the complications of subarachnoid hemorrhage? Complications include hypertension, cardiac rhythm and function disturbances, pneumonia, aspiration, ARDS, DVT, SIADH, and electrolyte disturbances. Left ventricular function usually improves over time.

6. With a subarachnoid hemorrhage, where do you keep the CO_2 level? Normal, you do not want to exaggerate the vasoconstriction.

7. If you use pentathol for cerebral protection, what is the end point? The end point is deep burst suppression or an isoelectric pattern on the ECG.

8. Disaster strikes, and the aneurysm pops. What do you do? Compress the ipsilateral carotid, and drop the pressure to a mean of 40 to 50 mm Hg to facilitate clipping.

CASE 18: PREGNANCY, INFECTION, AND PREECLAMPSIA

An 18-year-old, 100-kg woman is 32 weeks' pregnant and toxemic, and she presents with ruptured membranes. Two days later, she has chorioamnionitis and is scheduled for a cesarean section. She has gotten labetalol, Demerol, hydralazine, and magnesium. Her blood pressure is 170/100 mm Hg, pulse is 100 beats/min, temperature is 39.7°C, and hematocrit is 35%.

Intraoperative Questions

1. What is preeclampsia? What is eclampsia? What physical signs do you see? What laboratory results do you expect? How do hydralazine, magnesium, and labetalol work? Why not use nitroglycerin or sodium nitroprusside? What are the risks to the fetus? What does magnesium do, and how does it interact with anesthetics? What are the major complications and complications from anesthesia associated with toxemia? How do you monitor fetal well-being throughout the process? Describe the patterns seen on the fetal heart rate monitor.

2. Should you get the temperature down before doing anesthesia? Can you place a regional in the setting of an infection? What is the risk of abscess or seeding the CSF?

3. How does the patient's obesity affect your plans? Describe the effects of obesity on the lungs, airway, heart, and psychological status. Do you need an arterial line to get more accurate blood pressure readings?

Intraoperative Questions

1. What if the surgeon says, "I always do them under general." What are the pros and cons of regional and general anesthesia? What do you do if the patient is becoming psychotic?
2. You attempt intubation but get a grade 4 view. The fetus is still stable. Do you place an LMA? Do you wake up the patient? Do you perform a cricothyrotomy? What are the landmarks for doing a cricothyrotomy? How do you do insufflation? What are the dangers of insufflation? If you place an LMA, do you live with that, or get a fiberoptic scope and place ETT through it?
3. Describe how you will place the epidural. What are the pros and cons of a sitting position compared with being on her side? Which drug do you use? Do you use levobupivacaine? Why is bupivacaine so dangerous? Describe the treatment of a catastrophic intravascular injection of bupivacaine. How does an epidural cause hypotension?
4. At delivery, the neonate is floppy and cyanotic. Go through the resuscitation priorities, and explain how you would deliver drugs in a code. How do you do cardiopulmonary resuscitation (CPR) on a newborn? What is the risk of liver laceration? Do you give Narcan if you gave some epidural fentanyl? How is resuscitation different in the setting of meconium?
5. The surgeon tells you to hang oxytocin. Bleeding is brisker than brisk. What is the dose and route of oxytocin administration? How does it work, and how does it slow bleeding? Bleeding continues. What laboratory tests do you order? Do you place an arterial line? How will you treat a coagulopathy of unknown origin?

Postoperative Questions

1. In the PACU, the patient has a seizure. What is the differential diagnosis, and what is the treatment? What if she is still hard to intubate? Can you manage this without intubating by giving pentathol and stopping the seizure? When you intubate her, she is postictal and fighting the tube. Her blood pressure is 190/130 mm Hg, and you are worried about an intracranial bleed. Do you "put her to sleep" and go to CT just in case? Is this overreaching?
2. Two hours postoperatively, the heart rate jumps to 160 beats/min. What is the differential diagnosis, and what is the treatment? What are the mechanisms of tachycardia? What are the risks of leaving it untreated? What would you look for in a blood gas determination?

Grab Bag

1. A 4-year-old, 17-kg girl is scheduled for laser excision of laryngeal polyps. How do you induce anesthesia? How do you guard against an airway fire?
2. An OR nurse is spooked about all the N_2O that spills with all of our LMAs. How do you advise? Should she leave the OR? Do you tell people in that room to intubate more?
3. A veteran from Iraq got shrapnel in his left hand 2 months earlier and now has unremitting pain and hair loss in his left forearm. What is the differential diagnosis, and what is the treatment? After one stellate ganglion block, he still hurts. What is your advice? What are the risks of a stellate block compared with the risk of letting the arm get worse.

Update: Lactic Acidosis with β₂-Inhaler Treatment

1. What are the two mechanisms of lactic acidosis? In type A lactic acidosis, oxygen delivery to tissues is compromised. In type B lactic acidosis, lactate production is increased, or removal is decreased.
2. How can β-adrenergic inhalers do this? The β₂-agents produce excessive glycogenolysis and lipolysis, which can lead to lactate overproduction.

CASE 19: ABDOMINOPERINEAL RESECTION IN A PULMONARY PATIENT

A 68-year-old, 82-kg man is scheduled for abdominoperineal resection for cancer. He has had a left upper lobectomy and a lumbar laminectomy. He takes Valium to sleep and continues to smoke. The patient has a blood pressure of 150/90 mm Hg, heart rate of 85 beats/min, and respiratory rate of 18 breaths/min. The ABG determination shows partial pressures of 60 mm Hg for O_2 and 60 mm Hg for CO_2. Results of his PFTs all hover around 50% of the predicted marks.

Preoperative Questions

1. Discuss the significance of the ABG results? What does CO_2 retention tell you? What will his HCO_3 level be and why? Do you need split-function lung studies? In what case would you need these? Should you put him on bronchodilators as an inpatient or an outpatient? Do you need a pulmonary consult if the patient says, "I am as good as I get?" How will you define *optimization*?
2. The patient is nervous. Will you give him a sedative, Valium the night before, Versed the morning of the operation, or a narcotic? Will an anti-sialagogue help? How about scopolamine?

Intraoperative Questions

1. How does an arterial line measure blood pressure? How does a blood pressure cuff work? Which is more accurate? Should you place an arterial line before or after induction? Where? What if you blow both radials and the patient is howling like a madman? What if you place a brachial line and the hand gets dusky? Can you get complex regional pain syndrome (CRPS) from an arterial line? What is the treatment for that? Should you do a prophylactic stellate ganglion block?
2. How do you induce? Compare and contrast etomidate, pentathol, propofol, and ketamine. How about a straight narcotic blast if you are planning on keeping the patient intubated anyway? How do you avoid recall in a narcotic case?
3. What is the best anesthetic from a cardiac or respiratory standpoint? Will deep inhalation keep airways free of bronchospasm? If so, what do you do as the case draws to a close? What are risks of deep inhalational anesthesia? Is it worth switching to that blast from the past, halothane, at any time?
4. Which muscle relaxant do you use? Does any one of them cause bronchospasm? Is using suxamethonium a good idea to start? Do you need to check with the surgeons to make sure the patient is relaxed enough? What if surgeon says, "He is tight," even though you are at 0/4? How does the twitch monitor work?

5. You hear wheezing. What is the differential diagnosis, and what is the treatment? How do you determine the cause, because "all that wheezes is not..."?

Postoperative Questions

1. The patient is intubated and unresponsive in the PACU. How will you manage the ventilator? Explain the significance of the I:E ratio. Are any different techniques (e.g., pressure support) a good idea? How will you manage the CO_2 given his starting ABG values? What is the significance of the hypoxemic drive to breathe? How will you extubate him, yet allow him to keep breathing?
2. The heart rate jumps to 150 beats/min. What is the differential diagnosis, and what is the treatment? How will you tell atrial flutter from ventricular tachycardia? What will you do if the blood pressure is 100 mm Hg or 50 mm Hg? Which drug treatment will you use? Why? How does amiodarone work?

Grab Bag

1. Yikes! A surprise breech delivery starts to happen, and the obstetrician says, "Sorry, I thought it was the baby's face, but it is his butt!" How do you provide anesthesia for this emergency? Is there time for a spinal? What is the risk of general anesthesia?
2. Do you give Versed before an axillary block for prophylaxis in case you go intra-arterial? You give a whopping dose of lidocaine, and the patient says he hears ringing in his ears. What do you do?
3. What are the advantages and disadvantages of using a cell saver? Can you use it in a cancer case? If "the blood is already coagulopathic," do you avoid Cell Saver blood because it is "no good anyway"?

Update: Recall and the BIS Monitor

1. What is incidence of recall with a BIS monitor in place? The incidence is 1 case in 40,000 operations.
2. When does it most often occur? It occurs when the BIS value is greater than 60, during cardiac surgery, and in patients younger than 60 years old, 60% of whom are women.
3. What common instrument can falsely elevate the BIS measurement? The Bair Hugger can falsify the measurement.
4. What is the best prophylaxis for post-traumatic stress disorder (PTSD)? Acknowledge, apologize, and get counseling for the patient.
5. How does the BIS monitor work? It integrates EEG data by means of a proprietary algorithm based on empirical data. A value of 100 represents the awake state, and 0 is the isoelectric EEG.

CASE 20: CLIPPING AN ANEURYSM

A 29-year-old, 115-kg woman is scheduled to have clipping of the anterior communicating artery. She has an aneurysm that has not proved amenable to coils in the catheter laboratory. She had a subarachnoid hemorrhage 2 days before admission. She has not sustained cerebral vasospasm. She used to weigh 220 kg before she had laparoscopic gastric stapling. Her blood pressure is 170/95 mm Hg, pulse is 95 beats/min, respiratory rate is 18 breaths/min, temperature is 37.5°C, and hemoglobin level is 11 g/dL. She says she never has sex.

Preoperative Questions

1. Does the patient need a pregnancy test? What if she insists she does not want it and starts to get upset?
2. What is cerebral vasospasm? How is it treated? What can you do to prevent it? Should you attempt to reduce her blood pressure now? What are the risks of dropping the blood pressure compared with the risks of not dropping the blood pressure?
3. Detail the physiologic changes of obesity. What are the changes associated with gastric stapling? Does rapid weight loss pose a risk? She is still obese; how do you detail the risks of anesthesia to her?
4. Do you sedate her, given her obesity, her cerebral status, and her possible pickwickian syndrome? What is that?

Intraoperative Questions

1. Deliberate hypotension and a 15-degree head-up operation are planned. How do these two things influence your monitor selection? Do you need a CVP or pulmonary artery line? Which kind and why? What if the surgeon says he is planning hypervolemic-hypertensive-hemodilution (HHH) therapy postoperatively? What is HHH therapy? Where do you put your transducers? How will you monitor for air embolus?
2. The patient is a full head and full stomach. Should you do an RSI? What do you look for in an old anesthetic record? What if you cannot get a hold of it, but the patient says, "I don't know if I was hard to intubate, but my throat was real sore afterward." Is using suxamethonium okay? What about awake intubation? If so, how would you do it? What is the danger to the aneurysm? If you have to perform a tracheostomy, God forbid, how long does it take to heal?
3. How do you manage controlled hypotension? Is 40 mm Hg too low for a mean blood pressure? Will BIS help? Can you get an EEG? What other organs are at risk? How will you tell if there is ischemia? Do you need TEE? What will wall motion abnormalities tell you?
4. The surgeon positions the chin right on the clavicle. Is this okay? How do you protect the spinal cord?
5. Airway pressures are all the way up to 50 cm H_2O. Is this too high? Is there anything you can do to reduce it? Can you use HFJV or a kind of HFJV? With all this, she still has a P_{O_2} of only 70 mm Hg on 100% O_2. What do you do? Will PEEP help or hurt? How about when deliberate hypotension happens?

Postoperative Questions

1. The blood pressure is 230/120 mm Hg on arrival in the ICU. How could you have prevented this? What do you do now? She is still intubated; do you extubate or sedate? Do you give Nipride bolus? What if you do but give too much? How do you treat central nervous system (CNS) toxicity? What are the risks? What is the role of an ABG determination in such a case?

2. The patient is blind postoperatively. Discuss the mechanism for this, and explain what you will do. How can you prevent this situation? What do you tell the next patient having the same procedure about the risk of blindness?

3. Six days after surgery, the patient has scleral icterus. Urinalysis shows bile. Is this desflurane hepatitis? How can you tell? What will you do? The gastric stapling surgeon is apoplectic, saying you killed his patient. What is your response?

Grab Bag

1. A 30-year-old firefighter has burns 1 month old on his face, neck, and chest. He is scheduled to undergo skin grafting. Are ketamine sedation, an end-tidal CO_2 monitor near his nose, and pulse oximetry okay? What if the patient is stoic and says, "I can take it." If you use general anesthesia, is there any advantage to spontaneous ventilation? What if you are in a developing country? Assuming a 20% burn area, can you use suxamethonium? What if his neck is thick and muscular?

2. A 2-month-old, 6-kg infant needs cleft lip repair. Do you intubate an awake patient or breathe down? Do you start an intravenous line? What are the special problems with cleft palates? The tube comes out in the middle of the operation. Do you use a mask or reintubate? Do you let the ENT specialist reintubate? Do you extubate deeply? What if the surgeon says he does not want his stitches "blown apart by a stormy wake-up"?

3. While operating on an intracranial aneurysm, it bursts, and you need instant, deep hypotension. How do you do this? Do you use barbiturates? What are the problems? How do you do controlled hypotension in this uncontrolled situation? Should you use isoflurane or sevoflurane? Should you use propofol or Nipride?

4. Nursing students want to know the idea behind universal precautions. Why does everyone use double gloves with known AIDS patients? Are some precautions more universal than others?

Update: Nerve Agents from a Terrorist Attack

1. How do most nerve agents act? Nerve agents are acetylcholinesterase inhibitors, leading to acetylcholine excess.

2. What are the nicotinic and muscarinic effects? The effects include miosis, rhinorrhea, salivation, bronchoconstriction, diarrhea, sweating, fasciculations and weakness, up or down blood pressure measurements, and convulsions.

3. What is the treatment? Patients need to be isolated. They require airway support (do not use suxamethonium), and you can use atropine and scopolamine (i.e., cholinolytics with central and peripheral effects).

4. You should titrate to what end points? Drying secretions and resuming spontaneous ventilations constitute the end points.

5. How do atropine and scopolamine work? They bind to acetylcholine receptors and block the action of acetylcholine.

6. Why is glycopyrrolate ineffective? It is a quaternary amine that does not enter the CNS.

7. What should you avoid? Avoid suxamethonium, Mivacron, or ester local anesthetics.

CASE 21: RUPTURED SPLEEN AFTER A MOTOR VEHICLE ACCIDENT

A 25-year-old man is scheduled to have a laparotomy for a ruptured spleen and débridement of an open tibial fracture after an MVA. He is on "some antidepressant" according to his wife, but she is not sure which one. He also takes "a lot of that herbal stuff." His blood pressure is 90/70 mm Hg, pulse is 120 beats/min, respiratory rate is 26 breaths/min, and temperature is 35°C.

Preoperative Questions

1. What is the highest priority when he arrives? How do you assess circulatory and respiratory adequacy? Is a blood pressure cuff enough, or do you need an arterial line right away? How do you look for other injuries (e.g., CNS, hidden punctures, pneumothorax)? How do you secure the ETT if the face is bloody or he has a big beard?
2. Which fluids do you use to resuscitate, or does it matter? Do you need laboratory test results before you proceed? How will you decide when to give blood or blood products? At what point would you use "trauma blood" (O negative) rather than waiting?
3. Do you need to know which antidepressant he takes? What are the implications of the various antidepressant medications? What about the herbals? What herbal preparations can have adverse effects on anesthetics? Bleeding can occur with ginseng, *Ginkgo biloba*, and garlic. Sympathomimetic exhaustion can occur with ephedra.

Intraoperative Questions

1. He arrives in the OR with two 18-gauge intravenous lines. Is this enough, or do you need more? Should you insist on a CVP line? How big should it be, and where should it be placed? What are the pros and cons of various sites? Is there any place for a cutdown in modern practice?
2. Do you give any medications to decrease the chance of aspiration? Is there any evidence-based medicine that proves such techniques work? How will you secure the airway? How will you do it if the patient is awake? If you do an RSI, which drugs will you use? What is ketamine?
3. Given the patient's tenuous status, colleagues suggest scopolamine for maintenance and no potent inhaled agents. Do you agree? Is BIS of any use? How do you control conversation when you have zero agents on board?
4. The liver is lacerated. Will you put in more lines or transfuse earlier? Blood loss is beyond massive. How will you keep up? Will you use a rapid infuser, all the way to the bypass machine?
5. The SvO_2 is 28%. What is normal? What will you do? What components go into an SvO_2? More FIO_2? What are the dangers of prolonged O_2 therapy or of PEEP? Detail the problems with PEEP.

Postoperative Questions

1. The patient has refractory hypotension 24 hours postoperatively. What is the differential diagnosis, and what is the treatment? How do you make the diagnosis of septic shock? What are the guidelines for inotropic support?

How does an intra-aortic balloon pump (IABP) work, and would it help in this case?

2. For pain relief after recovery, what are the options? Is it too late to give a COX-2 inhibitor? What are they, and how do they work? Is there any risk to the kidneys?
3. The patient is confused and restless after these bone fractures. What is the differential diagnosis, and what is the treatment? How do you make the diagnosis of a fat embolism? Do you send the patient for CT? What are the dangers of sending an unstable patient to the dark and dingy confines of the radiology suite?

Grab Bag

1. During a rocky labor, a 17-year-old multipara suddenly loses consciousness and becomes cyanotic. What is the diagnosis, and what is the treatment?
2. A 4-year-old child develops stridor in the PACU. How do you evaluate and treat her?
3. A year after an industrial accident, a man complains of unremitting pain in his right hand and hair loss on his forearm. Your move!

Update: Coronary Artery Spasm

1. What is Prinzmetal angina? It is coronary artery vasospasm in someone with normal anatomic coronary arteries. It can lead to MI and death.
2. How can a regional trigger this? Sympathetic nervous blockade can lead to parasympathetic dominance, and this leads to coronary artery spasm.
3. What is another mechanism? It can be caused by compensatory sympathetic hyperactivity above the level of the block.

CASE 22: LUMBAR LAMINECTOMY AT HIGH NOON

A 55-year-old, 110-kg man is scheduled for a lumbar laminectomy at noon. He has diabetes and hypertension, and he had an MI 5 years ago. He is afebrile and is on glyburide, metoprolol, and an ACE inhibitor. He has a sodium level of 142 mEq/L, potassium level of 5.5 mEq/L, glucose level of 320 mg/dL, hemoglobin level of 15.9 g/dL, blood pressure of 140/85 mm Hg, and pulse of 80 beats/min.

Preoperative Questions

1. What is diabetes? What is the significance of his glucose level of 320 mg/dL? Do you need other tests, such as the HbA_{1c}? How does insulin work? How do oral hypoglycemics work? Does he need to be tuned up or the case cancelled? What if his glucose level is always this high or the surgeon really wants to go? How does long-term diabetes affect the anesthetic? How does diabetic ketoacidosis (DKA) affect the situation if this were an emergency?
2. How do metoprolol and ACE inhibitors work? How do antihypertensive drugs interact with anesthesia? What if he were on a statin? Is muscle necrosis a concern? Do you need liver function tests, or do you trust the internal medicine guy to take care of that?
3. What ASA do you give? Why? Does it really matter? What does the Mallampati scale mean? Does that matter?

Intraoperative Questions

1. What is the significance of a prior MI? Do you need special monitors? What is the chance of a repeat MI and mortality if it occurs? What is the significance if he has had a stent? More safe? Do we need to do an echocardiogram or ask for another catheterization? What is the natural history of CAD? Maybe it has gotten worse, and his "silent ischemia" never showed up. What do you ask, specifically, of the cardiologist?

2. Do you need to follow blood sugar levels intraoperatively? Do you need to see if he is spilling glucose into the urine or look for protein?

3. What are your plans for muscle relaxants? Which ones will you use and why? What if the surgeon plans to use monitoring of the spinal cord—can you do a TIVA with no relaxants? What if he jumps intraoperatively? Do you rely on BIS monitoring in a case of TIVA? How do anesthetics affect the spinal cord monitor? Do you need to do a wake-up test? If not here, in which case and why?

4. Can you do this under a spinal? Why or why not? How would you redose or treat a high spinal in the prone position? What is important about the selection of the patient?

5. If you use general anesthesia, which anesthetic will you select and why? What are the pros and cons of sevoflurane and desflurane?

6. Discuss the respiratory, circulatory, and airway considerations for an obese patient in the prone position.

7. Discuss prone positioning of an obese, hypertensive, diabetic patient. Is blindness a risk? Why? Are other nerve injuries possible? How do you prevent them?

8. The surgeon cuts the iliac vessel on the other side, and the systolic blood pressure plummets to 60 mm Hg. Do you need to repair the iliac vessel? What will you do? Will you change to a laparoscopic method, pack, or rapid infuser? How do you place big lines while the patient is prone?

Postoperative Questions

1. The blood pressure in the PACU is 220/130 mm Hg. What are the surgical and cardiac risks? Why is the pressure so high? What is the differential diagnosis, and what is the treatment of dangerous hypertension?

2. The patient has eye pain. What will you do? How did this happen, and how will you fix it? How could you have prevented the problem? Discuss the pros and cons of eye ointment, eye goggles, and taping. Discuss tear production under anesthesia.

3. The oxygen saturation drops to 83% unless he is given a 3-L nasal cannula, and then it goes up only to 89%. Discuss the oxygen-hemoglobin dissociation curve. What is the differential diagnosis, and what is the treatment?

Grab Bag

1. A 6-year-old girl is scheduled for femoral hernia repair. A cousin had malignant hyperthermia (MH) at a Nova Scotia outpatient center and "died because they did not have some orange stuff." Do you need further tests on this kid? Can you operate on her at an outpatient center? Do you need a muscle biopsy? Should you pretreat with dantrolene? How do you conduct the case? What if it is an emergency, and no one can get an intravenous line placed?

2. You are doing a heart case and give the usual amount of heparin, but the activated clotting time (ACT) fails to climb over 400 seconds (goes from 120 up to 205 seconds). The surgeon says, "The hell with it. This is an off-pump case anyway. What do you do? Why did the ACT not climb? Does it really matter in an off-pump case?

3. An immigrant from Transylvania comes in for treatment of appendicitis. He has acute intermittent porphyria. What is porphyria, and how will you manage his anesthetic? What do you avoid? How do you treat an exacerbation?

Update: Intubating Dose of Succinylcholine

1. What is the traditional dose? The usual dose of succinylcholine is 1 mg/kg.
2. What works just as well? The dose is 0.5 mg/kg.
3. Even at a lower dose, can you intubate in 60 seconds? Yes.
4. What is the potential advantage of a smaller dose? You can attain a quicker return of spontaneous ventilation. You come back about 90 seconds sooner.

CASE 23: PANENDOSCOPY

A 57-year-old man is scheduled for laryngoscopy, bronchoscopy, and esophagoscopy for suspected cancer of the larynx. He has a history of asthma, smoking, drinking, and hypertension. He takes theophylline, albuterol, prednisone, and an ACE inhibitor daily. He is afebrile and has a blood pressure of 170/100 mm Hg, pulse of 90 beats/min, and respiratory rate of 22 breaths/min.

Preoperative Questions

1. What additional preoperative information do you need about his pulmonary status? The chest radiograph shows consolidation of the right middle lobe and a right pleural effusion. What is the significance of these findings? Should you cancel the case or proceed? If you proceed, what is the significance for the anesthetic? Do you need PFTs? Is a preoperative ABG determination or a preoperative pulse oximeter reading okay? How do you determine if the situation is optimized? Do you insist that he use the inhaler three times daily for 3 days and then come back? Do you increase the theophylline dose or take him off it? Do you add cromolyn?

2. Do you need to "cover him with steroids"? Why or why not? What are risks of an addisonian crisis? If that happens, what steroid would you give, or does it matter with steroids? What is the difference between the different kinds of steroids?

3. If the surgeon can do this under the MAC, how would you premedicate? Would it be different if general endotracheal anesthesia were planned? Why?

Intraoperative Questions

1. Which monitors do you use for a MAC? Do you use more if general endotracheal anesthesia is planned? Why? Do you need an arterial line? Really? What if you blow both radials—is it worth going all the way to femoral placement for this short case? What are risks of a femoral line compared

with the risk of short-lived hypertension? Isn't the big problem tachycardia? That you can see!

2. You use general anesthesia. Compare awake intubation, intravenous induction, and inhalation induction. If the tumor is big, is there any role for heliox? If not in this case, when? If you use awake intubation, detail how you would go through topicalization, and give alternative routes of topicalization.

3. Intravenous remifentanil and propofol are smooth and offer a nice wake-up process. Is this a good idea? Would you use sevoflurane or desflurane? Why? Discuss the pros and cons of each method. Is the use of narcotics a good or bad idea? What if the patient also has obstructive sleep apnea? Should the patient be placed in the ICU postoperatively?

4. How will you ventilate during rigid bronchoscopy. Will you use HFJV? How do you do that? How do you keep the patient anesthetized? Do you use a suxamethonium drip? How does the CO_2 absorber work?

5. You detect multifocal PVCs during bronchoscopy. What is the differential diagnosis, and what is the treatment?

Postoperative Questions

1. The patient is combative 30 minutes postoperatively. What is the differential diagnosis? The nurse suggests sedation with propofol, Precedex, narcotics, or Versed. Discuss each option. You consider aspiration. Will you confirm it with a physical examination or chest radiograph? When does aspiration show up on a chest radiograph?

2. The blood pressure is 220/100 mm Hg, and the patient complains of chest pain radiating down his left arm; the jaw also hurts. What is the differential diagnosis, and what is the treatment? Do you go all the way to the catheter laboratory?

Grab Bag

1. How is fetal well-being assessed? Differentiate late and early decelerations. What is the mechanism? When do you need to get a fetal scalp pH, or is that old-fashioned? Why is bradycardia in the fetus so worrisome?

2. The patient gives good history for MH. Do you give dantrolene prophylactically? Do you give it on an outpatient basis? Do you change the machine? When you go on break, how do you keep someone from turning on vapors? How do you do a TIVA? What if it is a kid who will not hold still for an intravenous line placement?

3. What is the mechanism for DIC? Where does it occur? How do you treat it? In what setting might you see an amniotic fluid embolus, a fat embolus, or a pulmonary embolus?

CASE 24: LASER FOR LARYNGEAL PAPILLOMAS IN A CHILD

A 4-year-old, 23-kg boy is scheduled for laser excision of laryngeal papillomas. At his first operation 2 months earlier, he had postoperative fever and delayed recovery. His blood pressure is 80/60 mm Hg, pulse is 100 beats/min, respiratory rate is 20 breaths/min, and temperature is 37°C.

Preoperative Questions

1. How will you examine the airway? Discuss routine examination compared with this case with papillomas. What information do you need from the old record? What if you cannot find it? What about information from the ENT specialist? Do you need airway radiographs or flow-volume loop? Can you get this information for a child? How will you pick up airway obstruction in your physical examination?
2. What is the differential diagnosis for the earlier febrile episode? What about the earlier delayed recovery? Is it iatrogenic? How would you tell if earlier episodes were MH? Would an old anesthetic record help? Would you talk with an anesthesiologist, obtain laboratory studies such as a creatine phosphokinase level, or get a muscle biopsy? Can you wait that long?

Intraoperative Questions

1. What circuit do you choose for a 4-year-old child? Is there any advantage with Bain or Jackson-Reese systems? Can you do jet ventilation to allow the surgeons room to get out the papillomas? Will you use a small ETT? What about concern for an airway fire? How do you prevent one? Do you need heliox? Can you run nitrous oxide?
2. If you found out the patient did not have MH, how would you induce? If you found out he did have MH, how would you induce? Would you use rectal Brevital? What are the pros and cons? What if you cannot get an intravenous line in the kid who is susceptible to MH? Do you need relaxants to do the case? How do you monitor? Which relaxant do you use and why?
3. Which fluids do you use? How much and why? Do you use glucose or colloid?
4. While you are using jet ventilation, the kid develops subcutaneous emphysema. What now? Is airway compromise a concern? Do you need an ICU bed? It becomes very difficult to ventilate, even with a regular ETT. Does the patient have a pneumothorax or airway distortion? Should you get a chest radiograph? Should you place a chest tube right away or use ECMO?

Postoperative Questions

1. Suppose the chest tube is placed after a pneumothorax. When do you extubate? What do you tell the parents? Do you need an arterial line? Where do you place it? You extubate, and the kid becomes stridorous. What now? Do you use racemic epinephrine, reintubate, or keep the head up and observe?
2. The child is thrashing all over creation. What is the differential diagnosis, and what is the treatment? Is the problem related to pneumothorax? Why? How do you manage the intense pain of the chest tube? Do you use an intercostal block? How, and how much local anesthetic do you use? Do you use a chest tube as a pleural catheter? How can you tell if there is local anesthetic toxicity?

Grab Bag

1. You have a 1200-g, 30-week gestational age infant scheduled for a ventriculoperitoneal shunt. On 50% oxygen, the patient's saturation level dropped from 95% to 88%. What do you do? What is the risk of retrolental fibroplasias?

2. The patient has near-drowning episode, and his temperature is only 31°C. Do you correct the blood gases? Why? What is the physiology of correcting compared with not correcting the blood gases?

3. A 5-year-old child is scheduled for a hernia repair. The mother says a cousin had real live MH. Do you proceed, get a muscle biopsy, or insist that the patient be operated on at an in-patient facility?

Update: Cardiac Anesthesia

1. What do we have for detecting ischemia? The ECG is the most powerful and cost-effective modality. It is confounded by left ventricular hypertrophy, LBBB, digitalis, Wolff-Parkinson-White syndrome, and baseline ST abnormality. Lead II alone detects 30%; leads II and V_5 detect 80%; and leads II, V_5, and V_4 detect 95% of ischemia. You can keep the leads on. TEE is great, but you have to have it in, and you have to place it after induction. It is thrown off by paced rhythm, LBBB, and stunned myocardium. The pulmonary artery catheter gives too global of a picture.

2. How do you prevent ischemia? Ensure good anesthesia, and maximize O_2 balance (e.g., blood, heart rate, preload and afterload). β-Blockers are most significant, however, any conclusion about β-blockers is tempered by the POISE study.

3. For treatment, use all of the previously described methods, and go to mechanical support, such as an IABP. Go all the way to involving cardiologist and opening vessels.

CASE 25: TRANSURETHRAL PROSTATECTOMY AND CHRONIC OBSTRUCTIVE PULMONARY DISEASE

A 70-year-old, 120-kg man with chronic obstructive pulmonary disease (COPD) is scheduled for TURP for BPH. He has a 1-year history of dyspnea on exertion, paroxysmal nocturnal dyspnea, and ankle swelling. He does not like to take medications, so he does not. He is afebrile, and his blood pressure is 160/95 mm Hg and pulse is 88 beats/min. He puffs and auto-PEEPs when he breathes.

Preoperative Questions

1. Explain the patient's constellation of symptoms. Is his cardiac status optimized? What about his respiratory status? The surgeon says, "To hell with canceling. They never get 'optimized' anyway! Give him some β-blocker, and let's go." What is COPD? How do you differentiate shortness of breath caused by a cardiac problem from a respiratory cause from a combined cause? What are the likely results of an ABG determination, chest radiograph, ECG, PFTs, stress echocardiogram, and regular echocardiogram?

2. The internist calls and asks for medical suggestions. How long does the patient have to be "better" before it is okay to go—a day, a week, a month? How long before the BPH will start causing problems? What is the danger of waiting?

3. What is cor pulmonale? What is right versus left heart failure? How can you tell them apart, or does it matter? A mitral valve regurgitation problem is discovered. Do you fix it before the TURP?

Intraoperative Questions

1. If the patient is optimized, which anesthetic is best? What are the pros and cons given his condition and the operation?
2. Do you use the same monitors for spinal or general anesthesia? Why?
3. For cardiac protection, should you give a β-blocker? What is your concern about triggering asthma compared with cardiac protection? Why is there so much emphasis on perioperative β-blockade? What is the physiology of CAD?
4. Thirty minutes after the case starts, the patient becomes confused, slurs his speech, and says his shoulder hurts. What is the differential diagnosis, and what is the treatment? How do you tell if TURP syndrome (discuss this) and bladder rupture (discuss this) occur at same time? What is the danger of rapid sodium replacement with hypertonic saline?
5. The surgeon has to open the abdomen to repair the bladder. Do you stick with your T8 spinal or induce? How, given the big sympathectomy? Do you supply cardiac protection at induction? How do you manage the airway in the setting of obesity and an emergent situation? What about diffuse bleeding on entering abdomen. What tests do you order? What is the treatment?

Postoperative Questions

1. The blood pressure drops to 70/40 mm Hg and the heart rate is 130 beats/min 1 hour postoperatively. What is the most likely diagnosis, and what is the treatment? How do you differentiate hypovolemic shock from septic shock or from cardiogenic shock? Do you need an echocardiogram?
2. You give blood to the patient in the PACU. The patient develops rash and lumbar pain. What gives? How do you diagnose a transfusion reaction? What is the treatment, and what are the dangers? What is the most likely cause? What if you have to keep giving blood? What is difference between a major and minor transfusion reaction?

Grab Bag

1. The patient received magnesium for toxemia. A colleague suggests general anesthesia for a cesarean section because "that is the way we do it here, I'll stick around until the tube is in." What do you say? How will the magnesium interact with the patient or the fetus? What if you have to do an emergent cesarean section? Do you use a spinal, single-shot epidural, or general anesthesia? If you cannot intubate, do you use an LMA?
2. How much heparin do you give for a femoral-popliteal line? Do you get an ACT? What is an ACT? How much more do you give for heart surgery? Why do we give more? How does heparin work? What if a heart patient has HIT? What is HIT?
3. How do β-blockers work? What is their role in cardiac protection? A colleague says he gives "esmolol with each intubation." Is this a good idea or a bad idea? Why? What is the proposed mechanism of cardiac ischemia (e.g., plaque rupture).

Update: Continuous Spinal Anesthesia

1. What is the concern about continuous spinal anesthesia? The concern is microcatheter-caused neurotoxicity.

2. What about a wet tap? Put in a big catheter, the regular one, and you can do continuous spinal anesthesia just fine. Do not use lidocaine.

3. Where might this be of benefit? The approach can be helpful in revascularization of the lower extremities (i.e., fewer thromboses with ongoing sympathetic block), orthopedic operations, lumbar laminectomies, and cases for which the duration is unknown.

CASE 26: LOBECTOMY OF THE RIGHT UPPER LUNG

A 60-year-old, 80-kg man is scheduled for thoracotomy for cancer of the right upper lung. He had an MI 3 months earlier and got a stent in his left anterior descending artery. He has no chest pain now and takes Metoprolol. You hear a right carotid bruit. Vital signs are all normal.

Preoperative Questions

1. Which laboratory tests do you need before proceeding with lobectomy? Do you need ABG or PFT results? Do you need a flow-volume loop, or is that used only for mediastinal masses? Does the patient need a bronchodilator before and after the procedure? Why or why not? What if all test results point to less than 50% values? Can you proceed with the case? Should you get split-function lung studies?

2. Do you need further cardiac workup? What if this were a minor case, such as a cataract operation; do you still need such an extensive cardiac workup? What is the risk of a dobutamine stress test? What is a stress test? Can you die during one of those? Do you need further workup of the carotid bruit? What is the significance of a bruit? Do you need an echocardiogram of the carotid? What if the patient were dizzy? Would you workup the carotid or look for a rhythm disturbance? What if he had transient ischemic attack (TIA) symptoms such as amaurosis fugax?

Intraoperative Questions

1. Which monitors will you use and why? What are the hazards of an arterial line? What is the treatment of complications such as a dusky hand after line placement? Is it surgery, or do you pull out the clot? Do you use a stellate ganglion block and cancel surgery? Do you use nitroglycerin in the artery?

2. Should you use a CVP or Swan-Ganz line? What evidence-based medicine can back one or the other? Where would you place it? Do you use the same side as the surgery in the case of a lung isolation during the case? How would you recognize and treat pneumothorax? If you use a Swan-Ganz catheter, which kind do you choose? Why? What are the problems with big, clunky, continuous-cardiac-output Swan-Ganz catheters?

3. How do you isolate the lung? Go through all the options. What is the differential diagnosis, and what is the treatment for the lung not going down, and what is the differential diagnosis, and what is the treatment for desaturation? You go to one lung, and you see no trace on the CO_2 monitor. What happened? How do you isolate the lung if the airway is difficult?

4. When you manage blood pressure intraoperatively with a carotid bruit, are you going to do anything differently?

5. Do you use or avoid N_2O? Give reasons.

6. The patient goes into bigeminy. What is the differential diagnosis, and what is the treatment? Now he develops ventricular fibrillation with the chest open. What is the management plan?
7. With lung manipulation, the patient bucks and coughs. What is the treatment? Should you paralyze? Is he underanesthetized? How do you deepen anesthesia if the patient is already hypotensive?

Postoperative Questions

1. Two hours postoperatively, the patient is unresponsive to all stimuli but deep pain. How will you evaluate this situation? Do you keep the patient intubated? How do you sedate if he is fighting the tube?
2. After a big case with a lot of blood loss, the surgeon wants you to change to a single-lumen tube. How will you do this safely? What are the problems with keeping the double-lumen tube in? You start an epidural at the end of the case. Can you do this with the patient intubated?

Grab Bag

1. If a patient has a known elevation in the ICP, how does it affect your anesthetic induction? What about an open globe or an open globe and a difficult airway?
2. Describe the different pediatric breathing circuits, including the circle, Jackson-Reese, and Bain systems. Which is best?
3. A 3-year-old child in the PACU after an examination under anesthesia sounds croupy. He was just masked but has no LMA or ETT. What do you do?

Update: Shock

1. Do you use delayed or immediate resuscitation? Delay until hemorrhage is controlled, because rapid resuscitation increases bleeding.
2. Do you use colloid or crystalloid? Intermediate studies show that colloid stays in the circulation longer, but the outcome is no different. Even albumin has never been shown to be better.
3. What are newer treatments for cardiac failure? Cardiac resynchronization with a biventricular pacer shows promise.
4. What is a newer treatment for septic shock? Vasopressin increases blood pressure but does not constrict the renal vasculature. It improves blood pressure and increases urine output.
5. Do you use steroids? If the patient demonstrates adrenal insufficiency (i.e., unresponsive to corticotropin stimulation test), steroids have some benefit.
6. Does activated protein C help? This is a complex anticoagulant and anti-inflammatory drug. If the acute physiology and chronic health evaluation (APACHE) score is less than 25, there may be some benefit.

CASE 27: TONSILLECTOMY AND ADENOIDECTOMY WITH HAY FEVER

A 5-year-old, 20-kg girl is scheduled for tonsillectomy and adenoidectomy and placement of bilateral tubes. She has a history of hay fever and wheezing when she has a cold. She has double joints, which serves as endless amusement to her classmates at school. Her vital signs are normal.

Preoperative Questions

1. Which laboratory tests do you need? Is there a minimum requirement? If she is healthy but she might lose a lot of blood, do you need a hematocrit? How about getting one after she is asleep? Do you need the PT and platelet count because bleeding may be a problem? How about a baseline TEG, baseline ECG because she may bleed, or baseline chest radiograph because she may aspirate?
2. Is MH a possibility? Does double jointedness mean she has Ehlers-Danlos or Marfan syndrome? Do these patients have more MH episodes? Should you get a muscle biopsy? How far do you dig in her family history? How far out does a diagnosis of MH have to go before it affects her? What is MH? What are the genetics of it? Do you order a baseline creatine phosphokinase level so you will be able to tell if there is an increase?
3. What is hay fever? What is its significance in terms of anesthesia? Do you need a chest radiograph or an eosinophil count? What do you look for in the history, in the physical examination findings, and baseline ABG values? If she has a history of this stuff, should you start her on prophylactic cromolyn, albuterol, aminophylline, or steroids?

Intraoperative Questions

1. The mother wants the child asleep when she leaves the holding area room so she does not see the "scary OR." What is your response? Do you use rectal brevital? If not, in what case would that be acceptable? Do you use oral Versed, a fentanyl lollipop, or intramuscular ketamine? Is it better to go into the OR?
2. You breathe down with sevoflurane. Discuss the uptake of this drug compared with the more-soluble halothane. Why does a more-soluble drug take longer to put the patient to sleep? What kind of circuit will you use and why? How do Jackson-Reese and Bain circuits work?
3. For maintenance, will you use N_2O, narcotics, or relaxants? Did you say yes to all of these? Why? How do you assess depth? What are the dangers of moving? Do you intubate with suxamethonium without a relaxant? What if the surgeon is really fast?
4. After intubation, the patient cannot move air at all. What is the differential diagnosis, and what is the treatment? Is the cause an esophageal intubation, asthma, endobronchial intubation, or carinal stimulation? How do you tell which it is? If tightness and wheezing is caused by asthma, will a muscle relaxant help? How will this affect the uptake of sevoflurane? Is desflurane a good idea? Will N_2O help? What is the second gas effect?
5. What fluids are needed and how much? For a blood loss of 400 mL, do you transfuse? What is acceptable blood loss? What is the end point if you do transfuse?

Postoperative Questions

1. The patient is having severe delirium in the PACU. What is the differential diagnosis, and what is the treatment? Should you give intramuscular morphine or Demerol? What if the kid pulled out the intravenous line at emergence?
2. The temperature goes to 38.5°C in the PACU. Is this MH? What else could it be? If it is MH, what next? If not, then what? How far do you cool down if you realize you overheated the child with the Bair Hugger system?

3. The kid had a loose incisor before, and now there is only a space. What is the treatment? Do you need to request a chest radiograph or a plain frontal supine radiograph of the abdomen (i.e., kidneys, ureters, and bladder [KUB])? Who pays for all these x-ray studies?

Grab Bag

1. How does a preemie differ from a term infant? Can you anesthetize a preemie as an outpatient? How about an ex-preemie? How do you handle the NPO status of a baby?
2. The patient has bad ARDS and needs to come to the OR. Do you get an ICU ventilator? Why or why not? How good are our anesthesia machine ventilators? What is the fail-safe mechanism? How will you pick up a line crossover?
3. A T4 paraplegic is scheduled for an open reduction and internal fixation (ORIF) of the femur after a fall out of bed. Is a spinal okay? Is an epidural okay? How about using nothing? What is the risk of autonomic hyperreflexia? What is this? How can you avoid it, and how do you treat it?

Update: Bradycardia and Asystole during Spinal Anesthesia

1. Who is at risk for bradycardia and asystole during spinal anesthesia? Patients at risk include those with a low baseline heart rate, first-degree heart block, on β-blockers, with high sensory level, and males.
2. What is incidence of bradycardia after a spinal? The incidence is 13%, which is not an insubstantial number.
3. What is the mechanism? A decrease in venous return with an increased inotropic state of the left ventricle triggers hypotension and bradycardia. It is possibly a variant of the Bezold-Jarisch reflex.
4. When does this typically occur? It occurs between 55 and 65 minutes after spinal placement, which is a time when vigilance may be waning.
5. What is the best treatment? Use epinephrine early.

CASE 28: ASPIRATED PEANUT IN A CHILD

A 3-year-old, 14-kg boy is scheduled to have bronchoscopy for removal of a peanut. He inhaled it 2 hours ago at Chuck E Cheese after he ate a hot dog (mustard only) and cake (white with chocolate frosting). He has a diagnosis of Wolf-Parkinson-White (WPW) syndrome and is on Inderal. He had strabismus surgery a year ago without incident. His blood pressure is 90/70 mm Hg, pulse is 100 beats/min, respiratory rate is 34 breaths/min (anxious breathing), and temperature is 37.7°C.

Preoperative Questions

1. What is WPW syndrome, and how does it affect the anesthetic? What rhythm problems can you foresee? How will Inderal affect the anesthetic? Do you need electrolyte test results (e.g., potassium level) for this patient because you are worried about the WPW syndrome? Does Inderal affect any laboratory values or the MAC? Does it interact with anesthetic or induction agents?

2. How do you prepare for full stomach? Do you use a nasogastric tube, Ewall tube, Bicitra, or Reglan? Is there proof that any of this works? Can you give Bicitra to an anxious 3 year old? Do you offer sedation per rectum, oral Versed, or a fentanyl lollipop? Do you administer intramuscular medications or try an intravenous line?

Intraoperative Questions

1. How do you monitor cardiac status? What if a kid playfully keeps pulling off leads? Do you need an arterial line in case the kid goes into some brutal rhythm? What pulmonary complications do you foresee? Does a foreign body throw off the end-tidal CO_2? How does the end-tidal sampling mechanism work?
2. How will you induce if you cannot place an intravenous line? Do you mask with a full stomach? How are you going to protect the airway, because they will be putting a rigid bronchoscope in and you will not have a tube in? If the kid is fighting, can you give intramuscular suxamethonium to break the laryngospasm? Go through all the different intravenous options, and assume the kid is obese and you cannot find any veins.
3. Which breathing circuit will you use? Are there better dead space considerations with Jackson-Reese or Bain systems? Is a circle less complicated? How will you humidify the air? How will you keep the kid warm? What is the risk for hypothermia?
4. Wide complex arrhythmia occurs. Is it ventricular tachyarrhythmia (VT) or SVT with aberrant conduction? What is the differential diagnosis, and what is the treatment? What if the patient is in shock? How can you tell if he is perfused if you do not have an arterial line? What are the roles of the end-tidal CO_2, pulse oximeter, pulse, and color? Is amiodarone a good choice? How much do you administer, and what are the side effects?

Postoperative Questions

1. The patient is stridorous postoperatively. Is this a normal finding, given what he just went through, or is it abnormal? What is the differential diagnosis, and what is the treatment? Do you send the kid home? Do you leave the intravenous line in and send him to the floor? Do you keep the pulse oximeter on him? Who will respond or see or hear the pulse oximeter alarm if he is at the end of the hall? Should you send him to the ICU?
2. Ninety minutes postoperatively, the patient's temperature rises from 35°C to 39°C. The patient is tachypneic, rigid, and mottled. Is this the effect of the procedure? Is it aspiration or MH? How can you tell, and what tests will you order?
3. The kid is rubbing his eye and crying. What is the differential diagnosis, and what is the treatment? What do you document, and what do you tell the parents?

Grab Bag

1. The patient is unresponsive 1 minute after you do a stellate ganglion block. What might have happened, and what do you do about it? How do you tell a successful ganglion block in the short term (e.g., Horner's) or long term (e.g., pain relief, trophic changes improve)?

2. You are planning an abdominal aortic aneurysm operation, and the patient has brittle diabetes. The surgeon wants tight control to help with wound healing. How do you manage diabetes in such a case? What is the danger of recognizing low glucose under anesthesia?

3. How is an anesthetic affected by renal failure? What other organ systems are involved? What are the platelets or cardiac effects? Do you need an arterial line and CVP line for renal transplantation? Defend both ways.

Update: Gum Bougie Goings-on

1. Can the gum bougie help with LMA placement? Yes. When digital techniques have failed, placing the gum bougie and threading it may help place the LMA.

2. Can it help with intubation? Yes. It has been shown to be an effective adjunct in case of an unanticipated difficult intubation.

3. Are there any concerns? If the patient had a fresh lobectomy, the gum bougie could poke through. You cannot ventilate through it.

CASE 29: BRONCHOSCOPY AND LOBECTOMY IN A SCHIZOPHRENIC WOMAN

A 69-year-old woman with schizophrenia has a coin lesion of the left upper lung. She had an inferior wall MI 1 yr ago, and she has had stable angina since. She takes her nitroglycerin tablets three times daily. She continues to smoke Virginia Slims, because she thinks this whole women's lib thing is here to stay. She is scheduled to have bronchoscopy, video-assisted thoracoscopic surgery (VATS), and a possible lobectomy.

Preoperative Questions

1. What more information do you need about her history as far as her heart, her lungs, and her psychiatric medications are concerned? Do you need PFTs or flow-volume loops? Do you really need to look at the radiograph, or is that a surgeon thing? Do you need a preoperative ABG determination?

2. She takes her nitroglycerin three times daily. She seems to have stable angina. How is this different from unstable angina? Do you need a more extensive workup? What is risk of a stress test? What is the cost? The surgeon says, "Just give her β-blockers—that is what your literature says." Is he right? Why or why not? Would you really go all the way to CABG before taking out this tumor? What is the risk of waiting?

3. Which psychiatric medications interact with our anesthetics and how? What happens with serotonin reuptake inhibitors, tricyclics, and MAO inhibitors? If the patient takes a bunch of herbal medications, how will that affect us?

Intraoperative Questions

1. What monitors will you use? Which lead is best for detecting ischemia and why? Is TEE more sensitive? How does a Swan-Ganz catheter pick up ischemia, and what are its shortcomings?

2. How do you induce if she has an ejection fraction (EF) of 60% or 20%? What is etomidate? Can you use pentathol and give less? Do you need an arterial line before or after induction? What if she does not cooperate? Do you need a CVP line before or after induction? Why?

3. How do you ventilate during bronchoscopy? If you do not have a good seal and the patient starts to desaturate, what do you do? Is it really a problem if the CO_2 level starts to climb? Contrast this situation with the danger of hypocarbia. Is metabolic acidosis worse, or does the pH remain the same no matter what happens? What if hypercarbia is associated with bigeminy?

4. What problems are specific to mediastinoscopy? How do you prevent stroke? What if they biopsy the superior vena cava? Should you have put in a femoral line to get access to the inferior vena cava?

5. What if the lung does not drop during VATS? What if desaturation occurs on one lung or if the end-tidal CO_2 trace disappears?

Postoperative Questions

1. One hour postoperatively, the patient's blood pressure is 230/100 mm Hg. What is the differential diagnosis, and what is the treatment? What if high blood pressure is associated with a sudden drop in the heart rate to 35 beats/min? Do you reintubate and hyperventilate? Do you send the patient for CT? How will you sedate if, after intubating, she is thrashing around?

2. The patient has severe, left-sided chest pain. How will you tell incisional pain from ischemic pain, because they are in the same "neck of the woods"?

3. Urine output drops to 20 mL/hr after putting her back on the ventilator, but nothing else has changed. Why the sudden drop in urine output, and what are you going to do?

Grab Bag

1. How do you reverse too much fentanyl, too much morphine, and too much Versed, or do you just leave the patient on the ventilator? Do you run an infusion of Narcan? What are the dangers?

2. You get a wet tap. What do you do? Do you use a saline infusion or continuous spinal? What are the risks? Do you go again? Do you administer a prophylactic blood patch through the epidural catheter? Can you do the blood patch later? Should you give caffeine drinks? What if the patient is a Mormon and does not drink Coke?

3. An inguinal hernia repair is planned in a patient with a pacemaker. How do you handle the magnet? Do you interrogate? How? Do you put on a Zoll pad? Is the situation different if the patient has an automatic implantable cardioverter defibrillator (AICD)?

4. When would you use HFJV? How about ECMO? What makes you go from inotropic support to an IABP or a left ventricular assist device (LVAD)?

Update: Chronic Pain Liability

1. What are most common concerns? Nerve injury and pneumothorax are common concerns.

2. The most serious injuries result from what? Injections with local anesthetics and opioids resulted in most cases of death or brain injury.

3. What problems occurred after the patient is home? Patients have problems with the maintenance of implantable devices. A pump programming error can deliver too much narcotic.

CASE 30: LARYNGECTOMY AND NECK DISSECTION

A 59-year-old, 65-kg man is scheduled for total laryngectomy and left radical neck dissection. The ECG shows left axis deviation (LAD), occasional PVCs, and nonspecific ST-T wave changes. The chest radiograph shows hyperlucency. He takes something for his blood pressure but he cannot remember what, and he takes it only if he gets a headache. His blood pressure is 160/90 mm Hg, pulse is 80 beats/min, respiratory rate is 18 breaths/min, temperature is 37°C, and hemoglobin level is 11 g/dL.

Preoperative Questions

1. How will you assess the airway? What are your concerns? Do you need the ENT specialist's indirect laryngoscopy report or at least a chat with him? Do you need the flow-volume loops or CT scan? What do you look for in his history and physical examination?
2. What is your interpretation of the PVCs, nonspecific ST-T wave changes, and LAD? Do you need a cardiology consultation? What do you ask the cardiologist? Explain a thallium test, a stress echocardiographic test, dobutamine echocardiography, and a stress test without echocardiography. Which is best and tells you the most? When do you need to go to catheterization? What are the dangers of catheterization?
3. What about the antihypertensive medication? Do you need to know it? Does it really make a difference, because the admonition is always the same: "Watch the blood pressure carefully at induction." Should you use a β-blocker or an ACE inhibitor? What is the patient's record of compliance or noncompliance? Do you cancel if you do not know or just forge ahead?
4. The chest radiograph shows a hyperlucency. What is the meaning of this? What is the impact on the anesthetic? What is the effect of positive-pressure ventilation? What is the effect of bleb rupture? How will the patient handle fluids? What is the difference between a pink puffer and a blue bloater? What is the definition of COPD, and how is this patient optimized?

Intraoperative Questions

1. How do you secure an airway that is coming out anyway? Do you go retrograde with a wire? How is this done? Do you perform an awake fiberoptic procedure or an awake tracheostomy? How do you conduct each of these procedures? Do you use a Bullard scope? When is the time and where is the place to employ new airway technology in your practice?
2. How do you maintain a man who has a stable pattern of PVCs that cardiologists do not want to treat? Is desflurane a bad choice with its sympathomimetic business? Because it is a long case, can you go with cheaper isoflurane? What is your concern about the renal system? Are you going to run N_2O or air to decrease long-term high F_{IO_2} exposure? Why?
3. Do you need an arterial line? If the surgeon is slow but meticulous, can you draw samples for laboratory tests from the CVP line? If he has bad peripheral vascular disease and Raynaud's, is the risk of an arterial line worth taking?
4. The ECG shows a 3-mm depression. What is the significance of this finding? What is the treatment? Do you forge ahead or cancel? Do you go to

the cardiac cath laboratory? Do you use MS or nitroglycerin? Do you call a cardiologist into the room? For ventricular tachycardia and ventricular fibrillation, how do you run your code? Why choose epinephrine over vasopressin? Why not choose Levophed? How did they come up with these algorithms, and how do you randomize in a code study?

5. After an hour, the blood pressure plummets suddenly. What is the differential diagnosis, and what is the treatment? Four hours later, the blood pressure drifts down. What is the differential diagnosis, and what is the treatment? Which pressor do you use in each case and why?

Postoperative Questions

1. On arrival in the PACU, the patient's temperature is 32°C. How can you prevent this? What is the danger of it? How do you treat a low temperature?
2. Four hours postoperatively, the patient is still unconscious. What is the differential diagnosis, and what is the treatment? At what point do you throw in the towel and say, "Go to CT!" How do you tell if the problem is pseudocholinesterase deficiency?
3. The neurologist wants to go over possible nerve injuries with a fine-tooth comb in a study she is doing. Go over all the possible nerve injuries in this patient, and explain how you would test them.
4. The patient's blood pressure goes to 70/40 mm Hg 2 hours postoperatively. What is your next move?

Grab Bag

1. Which local anesthetic is best for a labor epidural or for a cesarean section? What are the relative advantages and disadvantages of lidocaine, bupivacaine, and levobupivacaine? Should you add epinephrine? What is the idea behind a test dose?
2. Anesthesia is needed for a burn patient. The man has 50% burns on his body, including his face. He needs several débridements over many days. What is the best management? Do you use ketamine? Do you intubate each time?
3. Two days after a spinal for knee arthroscopy, the patient calls and complains of headache. What is the management plan? Do you bring him in? Do you pour Mountain Dew down him until he fibrillates?

Update: Diplopia after Dural Puncture

1. Does diplopia occur after a dural puncture? Yes. After dural puncture, patients can get bothersome diplopia, generating a million-dollar workup.
2. What is most often affected? The abducens nerve (cranial nerve VI) is most often affected.
3. Does a blood patch help? No. It is good for headache, but it does not help diplopia.
4. What do you do? Use conservative treatment with an eye patch or prism glasses. The situation usually resolves within 8 months. You can go all the way to corrective surgery.
5. When does it occur? It occurs 4 to 10 days after dural puncture, but it may be as late as 3 weeks. It resolves in 2 weeks to 8 months.

CASE 31: VAGINAL HYSTERECTOMY IN AN ARTHRITIC PATIENT

A 58-year-old, 50-kg woman with long-standing rheumatoid arthritis is scheduled for a vaginal hysterectomy. Eighteen months earlier, she had an MI complicated by congestive heart failure (CHF) and VT. She now has an AICD in place. She takes an ACE inhibitor, prednisone, and gold shots. (She has a gold cap with a champagne glass on her upper incisor, wears gold lamé to the preoperative clinic, and drives a gold Maserati—go figure.) Her blood pressure is 150/90 mm Hg, pulse is 80 beats/min, and respiratory rate is 12 breaths/min.

Preoperative Questions

1. Describe the systemic effects of rheumatoid arthritis and how it affects anesthesia. Is rheumatoid arthritis associated with any other autoimmune diseases? What is molecular mechanism of these autoimmune diseases? The patient is hoarse. Why?
2. What is the significance of an MI 18 months ago? Why is timing so important to us? How about timing after a stent is placed? Are these patients "good to go" the next day because the vessel has been opened? What do the CHF and VT tell you about the extent of the MI? Which vessel was likely involved?
3. Should you turn off an AICD, put a magnet on it, or ignore it? What is the risk from Bovie cautery? What if it is a middle-of-the-night emergency, and you cannot turn it off? How does an AICD work? How do you interrogate it?
4. Do her gold shots have any impact on our work? Do steroids, ACE inhibitors, or aspirin? Do you need a TEG or other coagulation study?

Intraoperative Questions

1. Is an epidural or a spinal a good idea? Why or why not? Does regional anesthesia duck the airway issue? What are the advantages of regional as far as her heart is concerned? Do you have any proof of this? How about the risk of CHF after the sympathectomy wears off?
2. Do you place an arterial line, even for regional anesthesia or even when using an epidural and increasing the dose very slowly? What is the cutoff for a transfusion? Why? Discuss the rheology of blood. Do you need a mixed venous Swan-Ganz catheter to tell you about oxygen delivery? Discuss mixed venous status in a more general sense. For example, what if the patient has an arteriovenous shunt, or what if the patient has methemoglobinemia?
3. Urine output is less than 10 mL/hr under general anesthesia. Load up the patient with volume, or let the patient resume spontaneous ventilation, and see if that helps. Provide the rationale for these approaches. You give 500 cc's of albumin, and then see frothy stuff in the ETT. How does Lasix work? How does dopamine work? How about using epinephrine to get the cardiac output up?
4. The ECG shows multifocal PVCs. What is the differential diagnosis, and what is the treatment? Do you treat with lidocaine or amiodarone? Why? Do you load or use a volume load plus drip? You are more familiar with lidocaine, so do you stick with that, or go with the newer and better but unfamiliar drug?

Postoperative Questions

1. The rectal temperature 33°C. Do you believe it? How do you double-check it? What is the effect of low temperature on drug metabolism, muscle strength, and O_2 consumption? We talk about shivering and O_2 consumption, but has anyone ever had an MI from this? How do you tell good evidence-based medicine from tall tales?
2. What are the options for pain relief? Are epidural narcotics a good idea? How about Duramorph once daily so you do not have to mess with a pump? Is it just as safe?
3. You used regional anesthesia to avoid a bad airway, but now she has pulmonary edema. How do you secure the airway with the patient in active distress?

Grab Bag

1. A 20-year-old woman is delivering a monster baby—11 pounds. In the middle of forceps extraction, the mother develops severe pain despite a good epidural, and her blood pressure becomes unobtainable. What is the differential diagnosis? The surgeon says he needs to do an exploratory laparotomy NOW! How do you resuscitate her? Do you increase the dose of the epidural? How do you induce general anesthesia? What if the airway looks bad? Do you use an LMA-Fastrach? What is the risk of aspiration?
2. After an MVA, the patient is in a halo, and his ETT has a cuff leak. He has a cervical spine fracture. The PaO_2 on 70% O_2 is only 71 mm Hg. You determine that the cuff is ruptured. How will you resecure this airway? Why not go right to a tracheostomy?
3. OSHA is pressuring your hospital to clean up trace anesthetic agents, and levels are particularly high now that LMAs are in such widespread use. How can you advise the OR committee? Should your hospital use fewer LMAs?

Update: Ropivacaine Toxicity

1. What is the proposed benefit of ropivacaine? Because of its different chemical formula, it should be less cardiotoxic than bupivacaine.
2. Is that really so? In reading case reports of resuscitation, people with ropivacaine overdoses have "come back" after relatively short periods of CPR (5 minutes), whereas bupivacaine victims require hours. From these results, ropivacaine looks safer.
3. Of course, use of lipid emulsions is fast becoming the treatment for local anesthetic overdose.

CASE 32: TONSILLECTOMY AND ADENOIDECTOMY IN A CHILD WITH A MURMUR

A 4-year-old, 15-kg boy with recurrent tonsillitis is scheduled for tonsillectomy and adenoidectomy. Mom says the kid has a "hole in his heart" that will be repaired after he is a little older. He cannot keep up with kids on the playground and sits out most games. Pulmonary examination reveals a loud systolic murmur. His blood pressure is 90/60 mm Hg, pulse is 110 beats/min, and respiratory rate is 24 breaths/min. His breathing is unlabored, but he puffs and huffs when you walk down the hall with him. His temperature is 37°C.

Preoperative Questions

1. What do you make of the "hole in the heart"? What are the possibilities? Compare VSDs with atrial septal defects (ASDs). Compare right to left with left to right. What difference does that make to the anesthetic induction and overall case? What about his functional capacity? Why does he get tired so easily? What is the ultimate end point of any cardiac problem? What catheterization data do you need? What if he has an endocardial cushion defect? What does that mean anatomically and physiologically?
2. Why do the tonsillectomy and adenoidectomy first instead of the heart operation? What is the timing of antibiotics? What is the risk of endocarditis? What problems can the tonsils pose? What are the possible intubation problems? Compare right heart failure with obstructive hypoxemia.
3. How do you premedicate the kid? What is most important: the preoperative visit, oral versus intramuscular medications, or going straight into the OR.

Intraoperative Questions

1. Will you use sevoflurane, halothane, or desflurane for inhalational induction? Why? Will you use N_2O for the second gas effect? Is it a bad idea given his heart defect? Are uptake and speed of induction affected by right-to-left shunt? Why or why not?
2. Can you do this as closed-circuit anesthetic? How and why? Which kind of circuit do you use and why? How can you tell if the machine is causing rebreathing? Explain valve function and malfunction.
3. The surgeon says he is super quick and needs no intravenous line placed. Do you agree? If intravenous access is tough, where will you go? What if the intravenous fluid infiltrates? Do you try again in the same arm or go elsewhere? Which fluid do you use and why? Do you employ colloid or crystalloid? How low can you go before you transfuse? Do you alter the numbers given his heart condition?
4. The disconnect alarm goes off, and you then see the hospital O_2 supply has vanished. What now? How long can you run on the cylinders? You turn one on, and it hisses loudly. What now? What is the fail-safe system? What powers the bellows? Does the order of the flowmeters matter?

Postoperative Questions

1. The patient develops a croupy cough in the PACU. What will you do? Will you use racemic epinephrine? Is that any better than just warmed saline? How about subcutaneous epinephrine? What is the danger given the heart condition?
2. The kid was going to go home but now has severe nausea and vomiting. What is the treatment? Do you drop a nasogastric tube? How will you know whether he has swallowed a lot of blood? Should you keep this kid longer than usual because of his heart?

Grab Bag

1. The obstetrician hands you a kid with meconium. What does meconium mean, and what do you do? How long do you suction before you mask ventilate? What if the chest does not rise? What are the doses, roughly, for a newborn code? How about a code for a 7-year-old child?

2. A local geriatrician wants you to talk to a senior group about the increased risk of anesthesia in the older population. What do you tell them?
3. Do you get a C-spine radiograph for all Down syndrome kids? How about if they come in a C-spine collar after an MVA? What is the risk of spinal cord injury?

Update: Airway Loss during Shoulder Surgery

1. How is the airway lost during shoulder surgery? During prolonged shoulder surgery, excessive infusion of the irrigating fluid can lead to so much swelling that the airway becomes compromised.
2. How bad is the effect? One case reported went to a tracheostomy.
3. How do you prevent this? You can do a block, but you should still use general anesthesia to have airway secured in case this happens.

CASE 33: MASTECTOMY IN A PATIENT WITH HEART TROUBLES

A 66-year-old, 85-kg woman is scheduled to have a left radical mastectomy because of breast cancer. She has a long a history of systolic heart murmur, with recent angina and dyspnea on exertion. Catheterization showed moderate aortic stenosis and diffuse but inoperable CAD. She has Raynaud's disease in the upper extremities. Medications include Lasix, metoprolol, and Cardizem. Her blood pressure is 110/70, pulse is 70 beats/min, respiratory rate is 16 breaths/min, and temperature is 37°C.

Preoperative Questions

1. She has already had a catheterization; do you need a more extensive cardiac workup? The surgeon says, "Hey, enough's enough!" What are risks of aortic stenosis and CAD? Is she on the right medications? How will you know? How do you define *optimized* in such a patient?
2. What is Raynaud's disease, and how does it affect the anesthetic? Do you use Doppler ultrasound or anything else to document flow in the radials? Do you perform Allen's test? Where will you put your pulse oximeter? Would the "clothes pin" pulse oximeter be a problem? How does a pulse oximeter work?
3. The chest radiograph shows an effusion on the side of her cancer. What are the possible causes? Can this result from metastatic disease? As an anesthesiologist, do you insist on a thoracentesis to rule out metastases, or is that not your place? Should you drain it anyway to help ventilation? Why or why not?

Intraoperative Questions

1. What monitors do you need before induction? Do you need an arterial line? Where and why? What about Raynaud's disease? Where will you put the pulse oximeter? What are all the pulse oximetry options? What if it does not pick up anywhere at all? Where do you place the blood pressure cuff? Is it as accurate on the leg? Is the blood pressure cuff a problem with Raynaud's disease? Do you need a CVP line? The Swan-Ganz catheter provides what extra information? Has it ever been shown to make a difference? Should you use TEE?

2. How does TEE work? What are the contraindications? What are the risks? Do you need a second person to look at it while you look at the patient?

3. Describe your anesthetic concerns for the patient with aortic stenosis and CAD. Walk through the exact drugs you would use. Would you use esmolol for rate control? After intubation, the blood pressure goes to 100/110 mm Hg, and the heart rate to 115 beats/min. What is the effect on the myocardium? What is the treatment?

4. For maintenance, the patient is on a β-blocker. Is there a problem with any of the potent inhaled agents? Should you avoid desflurane, or can you increase the dose slowly?

5. For pre-emptive analgesia, can you use a thoracic epidural? Can you do the whole case with a thoracic epidural? How about some intercostal or paravertebral blocks? Should you use COX-2 inhibitors preoperatively?

Postoperative Questions

1. In the PACU, the patient develops retractions, cyanosis, labored breathing, and rales. What is the differential diagnosis, and what is the treatment? How does Lasix work? Do you need an inotrope? Will an inotrope and its attendant tachycardia adversely affect the heart? Will milrinone help?

2. You had the blood pressure cuff on the right arm, and now that hand is dusky. What is the diagnosis? Does the patient need an arteriogram or surgical repair? Are there any conservative options? Should you place a stellate ganglion block? How would you do that, what would you use, and what are the complications?

3. You had a hard time with the lines, and you have a Cordis in the right internal jugular. Do you send her to the floor with this?

Grab Bag

1. You are placing an epidural for labor, and the patient says she feels funny and has a metallic taste in her mouth. What is the differential diagnosis, and what is the treatment? At the same time, the fetal heart rate drops to 75 beats/min. The patient is sitting up. Do you place in left uterine displacement, give O_2, go right to a cesarean section, or treat the seizure? What if the patient aspirates?

2. A policeman was shot in the right foot 3 months earlier, and it now shows trophic changes. He cannot sleep because of the pain. What is the differential diagnosis, and what is the treatment? What are the complications of a lumbar sympathetic block? What if he is no better after two or more? Do you need to do this under radiographic guidance?

3. A 300-pound man had a fork stuck in his eye during a fight at a pie-eating contest. Do you wait 8 hours for his stomach to empty? Do you place a nasogastric tube? Do you give him ice cream so he now has pie á la mode? How do you induce? Do you use suxamethonium? What is the effect on intraoperative pressure?

Update: Dexmedetomidine

1. What is the advantage in the asthmatic patient? α_2-Blockade blocks neurally mediated bronchoconstriction. It is perfect for the intubated patient with COPD or the asthmatic patient.

2. What are the other benefits? It prevents hypertension and tachycardia. It provides anxiolysis and produces only mild cognitive impairment, allowing the ICU staff to talk with the patient.
3. What is its half-life? The half-life is 40 minutes.
4. What are the side effects? The side effects are hypotension and bradycardia.

CASE 34: EVACUATION OF A SUBDURAL HEMATOMA

A 75-year-old, 85-kg man is scheduled for evacuation of a subdural hematoma. He was "found down" with a scalp laceration. He has cirrhosis and was drinking heavily before this event. He is not intubated, is breathing with some snoring, and is barely arousable. He has an abdomen compatible with ascites. His blood pressure is 90/60 mm Hg, pulse is 70 beats/min, respiratory rate is 22 breaths/min, temperature is 38°C, sodium level is 123 mEq/L, potassium level is 3.2 mEq/L, glucose level is 60 mg/dL, and hemoglobin level is 10 g/dL.

Preoperative Questions

1. What additional laboratory tests do you need to assess liver function? What is cirrhosis? How does it affect anesthesia? What is the cytochrome P450 system? What related organs are affected in the alcoholic? Do varices mean you cannot place a nasogastric tube or a TEE probe?
2. What determines cerebral perfusion? Discuss the effects of a subdural hematoma on the mechanics of the brain. How do you determine whether the patient has increased ICP? Do you need to measure it preoperatively with a bolt?
3. Why is his temperature increased? Is it related to aspiration or a preexisting infection? Do you need to decrease temperature to help cerebral perfusion? Why is the glucose level low? Do you need to replace it, or is an excessively high glucose level even worse?

Intraoperative Questions

1. Given the emergent nature of the patient's course, do you induce without an arterial line? How accurate are you at palpating a pulse and reacting to a strong, medium, or weak pulse? What are the problems with arterial lines?
2. Do you need to obtain an ABG determination, or can you go on end-tidal CO_2 alone? Why or why not? Why is end-tidal value different from the arterial value? Do you need ABG values to determine oxygenation, or is the saturation monitor okay?
3. Discuss the sequence of induction, including handling an unanticipated difficult intubation. How does cirrhosis affect blood gases? How does ascites affect ventilation? Do you need to drain this? Are there any circumstances in which you might?
4. For maintenance, can you use a potent inhaled agent with the ICP considerations? Is it better to use remifentanil or propofol? What are the problems with each of these agents for infusion? Do you need a relaxant? Which one and why?
5. Before incision, the blood pressure goes up to 230 mm Hg, and the heart rate drops into the 30s. What is happening, and what should you do about it? What are the dangers of a dropping blood pressure?

6. After 2 hours, the end-tidal CO_2 is 52 mm Hg. Why? How can the level be affected by fever, thyroid disease, aspiration, MH, or bad ventilation? What will you do? Why is there a special concern here? How will you "shrink the brain"?

Postoperative Questions

1. Two hours postoperatively, he is not breathing, not moving, not anything. What is the differential diagnosis, and what is the treatment? Do you give Narcan or Romazicon? How do these drugs work?
2. Two days later, he is in the ICU. How do you provide nutrition? Do you use a CVP line or his gut? What is the danger if he comes back for a tracheostomy and he is on hyperalimentation? Do you stop it?
3. In the ICU, the patient has a grand mal seizure. The nurse suggests you paralyze the patient because he is on a ventilator anyway. Do you agree? What are the adverse effects of an "invisible" seizure?

Grab Bag

1. You just finished a renal transplantation, and the patient looks like a floppy fish. How will you proceed? How will you determine whether the patient is reversed? What if, after reversal, the patient has only 3/4 twitches? How will you sedate? Are there any special concerns about the "fresh transplant"? After placing the patient on the ventilator, the urine output drops to 0. What is the differential diagnosis, and what is the treatment?
2. Do you need to monitor the OR for trace anesthetics? What is the danger? What do you say to staff when you spill some desflurane? OSHA says to stop using N_2O. Can you get by without it? Why or why not? What are the pros and cons of N_2O?
3. A man with severe COPD is scheduled for a thoracotomy. Is a thoracic epidural indicated? How about giving intrathecal morphine or intercostal blocks? Will you use an intrapleural catheter or patient-controlled analgesia (PCA)? Describe how you place such a catheter and what the risks are. How will you diagnose and treat an epidural hematoma?

CASE 35: MITRAL VALVE REPLACEMENT

A 41-year-old woman is scheduled for mitral valve replacement because of mitral stenosis. She is weak and easily fatigued. Four months earlier, she had a cerebrovascular accident (CVA) with left hemiplegia and has residual slight weakness there. She takes digoxin, Coumadin (stopped 3 days ago), and Lasix. Her blood pressure is 110/75 mm Hg, pulse is 100 beats/min and irregular, respiratory rate is 18 breaths/min, and temperature is 37°C. The prothrombin time is 14 seconds, which is the upper limit of normal, and she cannot lie flat.

Preoperative Questions

1. What does her dyspnea mean to anesthesia? Describe the Starling forces at work in her lungs. Do you need a preoperative ABG determination?

Interpret the findings of a pH of 7.42, Po_2 of 68 mm Hg, and Pco_2 of 33 mm Hg. How will this affect your anesthetic? Is there a hypoxemic drive to breathe here? When is there? Is the low O_2 or high CO_2 level worse?

2. What is the cause of the CVA? Are there anesthetic implications? How long should you wait after a CVA to do an elective case? Do you need a more extensive workup? Do you need a carotid study or an echocardiogram looking for a clot? Is there any risk of cardioverting her? Why?

3. Do you keep the digoxin going? Do you give it on the morning of surgery? How does digoxin work? Is it just as good to manage the heart rate with β-blockers? What is digoxin toxicity? What is the treatment for digoxin toxicity?

Intraoperative Questions

1. Do you use a pulmonary artery or CVP line and why? If you use a pulmonary artery line, which kind? Is it okay to place a Cordis and assume you can always put a pulmonary artery line in later? Should you use TEE? Has TEE replaced the Swan-Ganz catheter? Why or why not? What if you need TEE in the ICU and cannot keep it in all the time? You put in a Swan-Ganz catheter, and the wedge pressure is 22 mm Hg. Interpret this finding. Do you need more information? What are the risks of using a Swan-Ganz catheter?

2. Is pentathol or paneuronium okay for induction? Why? What is the risk of tachycardia? Which induction drug is better? Does it matter? Can you just adjust the dose? You intubate, and the pulmonary artery pressure goes from 45/19 to 75/50 mm Hg. Do you use more anesthetic? Do you use nitroglycerin or an inotrope? What if the patient crashes on bypass? What if the heart rate goes to 120 beats/min. Now what?

3. Is a high-dose narcotic as used in 1980s anesthesia okay? What is the risk of recall? How do you prevent recall if you are using a narcotic-based anesthetic. Do you use BIS? How does it work?

4. During CPB, where should you keep the blood pressure? How do you provide anesthesia during CPB? Do you need relaxation? What if urine output drops while the patient is on CPB? Are there any physiologic consequences of pulsatile flow compared with CPB flow? Do you need to do an epiaortic echocardiogram to look for plaques in the aorta?

5. The patient cannot be taken off CPB because of low blood pressure and high pulmonary artery pressures. What is your next move? Do you use an IABP? Explain the contraindications and complications of using an IABP.

Postoperative Questions

1. In the ICU, blood drainage is 300 mL/hr for 2 hours. Do you need more protamine? Which laboratory tests do you order? Will a TEG help? Do you give FFP, platelets, or cryoprecipitate? How will you recognize tamponade? Is TEE necessary for the diagnosis?

2. Twelve hours later, ABG values on 50% oxygen are a pH of 7.35, Po_2 of 75 mm Hg, and Pco_2 of 48 mm Hg. Is it okay to extubate the patient? What else do you need to know? What if she had been hard to intubate? Is there anything you can do to hedge your bet? What is the risk of extubating if the patient is unstable or bleeding?

Grab Bag

1. The night of a shoulder surgery, the patient complains of pain, and you see a burn on his skin. What is the cause? How does the grounding pad work? Whose responsibility is it? Explain the concept of current density. What do you tell the patient, and how do you treat this?
2. What special precautions are needed when a patient has sickle cell trait or sickle cell disease? Do you insist on 50% hemoglobin S? What is a sickle cell crisis? How can it lead to a fat embolism?
3. Three hours after an abdominal aortic aneurysm resection, a 70-year-old man has a urine output of 10 mL/kg. The operation was above the renal arteries. What is the differential diagnosis, and what is the treatment? Do you insist on re-exploration?

Update: Vagal Nerve Stimulators

1. What is a vagal nerve stimulator? It is a device placed to encircle the vagus nerve on the left side of the neck. These devices are used to control intractable seizures.
2. How do they work? Retrograde conduction up the vagus stimulates areas of the brain known to control seizures.
3. How does that action affect anesthesia? The superior and recurrent laryngeal nerves are also stimulated. Patients report voice changes, and the left vocal cord and arytenoids are displaced medially.
4. What do you do then? Turn the vagal nerve stimulator off because it can cause airway obstruction with an LMA and it can cause vocal cord damage if the patient is intubated.

CASE 36: OBESITY AND EYE INJURY

A 45-year-old, 120-kg man is scheduled for emergent removal of metal from his left eye. He has recurrent asthma. He is on daily inhalers, visits the ER about once each month, and takes prednisone (10 mg/day). He is afebrile, and his blood pressure is 145/85 mm Hg, pulse is 100 beats/min, respiratory rate is 20 breaths/min, and hematocrit is 49%. He ate line-caught tuna, union-picked grapes, and shade plantation-grown coffee 2 hours earlier and cannot understand why bad things happen to good people.

Preoperative Questions

1. Why is a history of asthma important to you? What are long-term effects of asthma? Contrast them with the short-term effects and with COPD. What laboratory tests do you order, and what would you expect to see? How do kidneys compensate for CO_2 retention? Would you add more bronchodilator therapy, increase the steroids, admit the patient, or get another pulmonary consultation? What will you do if the patient is wheezing in the preoperative area?
2. The patient has a full stomach. Are you going to give anticholinergics? How might that help or hurt? Will you give H_1- or H_2-blockers?

Intraoperative Questions

1. What are your major concerns about induction? What are the risks of awake intubation and RSI? What is the effect of obesity? Will hyperventilation help or hurt? Can you attenuate the effect of suxamethonium with a defasciculating dose?
2. Is TIVA or inhalation better to keep bronchi quiet? If the patient was on aminophylline, do you have any concerns about rhythm?
3. Do you need muscle relaxants? Which ones and why? How will you monitor? What is the risk of bucking in this case? Do you use Norcuron, rocuronium, or cisatracurium?
4. Do you use an arterial line because his arm is too big for an accurate blood pressure cuff reading? How do we get accurate blood pressure readings from cuffs? How does the Dinamap blood pressure monitor work?
5. The patient develops wheezing in the middle of the case; the tube is at 27 cm. What is the differential diagnosis, and what is the treatment? What is innervation of the trachea? How about innervation above the trachea?

Postoperative Questions

1. A colleague says to extubate deeply to avoid bucking. Do you agree? How do you awaken the patient in a smooth fashion? How does obesity affect your decision?
2. In the PACU, the blood pressure is 210/110 mm Hg. What is the differential diagnosis, and what is the treatment? Does a high diastolic pressure increase perfusion? What is the mechanism of endomyocardial ischemia in the hypertensive patient?
3. Postoperative nausea and vomiting are big problems with a fresh eye. How do you prevent it, and how do you treat it? Do you use a nasogastric tube intraoperatively to prevent it? Do you not use N_2O or Decadron? Why? Do you use granisetron or ondansetron? Which one and why?

Grab Bag

1. A medical student is staring at the fetal heart monitor like a Cro-Magnon staring at a disassembled 747 airplane. What do you tell him about fetal well-being as measured by the fetal heart rate?
2. Do you use an EEG when you do a carotid endarterectomy? If not, why? How else can you tell that cerebral perfusion is okay? Awake? Shunt? Does *shunt* mean there is never ischemia?
3. A 40-year-old woman with myasthenia gravis is scheduled to have a laparoscopic cholecystectomy. How do you determine whether she is in good enough shape to undergo the operation? Do you adjust her medications? What is the danger of too little medication or too much?

Update: Direct Laryngoscopy Complications

1. What is the most common cause of claims against anesthesiologists? Patients most often sue because of dental trauma.
2. Provide a complete list of other structures that can be damaged. Other complications include mucosal tears, dislocation of the temporomandibular

joint (TMJ), injury to the hypoglossal and lingual nerves, and osteomyelitis of the mandible.

3. Who is at most risk? Patients with immunosuppression or after irradiation are most at risk for complications.

CASE 37: CLOSING A BRONCHOPLEURAL FISTULA

A 45-year-old, 75-kg man has emphysema and a massive bronchopleural fistula after a lobectomy a week earlier. He needs emergent thoracotomy to close the fistula. He is on a ventilator with a huge leak that is evident. Purulence is seen in the ETT and around the chest tube. His blood pressure is 75/50 mm Hg, pulse is 120 beats/min, respiratory rate is 40 breaths/min (breathing over the ventilator), temperature is 39.9°C, and hematocrit is 29%.

Preoperative Questions

1. Why is the patient hypotensive? Is it the result of septic shock, cardiogenic shock, or hypovolemia? How can you tell? Can any laboratory tests help? Do you need a chest radiograph, blood gas determination, or HCO_3 level?

2. For treatment of hypotension, should you go straight to the OR? Should you give fluids and pressors first? Which fluids and which pressors? How do you guide this therapy? Do you use steroids? Why?

3. What type of monitoring do you need before induction? Because he is already intubated, is the "induction" already done?

4. Preoperatively, the CVP is 15 mm Hg, the pulmonary capillary wedge pressure (PCWP) is 18 mm Hg, and the blood pressure 70/40 mm Hg. Is the patient in shock? What is shock? What diagnosis corresponds to these values? What do you do with this information?

Intraoperative Questions

1. The patient has a single-lumen tube in place. Do you change to a double-lumen tube, use a bronchial blocker, or change to a Univent? Why? What are the risks of changing the tube? What are the risks of using the tube changer? What is the risk of the tube changer poking through the lung?

2. What agent will you use? Can you use only an intravenous line because he is going to be on the ventilator anyway? Can you use N_2O for inhalation? What is the risk for hypoxemia or pneumothorax? Can you work this so he gets extubated soon, and you can get the pressure off the bronchopleural fistula?

3. The patient goes onto his left side and becomes cyanotic. What is the differential diagnosis, and what is the treatment? The Pao_2 is 50 mm Hg, and the $Paco_2$ is 60 mm Hg. Should you increase the tidal volume? Should you use PEEP or continuous positive airway pressure (CPAP), or both? Should you ventilate both lungs and reposition the patient on his back?

4. You place the double-lumen tube, but the lung is not going down. How do you fix this? Now the lung goes down, and he is still desaturated. At what point do you go all the way to ECMO or even a femoral-femoral bypass? What are the risks of doing that compared with the risk of doing nothing?

Postoperative Questions

1. At the end of the case, the surgeon asks you to change back to a single-lumen tube. Explain why you should not do this, and then explain why you should do this. Now decide what you will do.
2. The patient is on a T-piece and 50% O_2 to keep positive pressure off the stump. The saturation level is only 85%. Should you put him back on a ventilator? Should you use HFJV? How does this work, and when do you use it?
3. The patient is on a ventilator and wheezing. What is the treatment? How can you be sure it is not a pneumothorax?
4. You give a lot of albuterol. Can you give this intravenously? The patient develops multifocal PVCs. What do you do?

Grab Bag

1. You fill the vaporizer and spill some. A housekeeper comes in and smells the stuff, and she tells you she is pregnant. What do you tell her?
2. A hospital administrator thinks you are wasting money on all these urine tests for human chorionic gonadotropin (hCG). She says, "Can't we just go with the history?" What do you tell the administrator?
3. How do you give electroconvulsive therapy to a man with inoperable CAD?

Update: Management of Right Ventricular Failure

1. Describe the tiered approach to treatment of right ventricular failure. Use hypocarbia, hyperoxia, and inotropic support, and further afterload reduction with milrinone. Use selective pulmonary vasodilation with nitric oxide or prostacyclin ($iPGI_2$) and a right ventricular assist device (RVAD).
2. What is a typical dose of prostacyclin? The usual dosage is 50 ng/kg/min.
3. What are the advantages of prostacyclin compared with nitric oxide? It can be infused intravenously, whereas a clunky respiratory setup is needed for nitric oxide. Prostacyclin costs less. It has a short half-life (2.7 minutes), and the patient does not develop systemic hypotension.
4. What is the disadvantage of using prostacyclin? Rebound pulmonary hypertension occurs on withdrawal.
5. How about using inhaled Iloprost (prostacyclin)? It lasts 2 hours, but it is not available in the United States.

CASE 38: SMALL BOWEL OBSTRUCTION AND DEHYDRATION

A 75-year-old, 42-kg woman has been vomiting for a week. She has cancer of the colon and has lost 35 pounds in 2 months. She now has a small bowel obstruction. Her blood pressure is 130/70 mm Hg, pulse is 100 beats/min, respiratory rate is 20 breaths/min, sodium level is 130 mEq/L, potassium level is 2.5 mEq/L, bicarbonate (HCO_3) level is 32 mEq/L, and hematocrit is 42%.

Preoperative Questions

1. What is the patient's volume status? Contrast fluid loss from sweating, from NPO for a long time, from vomiting, and from blood loss. Do you need volume measurement preoperatively? Will you sit her up and see if she gets

hypotensive or tachycardic? Should you put in a CVP or Swan-Ganz catheter? Should you get an echocardiogram or just proceed?

2. Surgery is in 4 hours. Do you go to the holding area and hydrate the patient? Do you go to the ICU and measure CVP as you hydrate? Do you let her stay on the floor? If she is nervous, do you sedate her? With what? Do you observe her? What is the effect on protein binding of drugs?

3. Explain her electrolyte findings. What would her blood gas determination look like?

Intraoperative Questions

1. Do you give her Reglan as you roll into the room? Why or why not? Do you give Bicitra? What is the risk of feculent aspiration?

2. Do you place your monitors before or after induction? Why?

3. What will you use for maintenance? Because she is cachectic, how do you adjust your medications?

4. If she comes down on hyperalimentation, do you continue it? Do you access the line giving the hyperalimentation? What is the risk if you stop the hyper-alimentation?

5. The patient's blood pressure is 70/50 mm Hg intraoperatively, and her CVP is 15 mm Hg. What now? How long can you allow the blood pressure to stay this low? Because the CVP is already high, do you give more fluids? Do you give blood or Lasix to get rid of free water and then give blood to replace it? Do you place a Swan-Ganz or TEE line? Do you start inotropes? Which ones and why?

Postoperative Questions

1. Postoperatively, the patient has floppy-fish movements. Her train of 4 is 3/4, but she has not yet been reversed. What do you do? After reversal, she is doing only 200 mL tidal volumes. Do you extubate? There is no room in the ICU, and the PACU is closed. What do you do?

2. The arterial line stopcock got twisted, and she bled 500 mL of blood onto the floor. Do you transfuse? Do you tell her husband or just document it?

3. The CVP line pulls out as she is moved over to the PACU cot. Because the operation is over, do you bother putting another CVP line in? If so, do you use the same side or the left side? What is the risk of thoracic duct damage or dropping the other lung?

Grab Bag

1. A medical student asks why we no longer use Allen tests. What do you tell the smarty-pants student?

2. Describe safety measures to prevent an airway fire during a laser vocal cord procedure.

3. An 80-year-old man scheduled for a transurethral resection of bladder tumor (TURBT) has a loud systolic murmur. Do you proceed or wait for an echocardiogram?

Update: History of the Laryngoscope

1. Who first observed the functioning glottis? In 1855, Manuel Garcia, a singing teacher, saw it using a device with two mirrors that used sunlight.

2. Who did the first direct laryngoscopy? Alfred Kirstein of Germany, prompted by the fact that Kaiser Frederick had died of laryngeal cancer, did the first procedure. The device had a proximal light source and a rounded metal blade. He called it the autoscope and described it in 1895.

3. Who first used a device to pass ETTs? The first was Chevalier Jackson of Philadelphia. He described it in a 1913 article, "The Technique of Insertion of Endotracheal Insufflation Tubes."

4. Who introduced the idea of intubating for anesthesia? Henry Janeway, who worked in Bellevue Hospital in New York City, introduced the battery in the handle of the laryngoscope.

5. What changes occurred during World War I? Ivan W. Magill and E.S. Rowbotham improved the techniques for endotracheal anesthesia.

6. In 1933, what percentage of cases used an ETT? The tubes were used in 7% of cases.

7. When did the first article pertaining to laryngoscope blades appear? The article was published in 1941.

CASE 39: THYROIDECTOMY

A 49-year-old, 75-kg woman is scheduled for a thyroidectomy because of cancer. She has hypertension that is treated by an ACE inhibitor and hydrochlorothiazide. Her blood pressure is 160/110, pulse is 95 beats/min, temperature is 37°C, and hemoglobin level is 13 g/dL. There are nonspecific ST-T wave changes on the ECG.

Preoperative Questions

1. How do an ACE inhibitor and hydrochlorothiazide work to drop the blood pressure? Is the blood pressure adequately controlled? Will you cancel the case, lower the blood pressure yourself right now, and optimize the patient? How long does it take to optimize the patient?

2. What do nonspecific ST-T wave changes mean? Do you need an old ECG, a Holter monitor record, or further cardiac workup? What if there are no old ECGs to compare with?

3. The patient's temperature is okay, but is there anything else that indicates she is clinically hyperthyroid? What are the results of the physical examination? Is there a risk to the eyes if she has exophthalmos? If she were in thyroid storm and the case were emergent, how would you proceed? What are you looking for in the thyroid test results?

Intraoperative Questions

1. Can you do this under a regional block, a cervical plexus block, or a cervical epidural? Even if you think this ridiculous, how would you attempt to do it? How would you make sure you had no intravascular or intrathecal injection? What is the treatment for both?

2. How do you examine the airway? Do you need C-spine films or CT scans? What do you look for in the physical examination? What are the pros and cons of an awake look? Does it really tell you anything? Will any induction drugs affect the thyroid gland?

3. You give propofol and suxamethonium, and you see only arytenoids. How do you proceed? Is mask ventilation okay? Do you use wake-up or LMA-Fastrach methods? Do you proceed with an LMA-Fastrach?
4. The blood pressure cuff alarms, a line drops off, and the end-tidal CO_2 disappears, but the ECG rolls merrily along. What is the differential diagnosis, and what is the treatment? The blood pressure later drops to 70/40 mm Hg. What do you do? How do you tell whether the surgeon is leaning on the arm? Should that affect the arterial line?

Postoperative Questions

1. Do you get a calcium level in the PACU? Do you order thyroid tests? Do you obtain serial ECGs and enzyme tests because the blood pressure dropped that one time? When would you see hypocalcemia from hypoparathyroidism?
2. The patient is having difficulty breathing in the PACU. What is the differential diagnosis, and what is the treatment? You see a big hematoma, and her tongue is sticking out. What do you do? Do you open the neck yourself? What if you attempt to intubate but cannot?

Grab Bag

1. A 3-year-old boy, who is scheduled for ear tubes, has clear rhinorrhea and a temperature of 39°C. Do you continue or cancel? Why? What if "he'll never get better unless he gets these damned tubes!" If you proceed, do you use an ETT, mask, or LMA? What are the pros and cons of each?
2. A new nurse is freaking because an AIDS patient is coming down. How do you explain the relative risk, universal precautions, and philosophy of dealing with AIDS patients?
3. Extracorporeal shock-wave lithotripsy (ESWL) is planned in a trailer behind the hospital. Explain how you would set up anesthesia in this relatively remote location. Would you use an epidural, MAC, or general anesthesia? What are the special risks associated with ESWL? What if the patient has a pacer or an AICD?

Update: Mechanism of Local Anesthetic Nerve Toxicity

1. What prompted the most concern about the direct toxicity of local anesthetics? Concern was prompted by microcatheter infusions of local anesthetics and by the fact that 5% lidocaine causes transient neurologic pain syndrome.
2. Can other local anesthetics also cause this syndrome? Yes. Highly concentrated tetracaine can cause nerve injury.
3. What is the proposed mechanism? Local anesthetics show a detergent nature that solubilizes the neuron, causing damage.

CASE 40: CESAREAN SECTION AND MASSIVE VAGINAL BLEEDING

A 30-year-old, gravida 5, para 3, 61-kg woman is scheduled for emergent cesarean section and has massive vaginal bleeding. Her blood pressure is 80/50 mm Hg, pulse is 115 beats/min, and hemoglobin level is 8 g/dL.

Preoperative Questions

1. What is the patient's volume status? Do you need further evaluation or a tilt test, or should you not bother? Is the patient in shock? What is shock? What else will you see in a shock situation?
2. Why is her pulse so high? Describe the compensatory mechanisms that go into our circulatory defense. When will acute tubular necrosis intervene, and how can you prevent it? Should you give mannitol now? Should you give Lasix?
3. What is on the differential diagnosis for massive hemorrhage? What is the differential diagnosis for a more generic problem, uteroplacental insufficiency?
4. Discuss the physiologic changes of pregnancy and how they affect anesthesia.

Intraoperative Questions

1. Is using a regional technique a good idea? Why or why not? Is there time for a spinal or epidural? What is your concern about coagulation? What is the most likely abnormality? Compare dilutional thrombocytopenia, low-level of factor, and actual DIC.
2. Do you sedate before induction of general anesthesia? Do you place a BIS monitor? If you anticipate instability, how will you guard against recall?
3. Which induction technique do you use? Do you use ketamine or etomidate? What is the effect on the placenta at this point?
4. Which muscle relaxant do you use? What is the effect on the fetus? Explain why the fetus is not paralyzed. Discuss the ion trapping mechanism.
5. The baby is out, and the mother's blood pressure is unobtainable. Should you place an arterial line? What is the differential diagnosis? Can the cause be an amniotic fluid embolism, pulmonary embolism, bleeding, or an air embolism?
6. Go through the code of a patient in pulseless electrical activity (PEA). What is the differential diagnosis? Can you give vasopressin at any time? Do you suggest a hysterectomy to save the mother?

Postoperative Questions

1. The patient's urine output is low in the PACU. The uterus was cut out in a hurry. How will you determine the cause of low urine output? Do you get a pyelogram or just a fluid challenge? What is the dilemma if only one ureter is cut?
2. Prolonged relaxation occurs after administration of suxamethonium. What is the cause? What is molecular basis of this? What is the dibucaine number? Do you give her a medic alert bracelet or just blow it off and hope you do not see her again?

Grab Bag

1. A 19-year-old drug dealer with HIV is scheduled for a ganglion removal. No veins are available for a Bier block. He does not want to go to sleep. What is your suggestion? The guy is jumpy at the thought of a brachial plexus block. Do you thoroughly sedate him and just go for it? How do you conduct the arm block?

2. A 40-year-old woman in thyroid storm needs exploratory laparotomy for small bowel obstruction. How do you manage this emergent case with her in full-blown thyroid storm? Do you use propylthiouracil (PTU), iodine, or beta-blockade?

3. During a code, do you reach for epinephrine or vasopressin? Why? Name "shockable rhythms." What is the treatment of choice in systole or for PEA? What, besides hypovolemia, can give you PEA?

Update: Mediastinal Masses

1. What are biggest concerns for patients with mediastinal masses? They may have total occlusion of the airway and cardiovascular collapse.

2. When can these disasters occur? They can happen while placing the patient supine, at the induction of anesthesia, at extubation, and even a few days after extubation!

3. Children and adults can die from the effects of mediastinal masses. How do their modus morti differ? Children can have perioperative respiratory complications. Adults can have progression of the disease (e.g., solid tumor, lymphoma).

4. Why do kids have more respiratory problems? They have smaller airways that are more compressible.

5. When do adult respiratory complications usually occur? They occur immediately postoperatively or during the first 48 hours?

6. What heralds a cardiovascular collapse? In adults, one thing is pericardial effusion. Others are stridor, orthopnea, cyanosis, jugular venous distention, and superior vena cava syndrome. Kids can have a disaster with no preceding symptoms.

7. Does postural spirometry help? No one bothers getting it if they are symptom free.

8. What do you look for on CT? Look for tracheal compression of more than 50% and pericardial effusion. On PFTs, look for a combined obstructive, restrictive defect.

Béchard P, Létourneau L, Lacasse Y, et al: Perioperative cardiorespiratory complications in adults with mediastinal mass: Incidence and risk factors Anesthesiology 2004;100: 826-834.

CASE 41: NEPHRECTOMY, WHEEZING, AND ADULT-ONSET DIABETES MELLITUS

A 58-year-old, 87-kg woman is scheduled for left radical nephrectomy because of kidney cancer. She smokes a ton and has adult-onset diabetes mellitus. She takes 30 U of NPH insulin each morning. On examination, she is wheezing like a turn-of-the-century calliope. Her blood pressure is 160/90 mm Hg, pulse is 77 beats/min, respiratory rate is 12 breaths/min, temperature is 37°C, hemoglobin level is 10 g/dL, and glucose level is 225 mg/dL.

Preoperative Questions

1. How will you manage her insulin on the day of surgery? What would make you cancel the case? How high would the glucose have to be? What is the

danger of diabetic ketoacidosis (DKA)? What if the case were an emergency and the patient were in DKA? How will you manage intraoperative anesthesia and DKA?

2. If she is wheezing, should you cancel? The surgeon asks what you recommend; he does not like the pulmonologists. Should you start inhalers and aminophylline? How long should treatment last? What if she comes back and is still wheezing? Do you recommend she stop smoking? Insist on it? Do you refuse to do case until she mends the error of her ways? Do you start steroids? Discuss the risks of stopping smoking in the short term.

3. Discuss the risk of AIDS, hepatitis C, and other forms of blood-borne pathogens with the patient. What is biggest cause of transfusion reaction? What is the treatment?

Intraoperative Questions

1. She is placed in the right lateral decubitus position. How will you pad and take care of the patient in this demanding position? What are respiratory and hemodynamic problems with this position? If her arm plops off the armrest and no one notices, what injury may occur? How do you protect her eyes?

2. Do you recommend an epidural for the case or for postoperative pain relief? What level do you recommend? Do you place it before or after induction or in the PACU later? Why? Which drug do you use and what concentration? Do you add narcotics or not?

3. What invasive monitors do you need and why? You get two big intravenous lines. Is that okay? What if fluid from one infiltrates? What is the treatment? How would you know? What if an inotrope such as dopamine infiltrated?

4. Which kind of CVP line will you use—a Cordis, triple lumen, double lumen, or 12-French monster? Why? Which will work with a rapid infuser?

5. The oxygen saturation level plummets to 80% with kidney dissection. What is the differential diagnosis, and what is the treatment? How do you rule out pneumothorax or differentiate an embolus from tumor? Do you need TEE to see if the tumor is in the inferior vena cava? What would you see?

6. After 5 units of blood, the patient turns red, there is frothy stuff in the ETT, and the blood pressure drops. How do you diagnose a transfusion reaction intraoperatively?

Postoperative Questions

1. In the PACU, urine output drops to 15 mL/hr and is all red. What is the differential diagnosis, and what is the treatment? Was this expected from the operation? Is it a transfusion reaction?

2. The patient complains of incapacitating pain. Do you place an epidural, a local in the incision, or a spinal with only a narcotic? Do you use only parenteral medications? What if you are concerned that she may have a coagulopathy?

3. She has pain in her left eye. What is the differential diagnosis, and what is the treatment? She also has numbness in her left hand. How will you evaluate this?

Grab Bag

1. You are asked for a consultation by physicians in Tajikistan. They use traditional methods of pain control and never use epidurals. How do you explain the advantages of epidurals to them?
2. In the middle of a disk injection in a pain clinic, a patient has an allergic response. What is the mechanism? How do you treat it? What is the difference between an anaphylactic and anaphylactoid response? How will you treat a complete anaphylactic reaction (recall the patient is prone).
3. A neurosurgeon insists on no glucose whatsoever while clipping an aneurysm. Do you agree? What about a diabetic patient? What kind of fluid should you give? Will Hespan increase bleeding?

Update: Difficult Airway in the Anesthetized Patient

1. What is a groovy new algorithm? Use the gum elastic bougie, then use the intubating laryngeal mask airway, and then do a percutaneous cricotracheotomy.
2. What was the overall incidence of unanticipated difficult airways? The rate was about 1%.
3. What is the advantage of this over the more complex ASA algorithm? It is simple.
4. Has the gum elastic bougie proved more effective than just the stylet? Yes.
5. What percentage of patients is saved by the gum elastic bougie ? Eighty percent, and that is damned good!

CASE 42: HERNIA REPAIR IN A 6-MONTH-OLD CHILD

A 6-month-old, 6-kg boy is scheduled for right inguinal hernia repair as an outpatient. He was delivered at 34 weeks' gestation by cesarean section. Had an Apgar score of 4 at birth and developed respiratory distress syndrome requiring ventilation for 3 days. He has done well since. His blood pressure is 80/50 mm Hg, pulse is 120 beats/min, respiratory rate is 30 breaths/min, and rectal temperature is 37.5°C.

Preoperative Questions

1. Is this patient suitable for outpatient surgery? How does his history affect the risk of general anesthesia? How will you tell if he still has pulmonary dysfunction? You cannot do PFTs on a baby, so what do you do instead? What other factors may increase his risk?
2. Do you need any laboratory tests? If the surgeon wants a hemoglobin level, do you go along? How easy is it to get a blood test on an infant? Can you do the heelstick thing? Are these tests accurate? What if on the day of surgery, the technicians say the sample was lost—do you get another one and wait?
3. Do you need a chest radiograph? How about a baseline x-ray film in case something goes wrong?
4. Is premedication a good idea? If not, at what age do you start thinking about premedication? What routes are available?

Intraoperative Questions

1. How do you measure blood pressure in a 6-kg kid? How about temperature? Which monitors do you put on before induction? What should the kid's

NPO status be? What is the risk of hypothermia, and is that more of a problem in kids? The surgeon is overweight and hates the room warm. What can you do about this? Could this kid get MH?

2. Should you use intravenous, inhalation, or rectal anesthesia? Why? If you decide to go rectal, how do you do it? What are the risks? Once in, can you leave the kid alone? How long does it take to induce?

3. For inhalation, which agent do you choose? Why not halothane to start and then switch to sevoflurane? You are 3 minutes into the induction, and the kid is still awake. What is happening? You turn on the vaporizer, and you hear a hiss and smell tons of sevoflurane. What happened?

4. Two minutes into induction, the kid coughs, holds his breath, goes into laryngospasm, and desaturates. There is no intravenous line in yet. What do you do—oral airway, nasal cannula, wake-up, or intramuscular suxamethonium? What is the danger of giving suxamethonium to a kid? You give suxamethonium, and the complex widens and goes into ventricular fibrillation. What is the differential diagnosis, and what is the treatment?

5. Which kind of fluids do you give, and how much and why? Do you give glucose? What if he were a preemie?

Postoperative Questions

1. The infant is agitated, struggling, and crying in the recovery room. What is the differential diagnosis, and what is the treatment? If he is in pain, can you do a block now? Which one? How? Which local anesthetic would you use and how much? Do you use epinephrine?

2. The boy has inspiratory stridor in the PACU. Compare the mechanisms for inspiratory and expiratory stridor. How do you manage this? Do you use racemic epinephrine or reintubate? If you reintubate, then what? What do you tell the parents?

3. The nurse calls out that the child is completely apneic. Why? Is he reacting to the narcotics? Should you have avoided them? Is it a case of post-prematurity? Do you mask, reintubate, or give caffeine? Should he be moved to the ICU or sent home?

Grab Bag

1. A 34-year-old woman with mitral stenosis needs an urgent cesarean section because of fetal distress. When the epidural is placed, the blood pressure drops to 60/40 mm Hg when she is on her back, and the heart rate is 140 beats/min. What is the differential diagnosis, and what is the treatment? Are there special considerations because of the pregnancy? Is she experiencing shock or syncope?

2. A 20-something road warrior with multiple injuries requires exploratory laparotomy for a splenectomy, but he is out of it. There is no obvious head trauma. Should you delay for head CT or go right to surgery? How do you induce if you suspect an intracranial injury but do not have the time to confirm it?

3. The preoperative clinic is getting hematocrit values for all tonsillectomy patients because "they may bleed." The hospital wants to cut costs. What do you tell the hospital administration? How do you respond to the ENT specialist's concern?

Update: Factor VIIa

1. Is factor VIIa acceptable for Jehovah's Witnesses? Yes. No human proteins are used in the manufacture or purification of this stuff from baby hamster kidney cells.
2. What do we routinely use if we are trying to prevent bleeding? Use desmopressin.
3. Where else has factor VIIa (NovoSeven) been used besides cardiac surgery? It is used in cases of trauma, liver treatment, and prostatectomy.
4. What is the dose? Use 90 μg/kg.
5. How does factor VIIa work? It initiates thrombin generation by binding to tissue at injury sites, activates platelets, and stabilizes fibrin polymerization.
6. Does it work in hemophiliacs? Yes. That is the only recognized indication.
7. Are there any complications from factor VIIa? Yes. As expected, thrombotic complications, such as cerebral sinus thrombosis, MI, DIC, and DVT can occur.

CASE 43: CESAREAN SECTION IN AN ASTHMATIC

A 30-year-old, 75-kg woman with asthma is scheduled for repeat cesarean section. She uses a nebulizer for "cough-only asthma." She is wheezing and "not feeling too well." Her blood pressure is 120/60 mm Hg, pulse is 100 beats/min, respiratory rate is 24 breaths/min (breathing is wheezy), and temperature is 37°C. The platelet count is 120,000/mm^3.

Preoperative Questions

1. What physical findings are important? What is wheezing? Does a lack of wheezing mean there is no asthma? In what circumstance? What other things do you look for in severe asthma? If the patient is having problems with the accessory muscles, cannot talk, has a haggard look, or is unconsciousness - that is a BAD thing!
2. What are the physiologic changes of pregnancy, and how do they affect your job? Does this patient have preeclampsia or pregnancy-induced hypertension? How would you know if she did?
3. What is the best nebulizer, or does it make a difference? Theoretically, can you give albuterol intravenously?

Intraoperative Questions

1. Would you use regional or general anesthesia? Why? What are the hazards of each? What is the primary concern and danger of opting for general anesthesia? What effect does regional anesthesia have on placental blood flow? What effect does general anesthesia have on placental blood flow? What effect do these forms have on the mother's respiratory system, given her asthma? Does the epinephrine in the epidural help the mother's asthma or hurt the placenta, or does it not matter?
2. After levobupivacaine injection, the mother seizes. What is the cause? What is the treatment? Compare this with intravascular injection of bupivacaine and with lidocaine. After 15 minutes of coding, the mother's ST segments are depressed 3 mm. In the excitement, the fetal heart rate monitor detached, and when you put it back on, the rate is 60 beats/min, and no one knows how long it has been that way. The mother is now intubated. Should she be moved to the OR?

3. In the middle of the case, the mother becomes very difficult to ventilate. A subclavian line was placed during the code. What is the differential diagnosis, and what is the treatment? Determine whether the problem is asthma. Do you give more of the β-agent? What about the ST-segment depression?
4. The kid comes out flaccid and meconium stained and has an Apgar score of 3. The pediatrician panics. What do you do? The mother is under anesthesia. How do you take care of both?

Postoperative Questions

1. The pediatrician says he cannot pass a nasogastric tube. The kid obstructs when his mouth is closed. What is the differential diagnosis, and what is the treatment? The pediatrician says the kid looks "funny," and there is a loud murmur. You intubate, but the kid is still blue. What is your next move?
2. Mom awakens with crushing chest pain radiating down her left arm. You are afraid she had an MI from the code. What now?
3. In the PACU, she starts bleeding heavily, and the obstetrician wants to go back for a more vigorous evacuation of the uterus. Do you place the spinal or epidural now? Do you sedate or use general anesthesia?

Grab Bag

1. How do you monitor fetal welfare? What does variability mean? Why is bradycardia such a concern? Do epidurals cause cesarean sections? Explain the concept of ion trapping.
2. Right after a wet tap, do you do a blood patch? What if the patient does not have a headache yet? Can you do a blood patch through the epidural catheter? What other options do you have?
3. You do a caudal, and the patient develops tinnitus and bradycardia and then seizes. You just gave a big bolus of levobupivacaine. What do you do? How could you have prevented this? Are you "safer" because you did not use bupivacaine? Why do you have to do CPR so much longer than if you used lidocaine? Discuss lipid emulsion therapy.

Update: Lung Isolation

1. List all the techniques available for lung isolation. You can use a double-lumen tube, Univent tube, Arndt bronchial blocker, separately placed Fogarty catheter, main stem intubation, going on bypass, and intermittent apnea. You can also throw up your hands and do a type of HFJV, hoping the surgeon does not get too mad.
2. Is there any trial demonstrating one method is better than another? No.
3. What are the indications for one-lung ventilation? One-lung ventilation is done to facilitate exposure in thoracic surgery, for surgery on the bronchus, to prevent contamination, and to facilitate the use of differential lung ventilation and PEEP.
4. Is auscultation good enough to confirm the position? No. Most need repositioning after you look with the scope.
5. Why not use right-sided double-lumen tubes? There is a higher incidence of right upper lobe collapse and obstruction. With the newer tubes and visualization, this is less of a problem, so a blanket "never use a right-sided tube!" is not true.

6. What size Fogarty should you use? Use an 8-French Fogarty catheter. Its disadvantage is that it has no central lumen to allow egress or ingress of air.

7. What are some complications of the Univent tube? The bronchial blocker can be stapled into the right upper lobe during a right upper lobectomy. If it falls back, it can occlude the trachea entirely. The blocker can also poke through somewhere and cause a pneumothorax.

8. What is an advantage of the Arndt blocker? Can you put it in a regular tube. Plus, I trained with George Arndt, and I get a kick out of saying, "I know the guy who invented this!"

9. What is the disadvantage of the Arndt blocker? After you close the loop, you cannot reposition it. The loop can get stapled into something. You need at least an 8.0-French tube to make it happen.

CASE 44: CATARACT IN A SMOKER

An 80-year-old, dotty, 70-kg woman refuses a block for a cataract procedure. She says, "If you perverts are going to molest me anyway, I would rather be asleep."

Okay.

She takes aspirin, Persantine, and *Ginko biloba* ("to keep me sharp, unlike you rat bastard idiots").

Fine.

She has smoked 2 packs per day for 60 years ("what, because I smoke and you don't, you think you are not going to end up doing the dirt nap too? Ha!"). Her blood pressure is 170/90 mm Hg, pulse is 88 beats/min, and respiratory rate is 16 breaths/min.

Preoperative Questions

1. What is COPD? How can you optimize it? What do you do with a gem like this patient, who will not take the medications anyway? Should you cancel the case or admit her and force her to take the medications? Should you tell her to stop smoking (right!).

2. Is she hypertensive? Is she adequately controlled? What is too high, what is the risk, and what evidence is there that it makes a difference? Can we just control everything with our short-acting medications?

3. What are the implications of her aspirin use for us? Answer the same question for Persantine. How about *Ginko biloba*? How are herbal medications made, regulated, and controlled for quality? What are the specific risks of the "G" herbs (garlic, *Ginko biloba*, ginseng)? What are the risks associated with *Ephedra*?

Intraoperative Questions

1. What is the best technique, given her blood pressure and probable COPD? What is the effect of potent inhalational agents on bronchomotor tone? Are intravenous drugs better? Discuss how you would do an inhalation induction. Can you do it in one breath? Discuss the uptake and distribution of soluble versus insoluble inhaled agents.

2. Which muscle relaxant, if any, should you use? Is suxamethonium okay? Can you skip muscle relaxants altogether? Do you give lidocaine to suppress airway and hemodynamic reflexes? How does that work? Why not use

a laryngotracheal anesthesia (LTA) device? For that matter, why not use an LMA?

3. The surgeon does a block after induction. What are the dangers? What if the patient arrests after the injection? What if the eye bulges out after induction or the heart rate drops into the 20s. Do you give atropine? What is atropine, and how does it work? Why not use glycopyrrolate or scopolamine?

4. The blood pressure goes to 190/110 mm Hg, and the patient has multifocal PVCs. What is the differential diagnosis, and what is the treatment? Should you give lidocaine or amiodarone? What is the evidence for each? What is a type 1 recommendation compared with a type 2 or 3?

Postoperative Questions

1. How do you manage a smooth wake-up course without a lot of bucking? Can you perform a deep extubation? Explain how you would do this? Should you try an awake approach? How? Do you use sufentanil for a smoother wake-up course?

2. She aspirated, and you need to put her on a ventilator. What will your initial settings be? Do you need an arterial line, or can you manage her clinically? The ICU has an end-tidal CO_2 machine hookup.

3. As soon as you put her on the ventilator, the thing malfunctions, gives too big a breath, and you hear a pop. What is the differential diagnosis, and what is the treatment? If there is no time for a chest tube, what do you do?

Grab Bag

1. A 45-year-old man with intractable pain from pancreatic cancer presents for a nerve block. How do you advise him?

2. What special precautions do you take with a twin delivery?

3. What are the implications of morbid obesity for anesthesia?

Update: Heparin-Induced Thrombocytopenia

1. How do you anticoagulate someone with HIT for a cardiac case? You can use argatroban, danaparoid, lepirudin, ancrod, or bivalirudin. You cannot follow these well with standard tests.

2. What is argatroban? It is a thrombin inhibitor, and it has no specific reversal agent. At least it has a short half-life (40 to 50 minutes).

3. What dosage do you use? Use a bolus of 0.1 mg/kg and then infuse 5 to 10 µg/kg/min. Aim at an ACT greater than 400 seconds.

4. These cases are epic headaches, of note.

CASE 45: CHOLECYSTECTOMY IN A PREGNANT PATIENT

A 35-year-old, 78-kg woman is 6 months' pregnant and is scheduled to have a cholecystectomy and duct exploration for obstructive jaundice. She takes Theo-Dur (theophylline) for asthma and is very scared. She admits to smoking crack cocaine on weekends. Her blood pressure is 100/65 mm Hg, pulse is 90 beats/min, respiratory rate is 20 breaths/min, temperature is 37°C, and hematocrit is 34%.

Preoperative Questions

1. Do you need PFTs? Do the results make a difference, because you are going to do the case anyway? Are most inhalers used correctly? If not, show how they are used and then show how they should be used. How can you be sure the patient is actually doing what she is supposed to? How does Theo-Dur affect the placenta, the baby, the lungs, and the heart? Should you switch her to β-selective therapy? How selective is selective?

2. How do you relieve anxiety in a pregnant patient? Are there any special concerns given her cocaine use? What is mechanism of cocaine effect? What are the long-term effects on the patient? Can you give opioids, or will they cause spasm of the sphincter of Oddi? Can you give a pregnant patient Reglan, or will it hurt the fetus? Discuss the teratogenic potential at various stages of pregnancy.

3. Is a hematocrit of 34% normal? How does volume status change during pregnancy? If the hematocrit were 24%, would you get a workup, delay, or transfuse? What effect does transfusion have on baby?

Intraoperative Questions

1. Are pulse oximetry and end-tidal CO_2 values enough? Do you need ABG values? How about documenting a few ABG values "just in case" a malpractice lawyer says you did not take good care of the mother? Is that a valid argument? Do you document anything else, such as the fetal heart rate?

2. How do you monitor the fetus intraoperatively? Where do you put the fetal heart rate monitor? Who will watch it? Do you have an obstetrician on call?

3. You place a CVP line because she has no veins. What are the risks? Where do you place it? Can you just draw venous blood gases? Of what use are they? Is that the same as mixed venous blood gas? How?

4. Can you do this with a high spinal or epidural? Why?

5. Hypotension and hypoxemia occur as they explore the common bile duct. What is the differential diagnosis, and what is the treatment? Does she need to be in the left uterine displacement position? At what stage do you worry about supine hypotension syndrome? At what stage do you worry about a full stomach? When do you stop worrying about a full stomach?

6. The patient coughs on intubation and starts to wheeze at the end of the case. Should you extubate? Should you wait, deepen anesthesia, give inhalers, or keep on a ventilator? Why?

Postoperative Questions

1. How can you help with pain management? Should you use PCA? What dose and interval will you use? Do you worry about the kid getting narcotics, getting addicted, or jacking up his cytochrome P450 system? A colleague says, "Don't feed her addiction. She is already on cocaine!" What is your response?

2. Her urine output is 5 mL during the first hour in the PACU and 25 mL during the second hour. Do you wait and see if the trend continues or step in? A PACU nurse hangs a bag of water irrigation by mistake and runs in 2 L before she notices. What could happen now? What laboratory tests do you anticipate? What is the treatment?

3. The patient says her neck is sore, and she cannot move it at all. How will you evaluate this?

Grab Bag

1. A preeclamptic patient has an epidural in, and it is working. She needs an immediate cesarean section. Do you increase the dose of the epidural or go right to general endotracheal anesthesia. If you increase the dose, what do you use and how fast?
2. The patient has a pheochromocytoma. The surgeon asks for guidance in getting the patient ready for surgery. What is your advice?
3. How do you do closed-circuit anesthesia? What are the pros and cons? Where do you put the O_2 sensor in such a case? Is it different from a regular case? What do you do if the patient bucks and upsets all the calculations? Is there any danger in suddenly converting to regular anesthesia?

Update: ε-Aminocaproic Acid

1. How does ε-aminocaproic acid (Amicar) work? It inhibits fibrinolysis without suppressing thrombin generation.
2. Does it have a prothrombotic potential? Yes. Unheparinized patients have gotten excessive clots on pulmonary artery catheters. Intracoronary thrombosis is a concern.
3. Does Amicar reduce blood loss in cardiac surgery? Yes.
4. What dose does this? The loading dose is 150 mg/kg, and it is then run at 15 mg/kg/hr. In a double-blind, placebo-controlled study, this regimen decreased blood loss.
5. Does it matter when you give the Amicar? No. You can give it before or after anticoagulation; the results are the same.

CASE 46: EXPLORATORY LAPAROTOMY IN A DIABETIC WHO IS WHEEZING

An 18-year-old girl is scheduled for exploratory laparotomy for a twisted ovarian cyst. She ate a gyro (with tsatsiki sauce on the side) 4 hours earlier, has type 1 diabetes, and took 10 mg of prednisone for asthma 1 month ago. She is wheezing now. All vital signs are normal, but she is in a lot of pain.

Preoperative Questions

1. What further evaluation of her metabolic status do you need? Is it worth the delay? What are the differences among emergent, urgent, and elective cases? Is a blood gas determination needed, or is a HCO_3 level on a CHEM-7 panel okay? What findings would you see in DKA or pre-DKA (if such a thing exists)? Do you pursue tight control (explain the dangers) or loose control (explain the dangers)?
2. Does her recent steroid use matter? Do you cover her with steroids? Which, how much, and why? What is an addisonian crisis?
3. She is wheezing and cannot wait. What will you order in the holding area?

Intraoperative Questions

1. The patient saw a Montel show and knows about awareness. Explain the risk to her. She wants to be awake. Is that a possibility? What are the problems

with regional anesthesia and deep abdominal exploration? What are the problems with converting to general anesthesia in the middle of the case?

2. If you use a spinal, which drug, route, and place (midline versus para) will you use? As you inject, she coughs (i.e., barbotage), becomes flaccid, and collapses. What is the differential diagnosis, and what is the treatment?

3. Assume that did not happen, and you go with a spinal, but she is groaning and in agony. How do you convert with a sympathectomy in place? Do you use ketamine because she has asthma? You induce and cannot intubate.

4. You check the blood sugar level, which is 800 mg/dL. How do you treat? A few hours pass, and now it is a whiteout. What do you do?

5. With the spinal, the patient becomes bronchospastic. What is the treatment for a nonintubated patient?

Postoperative Questions

1. How do you decide to extubate? If you keep the patient on the ventilator, how do you adjust the settings in the face of her asthma? What are the dangers of PEEP? How do you diagnose pneumothorax?

2. What is the danger of undertreating low urine output? What is the danger of overtreating? What problems attend Lasix, mannitol, dopamine, and vigorous volume loading?

3. The patient asks about some comments she heard while "asleep, but I could not move." What is your response? What is the risk of post-traumatic stress disorder (PTSD)?

Grab Bag

1. What is the preferred anesthetic for a preeclamptic woman undergoing vaginal delivery? What is it for cesarean section? Suppose the blood pressure drops right after your first dose of a labor epidural. How will you manage this situation?

2. The surgeon complains of a bulging brain in the middle of a meningioma resection. How can you help the surgeon? What are your choices concerning position, barbiturates, CO_2, CSF drainage, and O_2?

3. You take over a case just as it is ending. A woman had a peritoneal abscess drained. Postoperatively, she cannot breathe well. What is the differential diagnosis, and what is the treatment? What tests and clinical methods do you use to determine a pseudocholinesterase deficiency?

4. The infection control committee is trying to determine why so many heart patients are getting mediastinitis. How can you help them? Could it be propofol or related to CVP line placement? Should you use gowns when placing lines? Do you use a Site-Rite pulsed-echo ultrasound probe so you do not fish around when you check the CVPs?

Update: Off-Pump Coronary Artery Bypass Grafting

1. What is the primary problem with cannulating the aorta? The high rate of calcification leads to emboli and neurologic injury. Off-pump cases obviate this problem.

2. What is the systemic advantage? Off-pump procedures avoid the systemic inflammatory response seen with extracorporeal circulation. This may help reduce neurologic, renal, and hematologic problems associated with traditional cardiac surgery.

3. Is mortality any better? No, although some studies lean toward it being safer. The jury is still out on this issue

4. What is a major concern? There is concern about whether the patients get revascularized well, and there is a concern about long-term graft patency, the rate for which does seem lower in off-pump cases.

5. What is major headache for anesthesiologists during these cases? Lifting the heart cuts off venous return, which drops the blood pressure.

6. Bottom line—the great "promise" of off-pump CABG ("It's better!") is yet to be proven.

CASE 47: ALLIGATOR TRAUMA IN A PREGNANT PATIENT

A 25-year-old, 50-kg aerobics instructor is scheduled for débridement and ORIF of a left femoral fracture after falling off her ATV. An alligator bit her foot, which will need amputation. She is 28 weeks' pregnant and has alligator snout–shaped bruises on her chest. Her blood pressure is 100/70 mm Hg, pulse is 115 beats/min, respiratory rate is 20 breaths/min, and hematocrit is 37%.

Preoperative Questions

1. Her hematocrit a year ago was 43%; why is it 37% now? What physiologic effects does pregnancy have? What are the effects of a femoral fracture, pain, or blood loss? Is she hypovolemic? Can you do a tilt test on a patient with a leg fracture? She has PVCs. Could she have an alligator snout–induced cardiac contusion? Is she likely to become a poikilotherm? Do you need further cardiac workup? Do you place defibrillator pads? Do you start a lidocaine drip or load with amiodarone?

2. What injuries might she have in her chest? Is dissection a possibility? How would you tell? What about pulmonary contusion? The chest radiograph shows a 10% pneumothorax. Do you need another chest radiograph? Is observation enough? What will positive pressure do to this approach?

3. Should you deliver the infant before you start the surgery? Should you call the obstetrician? Should you get a fetal scalp pH or place a fetal heart rate monitor? Who will watch and interpret it? Who is responsible if the obstetric nurse misses something—you or the obstetrician?

4. Should you call Animal Planet and tell them you have a story for them?

Intraoperative Questions

1. Do you need an arterial line, or are end-tidal CO_2 and pulse oximetry enough? Is a brachial line okay? Do you place a femoral line, or will it hurt the fetus? Where do the placental vessels come off? How is blood flow regulated in the placenta? What are the effects of pressors? Is there any danger if you hyperventilate and make the mother hypocarbic?

2. Is regional anesthesia safer given the pregnancy? Which route and which drug will you use? Will you use an epidural in case it takes a long time? What about the worry that the cardiac contusion will lead to arrhythmias? Will regional anesthesia be safer here, or is it better to have the airway secured?

3. The fetal heart rate goes from 140 beats/min with variation to 120 beats/min and no variation with the induction of general anesthesia. Is this good or bad? Should you proceed to cesarean section? Now the heart rate goes to 80 beats/min; should you look to the mother or go to cesarean section?

4. Thirty minutes after induction, the oxygen saturation level drops, the lungs become hard to ventilate, and the end-tidal CO_2 level drops. What is the differential diagnosis, and what is the treatment? Explain the physiology of a fat embolus and differentiate it from an amniotic or thrombotic embolus. Do you need a Swan-Ganz catheter or TEE? What would TEE show?

Postoperative Questions

1. Postoperatively, the patient has abdominal pains and premature contractions. Do you start tocolytic therapy? How much? Do you consult with the obstetrician? Discuss the dangers of prematurity, the lecithin-to-sphingomyelin (L/S) ratio, and the use of steroids to "help mature" the infant's lungs.

2. A 41-year-old woman is scheduled for a hysterectomy and says she has acute intermittent porphyria. How will you do the case? Will you use regional anesthesia? Discuss the molecular mechanism at play here, how you will prevent an exacerbation, and how you would treat one if it did happen.

3. A 60-year-old man with pancreatic cancer needs pain relief. Which block will you use? Describe the dangers of the block. Do you go straight to a neurolytic block? What are the dangers of that?

4. A 2-week-old child with pyloric stenosis presents for surgery. What are the anesthetic considerations? Is this an emergency? How does the neonatal kidney handle sodium?

Grab Bag

1. Does local anesthesia cause cesarean sections? Why or why not? Does it matter what local anesthetic you use? What about using spinal lidocaine? Does it cause a transient neurologic syndrome? How? How do you treat it? What is the disadvantage of always using bupivacaine? Are there other alternatives, such as procaine, for a very short case?

2. You are breathing down a kid, and he is still awake. Why? Will the addition of nitrous oxide help? How? What is the second gas effect? Contrast that with dilutional hypoxemia. How do you prevent that?

3. A woman had a breast biopsy under general anesthesia. She had a propofol/remifentanil anesthetic and "loved it." You are unfamiliar with these agents used as drips, but that is what she wants. Do you let your more familiar partner do the case, or do you go ahead and wing it? What are the dangers of unfamiliarity? What are the dangers of remifentanil infusion or propofol infusion? What is fat embolism syndrome, and can it happen with propofol?

Update: Complications of Noncardiac Thoracic Surgery

1. What is the most common complication of noncardiac thoracic surgery? Atrial fibrillation, especially after right-sided pneumonectomy, is a common complication. The traditional use of digoxin to "prevent" this has never been shown to be effective.

2. Because many patients develop MIs, should we be doing angioplasties on them? It has not been shown to be of benefit.

3. Is amiodarone a good idea? It is a good antiarrhythmic agent, but it can cause ARDS in post-pneumonectomy patients, so caution is the byword.

4. What is the primary cause of heart failure postoperatively? It is right-sided failure caused by an increase in right ventricular afterload.

5. Does postoperative nitric oxide have a place here? Maybe, because it would decrease right ventricular pressure and protect against right-sided heart failure. But expense and lack of proven benefit makes this a "not ready for prime time" idea.

CASE 48: TRANSURETHRAL PROSTATECTOMY AND THE HEART

A 72-year-old, 75-kg man is scheduled for cystoscopy for possible TURP to relieve BPH. He takes digoxin and nitroglycerin, and he has a holosystolic murmur (grade 4/6). He has a blood pressure of 140/110 mm Hg, pulse of 65 beats/min, respiratory rate of 14 breaths/min, and potassium level of 3.0 mEq/L. The ECG shows left ventricular hypertrophy and LBBB.

Preoperative Questions

1. Do you insist on an echocardiogram before you proceed? It shows tight aortic stenosis with a gradient of 90 mm Hg. What are the risks of anesthesia with this condition? Do you need to get valve replaced first, or do this procedure first? Can you interpret ischemia in the face of LBBB? Describe the normal path of conduction in the heart. Do you insist on catheterization?

2. Catheterization shows two-vessel disease. Do you need the heart fixed first? What if he is having chest pain at rest? Is this our decision to make?

3. The potassium level is 3.0 mEq/L. Do we cancel for this or insist it get replaced? What are the dangers of rapid replacement? How does potassium taste? Does it upset the stomach? Do you need a central line to give it intravenously, or can you give it peripherally? What are the problems with that?

Intraoperative Questions

1. Do you use a spinal anesthetic? What is the danger in the face of aortic stenosis? Is that an absolute contraindication? What about an epidural that you dose up ever so slowly? The PT is 14/12 seconds and PTT is 34 seconds. Do these values have any significance? Is a general anesthetic better? Why? Is spontaneous ventilation (a lost art) a good idea? What is the danger of a patient bucking with the cystoscope in place?

2. Can you do this without the usual litany of a CVP line or Swan-Ganz catheter? Why or why not? How about going right to TEE? What are the contraindications for TEE and problems with interpretation? What are the problems with the Swan-Ganz catheter and its interpretation?

3. The CVP starts out at 9 mm Hg, but an hour after dissection, the CVP is 20 mm Hg. Why? What do you do about it? How can you tell TURP syndrome with the patient asleep? How about awake? Answer the same questions for bladder rupture.

4. The patient is oozing like thunder. Why? Does he have DIC? How will you determine this? Will you give blood products? Which ones? What is the danger of this transfusion?

Postoperative Questions

1. Thirty minutes after arrival in the PACU, the PVCs progress to bigeminy. What is the differential diagnosis, and what is the treatment? Because he has an LBBB, how will you tell if he is ischemic? He goes into third- degree heart block. What do you do? What is the difference between lidocaine and amiodarone?
2. The Foley catheter is driving him crazy because of pain. What are the options? How about a Precedex drip? Can you send him to the floor with that? What are the dangers? Do you need an arterial line when you have that running? How does Precedex work?
3. You used 15 µg/kg of fentanyl for general anesthesia. His pupils are small, and he is not arousing. Do you use Narcan or wait? Do you use nalbuphine? Do you use Romazicon to get rid of the 3 mg of Versed you gave him at the beginning? Give your reasons for each decision.

Grab Bag

1. A woman presents in the labor and delivery suite with painless vaginal bleeding. How do you set up for and anticipate possible complications of this condition.
2. A child with congenital diaphragmatic hernia suffers low O_2 saturation after intubation. What specific to this child may explain this situation?
3. A diabetic asks about taking his morning insulin. How do you advise?

Update: Myocardial Ischemia

1. When do most perioperative MIs occur? The incidence peaks 24 to 48 hours after surgery (not the 3 days out that we were all taught).
2. What most often heralds this kind of MI:ST depression or elevation? ST depression often heralds the MI.
3. What is the mortality rate for perioperative MI? It is 10% to 15%, not the sinister 50% we were all taught. Such myths we grew up with!
4. What is the usual mechanism of an MI? Rupture of a vulnerable lipid-laden plaque leads to coronary thrombosis.
5. What is the scoop on intraoperative ischemia? The duration of the ischemia is important. You have to detect it and fix it right away. An elevated heart rate is a big no no.
6. What is the timing for beneficial β-blocker administration? No one knows and the POISE study calls the entire idea into question.

CASE 49: OBESE PATIENT WITH BURNS AND FRACTURES

A 20-year-old, 150-kg woman is scheduled for ORIF of an open tibial-fibular fracture and débridement of third-degree burns on her abdomen and back after a stunt on American Idol went all wrong. She takes thyroid replacement, digoxin, and a diuretic. She says she is allergic to barbiturates because she gets sleepy, and she refuses a spinal, because "Momma didn't raise her no fool." Her blood pressure is 190/90 mm Hg, pulse is 115 beats/min, respiratory rate is 22 breaths/min, temperature is 39°C, and hemoglobin level is 13 g/dL.

Preoperative Questions

1. How do you determine the percentage of burned skin, and why is this important? How do you calculate the fluid replacement needed? Which fluid do you give? What about the possibility of the burn involving the airway? What would you look for in the history and during the physical examination?
2. If she is allergic to barbiturates, can you give her pentathol? What would the medicolegal implications be if you blew it off and gave her pentathol anyway? What would you use and why? What about ketamine? Are there any risks when the patient wakes up?
3. What is Pickwickian syndrome? How does her obesity come into play here? What about her airway, right heart failure, and response to narcotics?
4. The blood pressure is high, and the patient is not too compliant. What are the results for your anesthetic? Does it matter if the blood pressure is all over the map for the case? Are there any outcome studies saying that railroad tracks are actually better for the patient? What does normal blood pressure do during the day?

Intraoperative Questions

1. What induction agent and technique do you use to secure the airway? The patient freaks when you mention awake intubation. How do you calm her, topicalize, and sedate? Is Precedex a good idea? Would you use intramuscular ketamine or suxamethonium? Is there any worry about hyperkalemia? If hyperkalemia occurred, what would you see on the ECG and why? What would you do about it?
2. For maintenance, do you use an inhalational (then you fight phase II of anesthesia as she wakes up) or intravenous method (then you worry that she has obstructive sleep apnea and will stop breathing later)? Do you use a propofol drip? What if you have to run gallons of propofol into her? What is the danger? Discuss cost and fat embolism.
3. You intubate, and 5 minutes later, the patient is cyanotic and bradycardic. What is the differential diagnosis, and what is the treatment? The nurse tries to set up the defibrillator when the code starts, but it will not fire. What do you do?
4. There has been large blood loss from débridement. How do you guide fluid replacement therapy? When do you transfuse? She is young; does that affect your decision? After 6 units, do you call for FFP, platelets, or cryoprecipitate? Why? Do you wait for blood test results?

Postoperative Questions

1. Do you keep the patient intubated? Why or why not? The ventilator takes 55 cm H_2O to get a 1000-mL tidal volume in her. Should you make a change? What is the danger of barotraumas? How do you make sure the tube is in the right place? Do you go to fiberoptic methods because she is so big?
2. The patient develops pulmonary edema 2 days later. Discuss the Starling forces at work in the lung of a burn patient. What is the treatment for pulmonary edema?
3. In the PACU, the patient temperature is 33°C, and she is shivering. What are the dangers of shivering? Do you treat or let it go?

Grab Bag

1. A 4-year-old boy, who just ate, comes in with an open eye injury. He is screaming like a banshee and will not allow an intravenous line. The eye

needs to be repaired. The surgeon says if the boy continues wailing, he will lose the eye for sure. Do you quickly breathe down the kid? Do you use intramuscular ketamine? Can you give suxamethonium? Is it dangerous in kids because of Reye's syndrome or something else?

2. Unexplained tachycardia occurs in a 23-year-old road warrior, who is getting his third washout of an open leg wound. How will you rule out MH as a cause of this worrisome finding?

3. When a patient arrives for an elective case, and no one thought about the AICD, do you have to turn it off? What else do you have to do? Can you use external paddles? Can you turn it back on when all is said and done?

Update: Methemoglobinemia

1. What is the primary concern about methemoglobinemia? Arterial desaturation occurs, scaring hell out of the anesthesiologist.

2. What is the treatment? You can give methylene blue intravenously.

3. What does the saturation go to? The usual level is about 88%.

4. Who might you see methemoglobinemia in? It occurs in patients on lots of medications that have oxidative properties (e.g., dapsone for *Pneumocystis*, Reglan, lidocaine). This overwhelms the cytochrome-b_5 reductase system that normally converts methemoglobin to hemoglobin; then methemoglobin builds up.

CASE 50: SCOLIOSIS AND ANEMIA

A 12-year-old, African American girl is scheduled for scoliosis repair. She has a family history of "blood trouble," and her own hemoglobin level is just 8 g/dL. Vital signs are all normal. She gets short of breath easily and cannot play softball with her friends.

Preoperative Questions

1. What effect does scoliosis have on anesthesia? It can affect respiratory function, positioning, and cardiac failure resulting from hypoxemia caused by restrictive disease. What kind of volume loss can you expect from a prolonged case requiring many levels of work?

2. The low hemoglobin level is a concern. What is the most likely cause? What other laboratory test results do you need for the sickle cell patient? Do you transfuse her? How much? If she has not had crises in the past, do you have to get her hemoglobin S level down to 50%, or is there leeway? Now that she is looking at a big blood loss, does that change things? Under what circumstances would you exchange transfuse her?

3. Given it is a prolonged case in the prone position, do you discuss the risk of blindness with the patient and parents? Why or why not? How do you answer their questions about the wake-up test?

Intraoperative Questions

1. What monitors do you place? How does an evoked potential monitor work? How do our anesthetics interact with those monitors? How can we ensure a good signal? What do you do if the signal starts to get worse?

2. Discuss the different major tracts in the spinal cord and how they are monitored. Discuss specifically the anterior cord with its motor supply.

3. Which anesthetic do you use to induce, which to maintain, and why?
4. How do you conduct a TIVA? Do you use a relaxant? Why or why not?
5. What are the special concerns about the prone patient with regard to nerve injury and respiratory insufficiency (especially if scoliosis is severe)?
6. The surgeon wants controlled hypotension to reduce bleeding, but you do not want a blind patient. How do you reconcile these views?
7. You move her into the prone position, and she starts to wheeze. What do you do next?

Postoperative Questions

1. In the PACU, she says her vision is blurry. Do you immediately get an ophthalmologic consult? Do you rub the goop out of her eyes?
2. Her temperature rises to 39.6°C. How will you tell if this is MH? What else could it be?
3. Two hours later, her blood pressure is 60/40 mm Hg and pulse is 150 beats/min, and you cannot get her to answer you. What is most likely going on? Do you wait for a hematocrit value or transfuse right away?

Grab Bag

1. You are comatose, covering the eyeball palace, when you are paged. After a routine retrobulbar block, the eye specialist and you look up and see a flat line on the monitor. What is the differential diagnosis, and what is the treatment? Should you go through the complete advanced cardiac life support (ACLS) protocol?
2. A 32-year-old woman with myasthenia gravis is scheduled for a thymectomy. What are the preoperative evaluation and optimization procedures for a myasthenic patient? Do you need an ICU bed? Do you need a muscle relaxant for intubation of this patient? How will you determine whether it is safe to extubate?
3. Which fluid is ideal for neurosurgery? What is your concern about glucose? Is colloid better? Should you use FFP? What are the dangers of FFP? What if the patient is a Jehovah's Witness?

Update: Bleeding in the Trachea

1. When spontaneous bleeding occurs in the trachea, what are your options? You can isolate the lung with a double-lumen ETT, place the patient "bleeding lung down," give medical therapy for diffuse bleeding (e.g., FFP, desmopressin), use angiography to see the bleeding vessel and embolize it (rare to see a vessel pumping so furiously), and use iced saline lavage with epinephrine in it.
2. What condition might cause this from both lungs? Goodpasture's syndrome can cause bleeding in the trachea.
3. What is the treatment option in this disaster? Believe it or not, bilateral nephrectomy works. Go figure.

CASE 51: FEMUR FRACTURE AND RESTLESSNESS

A 44-year-old, 48-kg, previously healthy woman was admitted to the hospital with a fractured femur from a car crash. No other injuries are found. Twenty-four hours later, she is scheduled for open reduction with internal fixation (ORIF). During the preoperative evaluation, she is restless and dyspneic. Her blood pressure is 100/60 mm Hg, pulse is 110 beats/min, respiratory rate is 34 breaths/min, and rectal temperature is 40.8°C.

Preoperative Questions

1. Why is the patient restless and dyspneic?
2. Discuss pulmonary embolus, and compare fat with blood clot thrombus.
3. Explain the differences among atelectasis, pneumonia, and aspiration. How does each cause dyspnea?
4. What other pulmonary findings might you anticipate?
5. Would you hear rales? What are rales?
6. What if you see bloody secretions?
7. What if you see an infiltrate on the chest radiograph?
8. What if the patient has cyanosis that is not relieved by O_2?
9. What other findings might you see? Are the neck veins distended?
10. What ECG findings might you identify? Does the patient have right axis deviation or right ventricular hypertrophy?
11. How is the diagnosis of fat embolism made?
12. What laboratory tests might help?
13. What physical findings might help? What does petechiae indicate in this setting?
14. What preoperative therapy do you suggest? Will you use oxygen, intermittent positive-pressure breathing, PEEP, steroids, or intubation?
15. Would you cool the patient before starting your anesthetic?

Intraoperative Questions

1. What is your choice of anesthesia after the patient is stable? Do you use regional or general anesthesia and why? What are the advantages and hazards of each in this patient?
2. You go with an epidural. What drug would you use and why? Would you include epinephrine? Why?
3. Thirty minutes after the block, the patient becomes restless and disoriented. What is the diagnosis? What would you do?
4. Is CVP monitoring important? Should you instead use Swan-Ganz monitoring or TEE? Defend your choice.
5. You need to convert to a general anesthetic, but the patient is on her side. What will you do?
6. While drilling through the marrow, the patient has a cardiovascular collapse. What is the cause? What is the treatment?

Postoperative Questions

1. Would you use epidural narcotics? Which one and why? How much? What are the complications?
2. The blood pressure drops to 70/40 mm Hg, and the pulse goes to 120 beats/min 1 hour after the patient is in the PACU. What is the cause? What is the treatment?
3. The surgeon asks if you should do a tracheostomy for postoperative care. What is your response?

Grab Bag

1. A 25-year-old woman, who is a roofer, is 2 days out from a decompression of an epidural hematoma after falling off a building. Now she has become drowsy and does not move her left side. CT shows a 4+ cerebral edema. She was extubated 4 hours ago. What would you do before her return to the OR? Would you intubate right now? How would you induce in the face of increased ICP? What if she was described as "hard to intubate" in the anesthetic record? After she is intubated, how will you reduce the ICP?
2. A 2-year-old boy is scheduled for ear tubes. Has a temperature of 37°C and a productive cough. Has been cancelled twice before, and the mother is going out of her mind. "He will not get better until he gets the damned tubes in; do not cancel him again!" Do you cancel? Do you perform a more extensive workup? Do you swallow hard and just do it? What dangers do you face if you proceed? What are the medicolegal implications?
3. A 20-year-old man had a large mediastinal mass resected. Soon after extubation, he is retracting with each breath and stridorous. What is the differential diagnosis, and what is the treatment? Is there anything special given the specific operation he had?

Update: Perioperative Hyponatremia

1. Why should perioperative hyponatremia be a special concern? Patients are allowed free intake of clear fluids until 2 hours preoperatively. With everyone drinking so much bottled water now, more people may be getting the equivalent of psychogenic polydipsia-induced hyponatremia. Not to mention all those plastic bottles are bad for the environment.
2. What are other causes of hyponatremia? Pregnancy, alcoholism, tumors causing SIADH, and TURP syndrome can cause hyponatremia.
3. Is the mortality rate higher for inpatients with low sodium levels? Yes. It is 7-fold to 60-fold higher!
4. How slowly should you correct the sodium level? No more than 25 mmol of sodium should be given in 24 hours.
5. What is the risk of rapid correction? Central pontine demyelinolysis can occur.

CASE 52: CHOLECYSTECTOMY AND JAUNDICE

A 56-year-old, 68-kg, severely cirrhotic man is scheduled for cholecystectomy for cancer. Physical examination reveals moderate ascites, jaundice, and spider angiomas. His blood pressure is 100/80 mm Hg, pulse is 100 beats/min, temperature is 36.8°C, and hematocrit is 28%.

Preoperative Questions

1. What tests (e.g., PT, albumin, enzymes, bilirubin) are important for the assessment of liver function? Why? Which, if absent, would make you delay or cancel the case? What values would make you cancel?
2. How does ascites affect anesthetic management? What is the effect of paracentesis? When and why does it work? Does cirrhosis alter premedication plans? How? Do you give vitamin K? Why?

Intraoperative Questions

1. Do you select pentathol, propofol, etomidate, or ketamine for anesthesia? What is the dose requirement? Is using desflurane a good idea? How about sevoflurane? What about risk of fires with sevoflurane? Is nitrous and a narcotic good? Why? What is the effect of hepatic blood flow on anesthesia? What is the effect of little arteriovenous malformations around the liver?

2. When choosing muscle relaxants, do you avoid suxamethonium? What is the effect of cirrhosis on cisatracurium or Pavulon? How is the volume of distribution altered?

3. During the procedure on 60% N_2O, the PaO_2 is 50 mm Hg. What is the differential diagnosis? Can intraoperative hypoxia be caused by traction, shunt, or tube malplacement?

4. What are the special fluid needs of a cirrhotic patient? Are the risks concerning glucose, sodium, potassium, albumin, FFP, and infections the same as for a patient without cirrhosis?

5. Is oliguria a special problem in this patient? Why? How do you manage low urine output in the middle of a case? Do you place additional monitors?

Postoperative Questions

1. What is the differential diagnosis (e.g., hepatic coma, anesthetics given intravenously or by inhalation, temperature, relaxants, glucose) for failure to awaken, and what is the management plan?

2. Vomiting and aspiration occur on emergence. The patient vomits and aspirates clear fluid, and wheezing starts with cyanosis. How do you manage this situation?

Grab Bag

1. A 28-year-old, gravida 4, para 3 parturient presents for emergency cesarean section because of abruptio placentae. She had wanted an epidural so she could see the baby. What do you tell her? What is abruptio placentae? What anesthetic is safest? What will you do if her veins are hard to stick? Can you use a leg vein? After delivery, the patient oozed from all over the place. What is the differential diagnosis, and what is the treatment?

2. A man with metastatic prostatic cancer presents with unremitting back pain. Parenteral opioids no longer work. What options can you present? What if he had pancreatic cancer? What are the dangers of a celiac plexus block? Can you treat by intravascular injection of bupivacaine? Why must CPR go on for so long?

3. An administrator asks you to use low-flow anesthesia to save money. Can you do this safely? What else can you do to cut costs but remain safe in the OR? How about skipping the PACU? Under what circumstances can you do that? Give guidelines.

Update: Laryngeal Mask Airway and the Prone Position

1. You are kidding, right? No. When the patient is prone, the jaw and tongue fall anteriorly, making LMA insertion easier.

2. When would you do this? It can be used for penetrating trauma posteriorly, such as a case in which a drill bit had stuck into the spinal column and the patient was prone.
3. How do you induce in such a horrific case? The patient is prone and kept en bloc, maintaining spontaneous ventilation.
4. What about aspiration? With the patient prone, the emesis would come out. In England, they do lateral and prone cases all the time with an LMA. And the English pound is kicking the American dollar, so maybe they are smarter than we are.

CASE 53: URETERAL REIMPLANTATION WITH BAD ASTHMA

A 7-year-old, 20-kg girl is scheduled to undergo bilateral ureteral reimplantation for vesicoureteral reflux. She has a history of long-standing asthma, with three ER admissions in the past 4 years, requiring intravenous steroids each time. At age 4, she had a tonsillectomy and adenoidectomy procedure and had postintubation croup. Medications include theophylline and cromolyn. Her blood pressure is 110/70 mm Hg, pulse is 100 beats/min, respiratory rate is 20 breaths/min, oral temperature is 37.5°C, and hematocrit is 35%.

Preoperative Questions

1. You perform a respiratory evaluation of her asthma before surgery? What additional history do you want? Do you need laboratory tests, PFTs, or ABG values? What medications do you continue or stop? Do you add medications? Does the patient need preoperative admission for optimization? How does Cromolyn work?
2. Which preoperative medications (e.g., narcotics, drying agents, Versed, rectal Brevital) do you select and why?
3. The parents ask to be in the room. The mother is a nurse, and she says, "I'll be okay." What is your response?

Intraoperative Questions

1. What is your choice of anesthesia? Do you avoid pentathol or ketamine if the child is still wheezing? What are the problems with both agents? What if the child is allergic to eggs? Do you employ mask induction? What if the parents are there for induction? What if the mother freaks out? Which inhalation agent will you use? Why? What are the advantages? What kind of system (e.g., Mapleson, Jackson-Reese) will you use? Why?
2. For airway management, how do you determine which tube size to use? Do you use a cuff? Compare the airways of children and adults. How do you humidify? Describe the reasons for postoperative croup, and explain how to prevent it. How do you control temperature in a child?
3. You place a tube but cannot ventilate. Is a plug, spasm, or esophageal intubation causing the problem? If it is bronchospasm, which agent do you give? Do you give steroids, theophylline, or inhaled agents? Explain the idea of β-agent specificity. How will end-tidal CO_2 help?
4. What is overnight deficit, and what is maintenance? Do you run "wet" or "dry," considering the patient's asthma? What is third space loss, and how do you

replace it? Do you use albumin? What is its cost compared with crystalloid? When do you give blood? What is the treatment for a transfusion reaction?

Postoperative Questions

1. Should the child be extubated at the end of the operation? Do you use deep or awake intubation in an asthmatic? If you keep her on the ventilator, what mode do you use, and how do you "wean to extubate in AM" without provoking bronchospasm? What are the standing orders for respiratory therapy?
2. One hour postoperatively, the urine output goes to 0. Is this a special problem in this patient? What is the differential diagnosis, and what is treatment?
3. Is PCA a possibility? The child is very mature. The mother tries to help by "pushing the button for her." What is your response?

Grab Bag

1. You put in an epidural for the senator's girlfriend, but she is getting only right-sided relief. Why? Discuss the anatomy of the epidural space. Should you take it out or pull back? What are the systemic alternatives if she is at 2 cm? What if she is at 9 cm? What if the senator's wife shows up?
2. Electrocautery unit is plugged in, and the line isolation monitor goes off. What happened, and what do you do about it? Why do you need line isolation? Contrast microshock with macroshock hazard.
3. How does epidural morphine work? How does intrathecal work? What are the risks of both? For thoracotomy, is a thoracic epidural better than PCA? What should you run in a thoracic epidural? Can they go to the floor? With what standing orders? Narcotics too? Do you need a pulse oximeter?

Update: ProSeal Laryngeal Mask Airways

1. What is different about ProSeal LMAs? They have a tube that allows for gastric suction. It also provides a better seal.
2. When might you use it? You use it in an obstetrics cases when you have a "cannot intubate, cannot ventilate" scenario. You can use it with a ventilator (e.g., LMA used in obstetric emergencies).
3. Does it protect against aspiration? In cadaver studies, it does better than traditional LMAs. But it's NOT an endotracheal tube, no way, no how!

CASE 54: RADICAL HYSTERECTOMY AND SUBSTANCE ABUSE

A 55-year-old, 65-kg woman is scheduled to undergo a radical hysterectomy for cervical cancer. She has a long history of alcohol abuse. She takes Valium nightly to help her sleep. Her blood pressure is 160/70 mm Hg, pulse is 76 beats/min, respiratory rate is 16 breaths/min, temperature is 37°C, hemoglobin level is 9 g/dL, and AST (SGOT) level is 45 U/L.

Preoperative Questions

1. Do the physical stigmata of liver disease make a difference? Which laboratory tests do you need? Do you need an ABG determination? What if the

patient refuses an ABG test because it hurts too much? Do you insist on a liver needle biopsy if the AST (SGOT) level is sky-high?

2. Why is she anemic? Do you transfuse preoperatively, transfuse early in the intraoperative phase, or skip transfusion if she is doing well? What if she is a Jehovah's Witness?

3. The surgeon puts her on a week of total parenteral nutrition. What are the implications for anesthesia? What are the glucose considerations? What is the physiology of hyperalimentation compared with tube feedings?

Intraoperative Questions

1. What intravenous drugs are "best" for liver disease? Discuss the cytochrome P450 system and its relation to anesthesia. Discuss a "revved-up" liver compared with a "burned-out" liver and the effects on metabolism of drugs. Is using N_2O a good or bad idea? Is regional anesthesia an option? What if the patient insists on a spinal?

2. Do you need an arterial line? Why? What are the risks? Where do you place it if you blow the radial artery? Is a CVP line adequate? Where should it be placed? What if you stick the catheter in the carotid? Is a pulmonary artery catheter better? If so, which kind?

3. Which relaxant will you use and why? What are the volume of distribution considerations? The surgeon says the patient is tight, but you see no twitches. What do you do?

4. The case will go for 10 hours. How do you keep the patient warm? What are the risks of using a Bair Hugger? What are the risks of hypothermia?

5. The surgeon says, "Hang blood from the very start!" What is your response? The patient loses 500 mL of blood, but the CVP is still at 10 mm Hg. Do you transfuse? What about the risks for AIDS and hepatitis?

Postoperative Questions

1. You extubate in the OR, and 10 minutes later in the PACU, the patient is gasping and cyanotic. What is the treatment? How do you determine the need for reintubation? What are the criteria for safe extubation? If the patient's intubation had been difficult, would you use a different approach for extubation?

2. Will you use epidural narcotics, intrathecal narcotics, or narcotics for both? What are the advantages and disadvantages of each? What is the treatment for delayed respiratory depression? Do you use local anesthetic infusion? What are the advantages? What are the risks?

Grab Bag

1. What mechanical devices in place help to ensure oxygen delivery? How would you pick up a line crossover? How would you manage it? What if, before the case starts, the line isolation monitor goes off? What if it occurs in the middle of the case?

2. The patient has herpes zoster of the thorax and is in intense pain. How can you help? What if zoster is on the face? If the patient had pancreatic cancer, what block would you use? What if the patient has complex regional pain syndrome (CRPS) of the arm?

3. How do you ensure adequate flow during CPB? Is flow the same as pressure? Give an illustration of the difference. What does the mixed venous blood gas

value tell you? What if acidosis develops on bypass? You are going to come off, and the patient's potassium level is 7.2 mEq/L. What is the treatment? If the hematocrit was 19%, would you come off?

Update: Paroxysmal Nocturnal Hemoglobinuria

1. What is paroxysmal nocturnal hemoglobinuria? It is an acquired hemolytic anemia characterized by activation of the complement system. Death results most often from thromboembolism.
2. How would you treat a pregnant patient? Use steroids, heparin, and blood and blood products. You want to avoid fulminant hemolysis and thrombosis. You avoid regional anesthesia because the patient has low levels of platelets, and you have to start heparin right away.
3. Is pain control problematic? Yes. If the patient gets respiratory acidosis, it could trigger hemolysis. If she gets stress from pain, it could also trigger hemolysis.

CASE 55: ACOUSTIC NEUROMA AND HISTORY OF FEVER

A 17-year-old, 50-kg boy requires intracranial and extracranial surgery for an acoustic neuroma. The intracranial portion will be done in the sitting position. He had a tonsillectomy and adenoidectomy at age 7 and apparently had a high temperature for several hours in the postoperative period. His blood pressure is 100/50 mm Hg, pulse is 68 beats/min, respiratory rate is 12 breaths/min, temperature is 37°C, and hemoglobin level is 12 g/dL.

Preoperative Questions

1. For routine assessment in a healthy patient, does a big operation require more preoperative testing than a smaller one? What laboratory tests do you need? What are the risks of doing lots of laboratory tests? What are the costs and medicolegal concerns?
2. What clues about MH do you look for in the history? Do you get old charts? What do you look for on an old chart? Do you get a muscle biopsy?
3. Do you use premedication for a nervous teenager? How do you explain the risk? He heard about "people waking up" in the middle of an operation. What do you tell him? Do you give Valium the night before?

Intraoperative Questions

1. Given this particular operation, what are special monitoring needs? Do you need an arterial line, CVP line, precordial Doppler, or TEE? What if the patient has a heart murmur? What is the best way to detect air emboli?
2. How does the concern about MH affect the anesthetic? What is the effect of inhaled agents compared with intravenous agents on ICP? Which muscle relaxants do you use and why? What is the importance of "no bucking" in an intracranial case? What about while sitting and in pins?
3. In the middle of a case, the patient makes a big gasping effort despite good muscle relaxation. What is the differential diagnosis? What is your response if you suspect air embolus?

4. "The brain is bulging!" exclaims the surgeon, who curses you and the next seven generations of your family for all eternity unless you can "unswell" the brain. What do you do?
5. What are the fluid requirements of a 12-hour operation? What are fluid needs in the face of mannitol, Lasix, or potassium replacement? What are the dangers?

Postoperative Questions

1. The patient is nonresponsive but breathing on arrival in the PACU. How do you manage ventilator support, and when can you safely extubate?
2. The patient is rigid, fighting, and hypertensive in the PACU. His systolic blood pressure is 200 mm Hg, and the surgeon does not want it to be more than 150 mm Hg. What is your management plan? Do you need more than one drug? Would you use Precedex, a narcotic, Versed, or propofol? How will you "unsedate" and do a neurologic evaluation?
3. The patient is hoarse 2 days later. How do you evaluate the situation? What do you tell the patient? Do you seek a consultation? What is the cost of that? The patient says, "I don't want to pay for another damned doctor!"

Grab Bag

1. What are anesthetic risks for a child with a tracheoesophageal fistula? Does the type of fistula matter? What are the different kinds of fistulas? How do you induce anesthesia in such a patient?
2. A 30-year-old man in end-stage renal failure presents with appendicitis. His potassium level is 6.5 mEq/L and hemoglobin level is 7 g/dL. What is the significance of the potassium level? Can you treat this acutely? Do you dialyze or transfuse? Can you do this with a spinal or an epidural? Are there any problems with coagulation?
3. In radiology, a man getting an intravenous pyelogram is fiery red, stridorous, and hypotensive. What is the cause, and how do you treat this? Differentiate anaphylactic from anaphylactoid reaction. How does epinephrine work? Because vasopressin works for codes now, why not use that instead of epinephrine?

Update: Mediastinal Lipomatosis

1. What is mediastinal lipomatosis? It is a benign condition with increased collection of adipose tissue in the mediastinum, leading to mediastinal widening.
2. Who gets it? People who are on long-term steroids who have developed Cushing's syndrome and people who are obese develop mediastinal lipomatosis.
3. What can it mimic? It can mimic mediastinal mass and cardiomegaly.
4. What practical difficulties can it present? The superior vena cava gets compressed, making central line placement difficult.

CASE 56: LABOR AND A LANGUAGE BARRIER

An 18-year-old, 62-kg immigrant from Laos is admitted in labor. She is 7 cm dilated and screaming, "Baby, baby!" Her blood pressure is 170/100 mm Hg, pulse is 100 beats/min, respiratory rate is 24 breaths/min, and temperature is 37.5°C.

Preoperative Questions

1. What laboratory tests do you want and why? Do you need the patient's bleeding time, a platelet function test result, or TEG information?
2. How do you get informed consent? No one in the department speaks Laotian. Can the husband be a translator? Who signs the forms? There is no consent form in her language. Now what?
3. Between contractions, her blood pressure is normal. Does she have preeclampsia? Differentiate preeclampsia from eclampsia.
4. She is positive for cannabis on her toxicology screen. Does that matter to you? On examination, she has a 2/6 systolic murmur. How do you know whether it is significant?

Intraoperative Questions

1. For epidural placement, what are the advantages and disadvantages of sitting or lying on the side? What if fetal heart rate drops when she sits up? What is uteroplacental instability, and how do you determine fetal well-being?
2. Which local anesthetic do you use and why? Do you use a combined spinal and epidural? Do you add narcotics to one or both? What are the risks of respiratory depression in the mother and fetus?
3. How can you tell if there is a wet tap? What is the treatment? Should you put in a catheter and do a continuous spinal? What are the risks of doing that?
4. At 8 cm, the fetal heart rate drops to 60 beats/min. What are the options? Should you proceed immediately to a cesarean section? Can the husband come along to the OR? If not, when?
5. Regional anesthesia fails at the cesarean section incision. What are the options? You use general anesthesia but cannot intubate. What now?

Postoperative Questions

1. In the PACU after a general anesthetic, you see a bloody stump of an ex-tooth. How do you manage this?
2. You had to do a tracheostomy intraoperatively to save the mother. What do you say to the husband?
3. The nursing supervisor asks for guidelines after epidural narcotic administration. What do you tell the supervisor?

Grab Bag

1. The roofer falls off—what else?—a roof and has multiple rib fractures. What are the options for pain relief? He has a chest tube. Can you use that for an intrapleural catheter? What are the pros and cons of intercostal blocks compared with a thoracic epidural and with PCA?
2. Where might DIC occur? How do you make the diagnosis? How do you treat?
3. You just gave 50 mg of rocuronium, and the surgeon says, "Oh, no!" and closes after only 10 minutes. Do you reverse? How do you assess? Do you put the patient on a ventilator? What do you tell the respiratory specialist? How do you sedate? Do you use propofol, Precedex, or narcotics? You have to leave and start another case? What do you tell the PACU nurse?
4. How do fluid guidelines differ in children and adults? What is the difference in NPO status, pain control, and airway management?

Update: Sickle Cell Disease

1. What are the most common clinical problems? Bony involvement is common, but any arterial bed can be involved, especially the spleen and the kidneys.
2. Can you use a tourniquet? Traditionally, people said no, but one group did an exchange transfusion on a sickle cell patient and then used bilateral tourniquets to do bilateral knee replacements. So in certain cases, you can use tourniquets.
3. Is sickle cell disease confined to blacks? No. It also manifests in people from south Italy, Greece, Turkey, and the Arabian Gulf, especially those from Saudi Arabia.

CASE 57: BLEEDING TONSIL AND SHOCK

A 5-year-old, 20-kg boy had a tonsillectomy and adenoidectomy at 2 PM. It is now 10 PM, and his mother came screeching into the ER in her Ford Expedition, almost hitting an emergency medical technician who was smoking a Pall Mall in the "this is a nonsmoking facility" area. The child's blood pressure is 80/50 mm Hg, pulse is 150 beats/min, and respiratory rate is 30 breaths/min. On physical examination, the child is listless.

Preoperative Questions

1. How do you evaluate the volume status in a child or in an adult? How do you estimate blood loss? What will the effect of positive-pressure ventilation be on a severely hypovolemic patient?
2. No one in the ER can place an intravenous line. How will you help? Can you place a central line in the ER? How about an intraosseous line? How will you get a blood sample for type and cross? Do you transfuse in the ER or run to the OR?
3. The mother is Jehovah's Witness and "refuses blood for my kin." What is your response? Do you accept the "watch tower" that she offers you?
4. Do you need any laboratory test results before going to the OR?

Intraoperative Questions

1. The intravenous line from the ER infiltrated, and the surgeon says, "We gotta go!" What do you do? The laboratory says they have only type-specific blood. Do you give it? Are there any special considerations if the patient is a girl? What is the effect on subsequent pregnancies?
2. How do you induce in the face of blood loss? Do you use ketamine or etomidate? Can you use inhalation induction with blood in the stomach? Can you use a relaxant only if the patient is moribund? What about using scopolamine?
3. After induction, blood pressure is unobtainable. What is the differential diagnosis? Do you feel a pulse? What are the hazards of waiting for a Dinamap blood pressure monitor? What about CO_2 production? Do you use a pulse oximeter? What is the treatment of PEA?
4. What is your end point for transfusion?
5. Near the end of the case, the child starts wheezing, and you get stuck in a washing machine cycle: lighten, wheeze, resedate, lighten, wheeze, resedate. How do you get out of this cycle?

Postoperative Questions

1. The chest radiograph shows fluffy infiltrate, and you are pretty sure the child aspirated blood. How do you manage this? It progresses to ARDS. What is the concept of the "best PEEP"?
2. The mother tells you later that her child had recall. What do you say to the mother and the child? What is the risk of PTSD in a recall patient? What are the medicolegal implications and documentation of a complication?

Grab Bag

1. A child with a congenital diaphragmatic hernia is intubated, but his saturation level is still 75%. What do you do? How do you reconcile the need for O_2 with the risk of retrolental fibroplasia?
2. A colleague never uses his nerve stimulator because he does not feel he needs it. At a hospital meeting, it comes out that he has the highest rate of reintubation in the department. What do you say to the hospital administrator, and what do you say to your partner?
3. A man inhales the glass stem of a crack pipe. The surgeon cannot place a large, rigid bronchoscope to fish it out. How will you oxygenate this patient as the surgeon finds a way to get that crack pipe out? Author tip: Think this is a good one? It's a complete exam question elsewhere in this book. And this is a case I DID MYSELF! (It was horrible.)

Update: Endoscopic Thoracic Sympathectomy

1. Describe the procedure of endoscopic thoracic sympathectomy. Through a scope, the surgeon sections the T2-4 sympathetic nerves. This procedure is used in the treatment of palmar or axillary hyperhidrosis.
2. What is the anesthetic concern? These are the cardiac accelerator nerves, so you worry that there may be a dangerous bradycardia or suppressed baroreceptor reflex.
3. Is it so? In a study of patients with bilateral sympathectomies, they had a poor response to decreasing blood pressure. If a patient lost a lot of blood, he might not be able to increase his heart rate in response.
4. What about someone after sympathectomy coming for another operation? The patient's heart is "denervated" from a response point of view.

CASE 58: LUNG RESECTION AND A BAD AIRWAY

A 70-year-old, 100-kg man with a hundred pack-year smoking history is scheduled for bronchoscopy and right upper lobe resection. His airway examination shows a thick neck and tongue, large teeth, and a Mallampati 4 view. The hematocrit is 54%, blood pressure is 150/90 mm Hg, and pulse is 80 beats/min. The patient is afebrile.

Preoperative Questions

1. How do you determine who has a difficult airway? Do you need C-spine films or ENT evaluation? What do you tell a patient with a difficult airway?
2. What are you looking for in the PFTs? What if the values are all less than 50%? Do you cancel the case?

3. The surgeon says he will be done quickly and that an ICU stay will be a "waste of hospital money." What do you say?

4. The patient fears getting "paralyzed from that needle in my back. I watch Oprah, you know." How do you explain this risk?

5. The ABG result shows the infamous "60/60" partial pressures of O_2 and CO_2. How will this affect your plan?

Intraoperative Questions

1. Do you put the arterial line, CVP line, or an epidural in while the patient is awake? Why or why not for each? What is the risk for neural injury compared with the patient's comfort and acceptance?

2. The patient has a difficult airway, but there is no way you can place a double-lumen tube for lung isolation. What do you tell the surgeon? What are the options? Is awake intubation possible? How does a Univent work or a bronchial blocker?

3. You drop the lung, but the surgeon said you did not. How do you manage this?

4. The saturation level drops for one lung. What is the differential diagnosis, and what is the treatment?

5. The surgeon enters the pulmonary artery, and massive bleeding occurs. What do you do?

6. With chest closure, the inspiratory pressures go to 60 cm H_2O, and alarms go off like crazy. What is the differential diagnosis, and what is the treatment?

Postoperative Questions

1. You placed an epidural, but 2 hours later, the patient is in agony. How do you evaluate and solve this problem before the pain service jumps down your throat?

2. You placed a double-lumen tube, but the surgeon wants it replaced with a single-lumen tube. How do you accomplish this safely? Do you use a tube changer or fiberoptic scope? Do you refuse to change the tube?

3. The patient arrests in the PACU. What are the most likely causes? What do you do?

Grab Bag

1. A 55-year-old, 110-kg woman presents for panendoscopy for a postpharyngeal mass. She is scared of an awake intubation, because she had one last time, and it was brutal. What do you do?

2. A healthy 3-year-old boy is scheduled for myringotomies. His mother relates that he is "a little muscle man" with very large gastrocnemius muscles. Do you proceed or pursue other diagnoses? Do you use suxamethonium?

3. A pregnant woman presents for an appendectomy. She is 27 weeks' pregnant. How do you manage her anesthetic and allay her fears about the baby? Do you involve the obstetrician? Do you use a fetal heart rate monitor? Where do you put it?

Update: Vasopressin and Shock

1. How does vasopressin work in relation to shock? Hypotension induces secretion of vasopressin from the hypophysis, contributing to blood pressure stabilization.

2. Why do vasopressin levels then fall? In septic shock, the vasopressin stores are depleted.
3. What does vasopressin do to splanchnic circulation? It redistributes the flow.
4. What is vasopressin's effect on the heart? Like all vasoconstrictors, vasopressin decreases cardiac output.
5. Is vasopressin the magic bullet? No. It did not show any improvement over norepinephrine.
6. Author experience: Vasopressin is handy when nothing else is getting the pressure up.

CASE 59: HYPERTENSION AND CAROTID ENDARTERECTOMY

A 60-year-old man with hypertension is scheduled for a right carotid endarterectomy. His blood pressure is 180/106 mm Hg. He takes glyburide "when he feels like it," and his blood sugar level is 240 mg/dL. The surgeon is concerned about any delay because the lesion is "ragged," and the patient could "stroke at any minute."

Preoperative Questions

1. Is a more extensive workup needed? How does carotid disease correlate with heart disease or with silent ischemia? What is the cost of the complete workup, including complications?
2. At what point is the blood pressure too high to operate? What is the danger of putting off the operation? What is the danger of dropping the blood pressure to "normal" in the face of carotid obstruction?
3. What laboratory tests do you need, given the small blood loss you face?
4. Do you use EEG intraoperatively? Do you use a local with sedation? Do you go for broke with a shunt? What is best way to monitor the brain?

Intraoperative Questions

1. How do you perform a block for a carotid endarterectomy? What if the patient becomes dyspneic in the middle of the block? What is the differential diagnosis, and what is the treatment?
2. In the middle of the case, a blocked patient suddenly gets agitated, but the neck is wide open. What do you do?
3. You pull back the drapes, and while the surgeon is screaming bloody murder, you see the patient has vomited. What is your next move?
4. You induce. How do you keep the blood pressure from getting too high?
5. The EEG technician says she sees a worrisome drop in the signal with cross-clamping. What can you do?
6. You give protamine to reverse the heparin, and the blood pressure drops to 60/30 mm Hg. What is the treatment?

Postoperative Questions

1. In the PACU, the patient suddenly develops unilateral weakness. What do you do?
2. Two hours postoperatively, an ICU nurse pages you and says the patient's tongue is "sticking way out." What is the differential diagnosis, and what is the treatment?

3. How would you diagnose whether the surgeon cut the recurrent laryngeal nerve?

Grab Bag

1. Five hours after CABG, how would you suspect, diagnose, confirm, and treat cardiac tamponade? What medical therapy do you use to buy time? When do you yourself open in the ICU? Compare the risk of infection with survival.
2. During a routine knee case, a young, healthy patient went nodal for a short time, but he had no consequences. He wakes up fine. Can he go home, or do you need to observe him?
3. Do you need to perform temperature correction for blood gases during CPB or when a patient comes in with severe hypothermia? Why or why not? What is the physiologic principle behind temperature correction, and does it make a difference?

Update: Laparoscopic Procedures in the Head-Down Position

1. What is the concern about laparoscopic procedures in the head-down position? With all that time with the head down, venous return may be impaired and cause cerebral ischemia.
2. Well, does it? No. Transcranial Doppler ultrasound shows that the cerebral perfusion is maintained.
3. What are the effects of the pneumoperitoneum? The intra-abdominal pressure increase causes an increase in the ICP. This should be done with caution in patients with intracranial pathology.

CASE 60: ARTHRITIS AND A VALVE REPLACEMENT

A 75-year-old woman with severe arthritis is scheduled for a mitral valve replacement. The airway appears difficult. Her laboratory test results are normal, as are her vital signs. As you are talking to her, the surgeon calls and tells you she will need "a few bypasses, too."

Preoperative Questions

1. What special dangers does "left main disease" pose? Compare it with run-of-the-mill CAD. Compare stable and unstable angina.
2. Does it matter whether the patient has regurgitation or stenosis? Why? How is anesthesia managed differently for these two conditions?
3. What organ systems are involved by arthritis, and how does that affect the anesthetic?
4. You cannot find an EF value anywhere on the chart. Do you insist they repeat the echocardiogram and get that damned EF?

Intraoperative Questions

1. How do you determine who needs an awake intubation? Can you do one in a CAD patient? The surgeon freaks and says, "Put her to sleep. No one *ever* does my patients this way!"

2. You cannot move her neck at all and opt against an intrajugular central line. What are your other options? Can you place a femoral or subclavian line? What are the risks and advantages of both?
3. The pulmonary artery pressures double, and TEE shows a dilating ventricle as the surgeon is taking down the internal mammary artery. What do you do?
4. How do you safely separate this patient from CPB?
5. Bleeding is problematic after bypass. What is the differential diagnosis, and what is the treatment? How do Amicar and protamine work?

Postoperative Questions

1. The surgeon wants the patient extubated as soon as possible. You want the difficult airway protected. How do you reconcile these two needs?
2. The ICU nurse cannot get the Swan-Ganz catheter to wedge. What do you do?
3. The ICU nurse gets the Swan-Ganz catheter to wedge, but now there is bleeding through the ETT. What is the differential diagnosis, and what is the treatment?

Grab Bag

1. A 5-week-old, 3-kg boy presents for pyloromyotomy for pyloric stenosis. He is listless and will not take milk. His blood pressure is 50/30 mm Hg, pulse is 120 beats/min, respiratory rate is 30 breaths/min, temperature is 36.5°C, hemoglobin level is 18 g/dL, sodium level is 143 mEq/L, and potassium level is 2.5 mEq/L. How do you proceed with this emergent case?
2. A 29-year-old woman who is 28 weeks' pregnant presents for evacuation of a subarachnoid hemorrhage. The surgeon plans to clip an arteriovenous malformation and needs controlled hypotension. The current blood pressure is 160/100 mm Hg. How do you manage this?
3. A 27-year-old man presents for resection of a pheochromocytoma. He has had headache, palpitations, sweating, and nervousness for 4 months. His current blood pressure is 170/110 mm Hg, and the pulse is 125 beats/min. Do you continue? If not, how do you optimize him and for how long?

Update: Atelectasis

1. How often does atelectasis occur in the anesthetized patient? It occurs in 90% of anesthetized patients.
2. What favors its formation? It is favored by the use of 100% O_2 and by not using PEEP.
3. What is your recommendation? Use PEEP. Avoid 100% O_2 if possible.

CASE 61: PREECLAMPSIA

A 30-year-old primigravida is at 39 weeks' gestation and has been admitted from the obstetrician's office with severe preeclampsia. She has a headache, blurred vision, edema, and a 6-kg weight gain. She took no medications during her pregnancy except vitamins and iron. Now she is on magnesium and just got 10 mg of hydralazine. She has a Foley catheter, which shows scant urine, and it is dark. Her blood pressure is 190/110 mm Hg, pulse is 90 beats/min, respiratory rate is 24 breaths/min (she is puffing), and temperature is 38°C. Laboratory results show a creatinine level of 1.8 mg/dL, and blood urea nitrogen (BUN) of 48 mg/dL.

Preoperative Questions

1. Is there anything else you want to do before going to the OR, such as more magnesium or more hydralazine? Do you start nitroglycerin or Nipride? Should you at least mix them up and have them ready? Do you really need to cover up sodium nitroprusside with a dark thing, or is that an urban myth? Do you need any more laboratory studies? If you could have one, which would you have to best assess coagulation?
2. How do you evaluate fetal well-being before going to the OR? What are you looking for? Explain the sinister and the not-so-sinister patterns of fetal heart rates. Do you need a fetal scalp pH? What is the risk of that?
3. Do you have a fiberoptic scope ready for an obstetric case? Why? What do you have on the difficult intubation cart? Do you have a separate light source? How do you train the nursing staff so they do not give you blank stares when you ask for the "difficult airway stuff"?

Intraoperative Questions

1. Do you place any invasive monitors? Based on what guidelines? Is there proof that any of this makes any difference? Is a critically trained finger on the pulse or a STAT setting on the blood pressure cuff just as good? The patient wiggles like thunder when you attempt to place an arterial line, and it is even worse with a central line. Do you sedate her? What is the risk to the fetus? What do you tell the pediatrician? What if the patient is truly honest-to-God psychotic and uncontrollable?
2. You place the pulmonary artery catheter, and the wedge pressure is 6 mm Hg, the cardiac output is 6, the CVP is 6 mm Hg, and the mean blood pressure is still sky high at 140 mm Hg. How will you manage this? Will you use an inotrope or a dilator? How do you mix, and how do you infuse? What if the pump fails, and the stuff runs in wide open? Should the "666" coincidence make your hair stand on end?
3. Do you use regional or general anesthesia? Why? If you use an epidural, how low will you go with the platelet count? Even if the count is low, is it better to not lose the airway or risk an epidural hematoma?
4. Do you add opioid to epidural? Which one and how much? Do you add opioid to a spinal? How much, what kind of needle, and what time do you expect to get from it?
5. The PT is 18 seconds, and the platelet count is 25,000/mm^3. You go with general anesthesia. What measures do you take to avoid an intracranial bleed? Which induction agents do you use? How do you blunt the sympathetic response to intubation but not hurt the fetus?
6. Thirty minutes after a tough intubation (three attempts and you possibly flaked an upper incisor), you see the SaO_2 is 91% on 50% oxygen. What is the approximate A-a gradient? How will you fix this? If she aspirated, is it a for-sure go to ventilation, or can you observe? How bad is bad when it comes to aspiration? What if you can still keep the saturation level above 90% on nasal cannula at the end of the case?

Postoperative Questions

1. At delivery, the child has meconium and a heart rate of 50 beats/min. Do you start CPR? Do you give bicarbonate through the ETT? What doses of epinephrine

are appropriate for a newborn or for shock? How do you prevent meconium from progressing to bronchopulmonary dysplasia (BPD)? What is BPD?

2. Twenty-four hours after surgery, the patient seizes. What is the treatment? Do you intubate or give pentathol and make the seizure go away? What if she just ate a celebration dinner?

3. The next day, she complains of back pain, and her legs feel weak. What is the differential diagnosis, and what is the treatment? Do you get a CT scan? How much time do you have before she is permanently paralyzed?

Grab Bag

1. You cannot wean a patient from CPB after mitral valve replacement because of hypotension. How will you diagnose the problem and get the patient off CPB?

2. A 65-year-old, 70-kg man with arthritis presents for total knee replacement. The surgeon does these operations under spinal anesthesia, but you are spooked about the airway. How do you proceed?

3. You are dozing off in the middle of an intramedullary rodding of the femur, when your CO_2 line fills up with yellowish fluid and occludes. The patient's hemodynamic status takes a dive. What happened, and what do you do? (Note: this, too, is a "full stem" elsewhere. And yes, it's another disaster I did myself.)

Update: Anaphylaxis

1. What does the Greek term *anaphylaxis* mean? It means antiprotection. *Prophylaxis* means protection.

2. What do you usually see under anesthesia? Because the cutaneous signs are under the drapes, we see respiratory and cardiovascular signs such as hypotension and bronchospasm.

3. What are the most common causes? Muscle relaxants and latex can cause anaphylaxis.

4. What is the treatment? Stop the offending agent, such as fluids or epinephrine.

5. Why epinephrine? Its α-adrenergic effect supports the blood pressure, and its β-adrenergic effect relaxes the bronchial tree.

CASE 62: CAROTID ENDARTERECTOMY AND HEART TROUBLES

A 70-year-old, 80-kg man is scheduled to have a right carotid endarterectomy. He has had several TIAs but has no residual. He has a long history of high blood pressure and high cholesterol. His blood pressure is 190/110 mm Hg, pulse is 55 beats/min, and respiratory rate is 18 breaths/min. The ECG shows sinus bradycardia and a left anterior hemiblock. He takes Lasix, digoxin, and metoprolol.

Preoperative Questions

1. Is the blood pressure adequately controlled? Why or why not? Do you need to increase his medications? The surgeon says, "The damned internist will not do anything anyway because the patient is on Medicaid, so we may as well go." Which antihypertensive would you add? Would you use an ACE inhibitor or vasoactive drip in the ICU, or will sedatives alone do the trick?

2. Do sinus bradycardia and left anterior hemiblock mean anything? Do you need a more extensive cardiac workup? What kind? Is cost a consideration?

Do you need a pacer? Do you test with atropine to see if anything loosens up? Discuss normal innervation of the heart in terms of conduction. What if the patient has a first-degree block in addition to the other maladies?

3. What is a TIA? What is the prognosis? How do you know the TIA is not "coming from" the heart? What if he were in atrial fibrillation? What is atrial fibrillation? Why does the heart not go into ventricular fibrillation when atrial fibrillation is present?

Intraoperative Questions

1. What special monitors will you use and why? Do you use the V_5 lead to monitor ischemia? Is that sufficient? What are the risks of an arterial line? What are risks of no arterial line? Has anyone ever looked at that? How would you design such a study?
2. You want a smooth wake-up process. You will be using an EEG, but you do not want to harm the patient with too low or too high of a heart rate, or too much blood pressure swing-osis. How will you do it? What are the two factors watched on the EEG? Is it better to do him awake so you can see for yourself that his brain is perfused?
3. Describe the organ systems at risk if the blood pressure goes to low. How long can a low pressure stay low and still not harm, for example, the kidneys? At cross-clamping, what do you do with the pressure and how? Do you need a central line if you are going to infuse all this inotropic stuff? What if the peripheral line infiltrates, and you had Levophed going?
4. Which muscle relaxants do you use and why? How will you monitor when you cannot get at anything, do not want to bump the head, and the arms are tucked?
5. At cross-clamping, do you give a slug of pentathol? Why or why not? What is your rationale for such a maneuver? Why not use propofol?
6. Should you keep CO_2? Where and why?
7. During dissection, the heart rate drops to the 20s. What next? How can you be sure the circle of Willis is doing its collateral thing and keeping the brain perfused? Is using the BIS monitor as good as an EEG?

Postoperative Questions

1. The patient fails to awaken at the end of the case. How long do you wait, and what do you do while you are waiting? Do you give a bolus of barbiturates for cerebral protection? Do you re-explore? Do you obtain CT or angiography? Do you get echocardiography for the neck? Do you hyperventilate or hypoventilate?
2. Swing the other way; the patient wakes up a Ragin' Cajun, coughing and sputtering, ready to pop open the stitches. What do you do in this case?
3. The nurse calls you over and asks if the ST changes are new. What are all the steps you take to ensure the myocardium does not suffer? What is the difference between ST depression and ST elevation?

Grab Bag

1. A 28-year-old woman is 14 weeks' pregnant, but her carpal tunnel disease is preventing her from sleeping at night, and she is going nuts. Do you do this elective case even though she is pregnant? How? What if you have to convert to general anesthesia? What do you tell her about the risk to the fetus?

2. The general surgeon says, "Do not use nitrous; it makes the guts swell up." Do you agree? Be a Talmudic scholar and argue that there is no place for nitrous in modern anesthetic practice. Now argue that there is a place for nitrous, and explain where that place is.
3. Compare the available arm blocks. Which is best for which procedure? Which is better than general anesthesia? What are the risks of each and the treatment for complications?

Update: Nitric Oxide

1. What is the theoretical advantage of nitric oxide in the treatment of ARDS? As a vascular endothelial derived relaxing factor, it should help with oxygenation and right ventricular off-loading.
2. What does it do? There is a transient increase in oxygenation but no improvement in outcome.
3. What, besides cost, are other concerns about NO? It inhibits the immune response and is a free radical that leads to toxic intermediates. It can cause methemoglobinemia at levels greater than 40 parts per million (ppm).
4. Has the U.S. Food and Drug Administration (FDA) approved it for treatment of hypoxic respiratory failure? No.

CASE 63: OPEN REDUCTION AND INTERNAL FIXATION OF THE HUMERUS

A 65-year-old, 45-kg woman is scheduled for ORIF of a compound fracture of the humerus. She fell off a roof 3 hours earlier. She is lethargic and hoarse. The woman is on thyroid replacement therapy, but she has not been remembering to take it lately. The patient's blood pressure is 90/50 mm Hg, pulse is 50 beats/min, respiratory rate is 10 breaths/min, hematocrit is 29%, and temperature is 35.9°C.

Preoperative Questions

1. Why is she lethargic? What about CNS problems, drugs, sepsis, and sedatives from the ER? How do you figure out the cause? Does it matter?
2. Is she on adequate thyroid replacement? What in her physical examination and vital signs tells you she might by hypothyroid? What other examination findings do you expect to see? What would her thyroid test results show?
3. She fell pretty far. What other injuries should you entertain? Do you need a head CT, or are you going with the presumptive diagnosis of hypothyroidism? What is the danger of not uncovering other injuries (e.g., pneumothorax, ruptured spleen, intracranial bleed)?

Intraoperative Questions

1. A colleague suggests an interscalene block. Do you agree? What are the pros and cons? Walk through how you would do an interscalene block, mentioning the landmarks and pitfalls. Just after you inject, the patient rolls her eyes back and goes limp. What is the differential diagnosis, and what is the treatment? After you snatch her from the closing jaws of death, the damned block does not work. What now? Discuss dosing for lipid emulsion in such a case.
2. Because she is hypothyroid, do you give her some thyroxine? Do you support her hemodynamically? How long will it take the thyroid replacement

therapy to do anything for her? Because she may be unstable, do you need a CVP or Swan-Ganz catheter?

3. While you are giving blood, she starts to ooze, her pressure drops, and red appears in the urine. What is happening? What is the treatment for a transfusion reaction? Should you alkalinize the urine? Do you need a CVP line? What, besides death, are the risks of a transfusion reaction?

4. The heart rate drops into the 30s. What is the treatment? How do you proceed? Do you put in a line and drop a wire? What are the risks associated with that? Do you place an external pacer? How do you set the buttons on the stupid thing after it is on the patient?

Postoperative Questions

1. Ten hours have passed, and the arm still is not moving. The patient is starting to panic. Is this a nerve injury, long block, or ischemia? What is the proposed mechanism of local anesthetic–induced neurotoxicity? How can you prevent it?

2. The surgeon asks for a continuous regional for pain relief. Is it a good idea? How do you do it? Who watches? What are the possible complications? What if the arm gets too numb, and the patient cannot protect it?

3. Oops! There are three little burns where the ECG pads were. What happened? Explain the concept of current density. How does a Bovie work? Why does it need to be grounded? What is a ground?

Grab Bag

1. Why do we electrically isolate the ORs? In a simple diagram, show how a line isolation monitor works. What is the difference between microshock and macroshock?

2. The patient has an open eye and full stomach. Do you avoid suxamethonium? What is the danger of using other relaxants? Do you need to paralyze the patient during eye surgery? How do you prevent coughing and bucking? What if you are asked by the state to review a case in which bucking led to blindness? Do you discipline the anesthesiologist?

3. Five minutes after placing a spinal, the patient becomes cyanotic, and the pulse is unobtainable. What will you do? What is the mechanism of a high spinal?

4. Meconium is seen at delivery. What does this mean? How will you manage a neonatal resuscitation if the pediatrician got in a car wreck on the way in? How do you manage choanal atresia?

Update: Esophageal Perforation and Intubation

1. What is the cause of the esophageal perforation? Usually, a styletted tube tears the mucosa during a difficult intubation.

2. What physical examination signs will you see? The patient will have subcutaneous emphysema.

3. What constitutes the best prophylaxis? Do an awake intubation—what else could you want?

4. What is the treatment? Use a nasogastric tube, drainage, and antibiotics.

5. Where are the most common sites of perforation? The piriform sinus and posterior esophageal wall are the most common sites.

6. What symptoms do patients complain about? They report neck, shoulder, chest, and back pain. Because it is so serious, do urgent endoscopy or water-soluble contrast radiography as soon as possible.

CASE 64: RENAL TRANSPLANTATION AND ANEMIA

A 45-year-old man is scheduled to receive a living-related renal transplant. He has edema, hypertension to 175/100 mm Hg, a potassium level of 4.8 mEq/L (dialyzed yesterday), and a hemoglobin level of 7.3 g/dL.

Preoperative Questions

1. How is dialysis performed? Compare the process through a shunt and through a Shiley? What are the risks of dialysis? It can be too dry, and aluminum toxicity can be a problem. The arteriovenous shunt bypasses the lung "filter," so the patient can get high output failure and sepsis. Because of the use of heparin, the patient can bleed if he goes right to the OR after dialysis. It is hard to get lines if they have just been "wrung out."
2. Why are renal patients so often hypertensive? What is a Goldblatt kidney? Why is the patient so anemic? Should he get cranked on erythropoietin before the case? What is the risk of that? Should he be transfused?
3. How do you know where a renal patient is from a volume standpoint? Is it all by guessing and by God's grace until you get a line in the patient?

Intraoperative Questions

1. How do you monitor this patient? Do you need an arterial line and CVP catheter for every renal treatment? Do you need a Swan-Ganz catheter? Why not use TEE and avoid all those big sticks?
2. Can you do regional if his platelet count is okay? Do you need a platelet function study because his plasma is uremic? Where is the kidney put? Would an epidural do the trick?
3. How will you induce? Will you use a modified or generic RSI? Do renal failure patients empty their stomachs well? What is the benefit of a modified RSI compared with the real thing? Does cricotracheotomy help?
4. It is an unexpectedly difficult intubation. Go through the steps you would adopt from the difficult airway algorithm. Describe use of the Eschmann intubating stylet. Has this been proved to make a difference?
5. How would you tell there is an anesthetic machine disconnect? What other alarms and safety mechanisms are on our machine? What is the diameter index safety system (DISS)?

Postoperative Questions

1. How do you manage postoperative pain? Do you administer an epidural? What if heparin is given during the case? What if the platelet count was only 120,000/mm^3 before the case? What are the advantages for the patient? Is it better than PCA? What are advantages of PCA? What do you put in it—sufentanil, fentanyl, MS, Dilaudid, or Demerol?
2. You ran in all kinds of anti-rejection drugs during the case, and the patient's lungs seem to be turning to wood. On 100% O_2, the Pao_2 is only 61 mm Hg. What do you do? Extubate? What are the absolute indications for intubation? For that matter, what are the absolute indications for lung isolation?
3. In the PACU, the CVP is 20 mm Hg, but there is still no urine output. The surgeon says, "Give fluids. That kidney looked good and will open up!" What is your response?

Grab Bag

1. Parents tell you their kid hated his last ear tube placement and is scared stiff now. How can you allay their fears? Do you premedicate? Which drug and route do you use? Does it vary according to age? Do you let the parents into the room? Both of them? What if the kid gets blue and the mother goes nuts?
2. During a case, the inspired CO_2 level is 12 mm Hg. How could that be? What is the danger of this level? How do you fix it? How does the soda lime absorber work?
3. A woman has had an intrauterine fetal death. She is far enough along to deliver. Do you place an epidural? If you were concerned about DIC, how would you rule this out first? Would you sedate or use narcotics? What if she wants to see the baby?

Update: Propofol in the Head-Injured Patient

1. Why use propofol in the head-injured patient? It is used often for sedation in the ICU. It has the added benefit of reducing the ICP and not accumulating, so you can turn it off and do a neurologic assessment.
2. How does propofol affect cerebral autoregulation in the healthy patient? Cerebral autoregulation is maintained.
3. What about the head-injured patient? There's the rub! Propofol can hurt cerebral autoregulation, and large doses should not be used in these patients.

CASE 65: CORONARY ARTERY BYPASS GRAFTING

A 66-year-old, 100-kg man is scheduled to have three-vessel CABG. He has a systolic murmur heard that is best over the left sternal border with the bell (third) attachment of a fancy cardiology stethoscope that only medical students seem to have. He is on an ACE inhibitor and metoprolol. The patient is afebrile, and his blood pressure is 145/85 mm Hg, pulse is 55 beats/min, and hematocrit is 13%.

Preoperative Questions

1. He has gotten the million-dollar workup already. What information do you want to extract from it? Does it really matter what vessels are involved, because we do these all the same? What is the special significance of left main disease? What if the catheterization laboratory data said he has an EF of 30%, but while obtaining his history, he tells you he does all of his normal activities and climbs stairs easily—two at a time, no less!
2. How is cardiac catheterization done? Why do catheterization laboratory EFs so often look bad, but they are better when we see them?
3. Is discussion or kick butt sedation better? Because everything is on the fast track, do you give MS and scopolamine, or what do you do?

Intraoperative Questions

1. The patient wants to be asleep before he even goes into the room. Is this feasible? How about setting the blood pressure cuff on STAT? Is that

good enough? What if the patient was mentally disabled and really could not hold still for an arterial line?

2. Would you use a CVP, Swan-Ganz, or TEE line? Why? Will you place central lines after induction? What are the pros and cons of that?

3. You put a Cordis in the carotid. What is your next move?

4. Do you induce with pentathol if the EF is good or etomidate if it is bad? Is that the way to go? Do you use high-dose narcotic maintenance or vapors as in a regular case?

5. The surgeon decides to do case off pump. What are the special concerns, and how do you manage them in an off-pump case? What are the advantages in avoiding the pump run?

6. You cannot get off bypass without inotropes. What do we have at our fingertips? Design a logical use of supportive drugs.

7. After the clamp comes off, the patient fibrillates. Four attempts to shock have no effect. What now? Do you shock again, use drugs, check gas, and check the temperature?

Postoperative Questions

1. It is all fast track now. Describe the pros and cons of extubating on the table. Would you do it? Under what circumstances?

2. Lay out the ventilator parameters and laboratory tests for a "wean to extubate in the morning" scenario.

3. How will you be able to tell whether the patient's bleeding is leading to tamponade?

Grab Bag

1. Do we need to use micropore filters when we give blood? Why or why not? What problems attend massive transfusion? How does a TEG help, and has a TEG ever been proved to help? What is a TEG?

2. What problems accompany hypothermia? What problems accompany hyperthermia? Why do we need to hook a Bair Hugger to the heating blanket? What do you do if you pull it back and see a second-degree burn on the leg? What if the blanket catches fire intraoperatively?

3. What is MAC, and how is it useful to us? Is MAC related to lipid solubility? What is related to lipid solubility? Is there a risk of airway fire with sevoflurane? How do you obviate that risk?

Update: Hypotension and Bradycardia during Shoulder Surgery with an Interscalene Block

1. What is the incidence of this maladaptive response? The incidence of hypotension and bradycardia during shoulder surgery is 13% to 28% in the sitting position.

2. What is the proposed mechanism? Venous pooling from the sitting position and increased sympathetic tone induce a low-volume hypercontractile ventricle. This results in sudden parasympathetic activation and sympathetic withdrawal (i.e., Bezold-Jarisch reflex).

3. What contributes to the problem? The use of epinephrine-containing solutions contributes to the problem. Surgeons should use epinephrine-free solutions.

CASE 66: MULTIPLE TRAUMA

A 52-year-old man in an industrial accident has a fractured jaw and three right rib fractures. He also has pain in the abdomen and is scheduled for an exploratory laparotomy. His blood pressure is 85/65 mm Hg and pulse is 140 beats/min. He is in distress. The ABG determination shows a pH of 7.22, P_{O_2} of 75 mm Hg, and P_{CO_2} of 34 mm Hg.

Preoperative Questions

1. What is the patient's volume status? Why is the blood pressure so low? Why is the heart rate so high? Besides hidden blood loss, what could account for this picture? How will you tell tension pneumothorax from cardiac tamponade from blood loss from cardiac contusion? How does cardiac contusion show up on the ECG?
2. What is pulsus paradoxicus? What is electrical alternans? Does the appearance of neck veins help? How?
3. Do you secure the airway now or go to the OR? What are the pros and cons of an off-site intubation? What if he vomits and the ER gurney will not go head down? Do you have extra stuff with you (e.g., intubating boogie, LMA-Fastrach), or do you just go with what they have in the ER? How does a Combitube work, and would you use it? If you got an LMA in, would you go up to the OR with just that or figure a way to get a fiberoptic scope down to the ER and secure the airway there? How about a cricotracheotomy? Would you use the Arndt kit? What are anatomic pitfalls of a cricotracheotomy and jet ventilation?

Intraoperative Questions

1. What is your choice of monitors? Why? The Cleveland Clinic physicians place all their arterial lines brachially, and they never seem to have a problem. Will you do what they do? Do you need a CVP line if the surgeon is anticipating a large-volume loss? Do you put the CVP line on the side of the rib fracture? Is this a good idea? Why? Compare the physiology of a tension and a nontension pneumothorax.
2. How would you induce? Because of the blow to the jaw, is the cervical spine at risk? How do you rule this out? The jaw is fractured, and after he is induced, will you be able to open it? What if a fragment is stuck in the TMJ? How will you know ahead of time?
3. For maintenance, do you avoid N_2O? Why? If the chest tube is in, is N_2O okay? Is N_2O a myocardial depressant? Is it better to go with all narcotics? What is the danger of recall? Do you use scopolamine to prevent recall if the patient is unstable? What is the danger of scopolamine?
4. The patient becomes hypotensive immediately after induction. What is the differential diagnosis, and what is the treatment? What volume do you use to resuscitate, and what is your end point? What are the problems with massive transfusions?

Postoperative Questions

1. You extubate at the end of the case. The patient makes a deep inspiratory effort but is obstructed. Shortly after that, he desaturates, and pink frothy

foam comes out of his mouth. What happened? Discuss the Starling forces at work. What is the treatment? What if his jaw is wired shut? Do you try blind nasal passage? What is the risk if he has a Le Fort fracture?

2. You opt for multiple intercostal blocks. How would you do it, and what is the risk? What is the maximum amount of local you can put in there? Is levobupivacaine safer? Is epinephrine safer?

3. Because the Foley catheter had no output, you gave another 3 L of fluid. The nurse goes, "AAG!" The Foley catheter was kinked, and the bladder is now huge. What do you do? Do you call a genitourinary specialist? Do you forget about it?

Grab Bag

1. A 40-year-old woman has burning pain in her left hand 2 months after fracturing her radial head. How will you evaluate this? What is the treatment? What are the options? What if there is no improvement after one stellate ganglion block? What are the potential complications of a stellate ganglion block?

2. You hang some penicillin for an oral surgery case, and the patient develops erythema, hypotension, and wheezing. What is the mechanism of this problem? How will you treat it? It progresses to PEA. What do you do?

3. A woman who was a difficult intubation is going for magnetic resonance imaging (MRI). She has an armored tube in, which will explode because there is metal in it. The surgeon asks you to change it to a regular tube. How will you do this?

Update: Anesthesia in the Civil War

1. How many anesthetics were delivered during the Civil War? The estimated number is 80,000.
2. Which anesthetic was used most? Chloroform was used most often. The flammability of ether was problematic.
3. How was it delivered? It was dripped onto a cloth or paper in the shape of a cone with a sponge at the apex.
4. Which famous cavalry general administered an anesthetic to a Union soldier? Nathan Bedford Forrest did this after his troops overran a hospital in the middle of an operation, and the anesthesia person fled.

Part IV

Suggested Topics

16

Make Your Own Exam

In this chapter, the provided topics should be used to make your own exams. Writing your own exam is the best way to prepare for the oral boards.

1. A Jehovah's Witness is a paraplegic from a motor vehicle accident (MVA). She has aortic stenosis with an aortic valve area of 0.6 cm², pulmonary hypertension, trace mitral regurgitation, and an ejection fraction (EF) of 20%. She is scheduled for an aortic valve replacement.

2. A 40-year-old woman with a presumptive diagnosis of lymphoma has progressive shortness of breath and is scheduled for mediastinoscopy. The chest radiograph shows a large mediastinal mass.

3. A 38-year-old, indigent man is scheduled for rigid bronchoscopy for removal of a glass stem of a crack pipe. Chest radiograph shows a 2-inch-long object in the right main stem bronchus. The patient is coughing like mad and has a long history of tobacco and ethanol use.

4. A 75-year-old man is scheduled mitral valve repair or replacement. He has a pacer in but cannot remember whether it is an automatic implantable cardioverter defibrillator (AICD) or a regular pacer. He was told, "Never put a magnet on this!"

5. A 35-year-old woman with Goodpasture's syndrome is coughing up bright red blood in the intensive care unit (ICU). She is scheduled for bilateral nephrectomy. She is in distress, and the surgeon asks if you can get a double-lumen tube in her.

6. A nervous, cachectic, 30-year-old woman with long-standing ulcerative colitis is scheduled for total colectomy. She takes steroids regularly.

7. A 4-year-old boy, described as "clumsy" by his father, comes in barely responsive for evacuation of an epidural hematoma. He has circular burns on his forearms.

8. A 65-year-old alcoholic needs an emergent transjugular intrahepatic portosystemic shunt (TIPS) procedure in the radiology suite. He has already lost 10 units of blood and is now receiving fresh-frozen plasma (FFP). His platelet level is determined to be 35,000.

9. A 20-year-old girl has been suffering from polydipsia, polyuria, and worsening visual field losses. She is admitted for excision of a pituitary tumor.

10. A 19-year-old Jehovah's Witness has a severe posterior nosebleed and is in shock. She refuses blood. Blood is pouring out of her mouth, and the surgeon needs the airway secured and the patient sedated so he can put in a posterior pack.

11. A 24-year-old Cambodian immigrant speaks no English. She is scheduled for a Harrington rod. She has scoliosis resulting from polio. She has marked curvature in her spine and needs home oxygen.

12. A panicked call comes from the radiology suite. A 65-year-old man was getting scanned for a ruptured abdominal aortic aneurysm (AAA), and he

just lost consciousness. They are mask ventilating the patient now and need to get him to the operating room (OR).

13. A 55-year-old former pro wrestler has gone to seed. He was getting treatment for "walking pneumonia" and now has herniated his L3-4 disk and has a footdrop. He needs emergent decompression, but his pneumonia is still there clinically and evident on the chest radiograph.

14. A 13-year-old boy is admitted with torsion of the testes and needs an emergent operation. He admits to huffing glue, paint, and Renuzit, and he was doing it just before he came in. He smells of fresh pine scent.

15. A 25-year-old man working at a shipyard crushed his hand and needs débridement. He prefers to be awake. He says he is allergic to lidocaine because his heart raced like crazy at the dentist once.

16. A 45-year-old do-it-yourselfer accidentally fired a paint gun into the tip of his left index finger, and there is discoloration all the way up to his axilla. Extensive débridement is planned.

17. A 50-year-old woman with renal failure is to have an arteriovenous fistula (AVF) placed in her left upper arm. She has had a half-dozen of these, and all the other sites are shot up. She has had bilateral femoral-popliteal grafts, and no one can get an intravenous line into her.

18. A man with ankylosing spondylitis develops an incarcerated inguinal hernia. He cannot lift his head at all, and it appears fixed on his chest. His back feels like one solid stone.

19. A 6-year-old boy with tetralogy of Fallot presents for repair. He frequently has to squat and bear down to feel better. His baseline oxygen saturation is 90%, and his growth is obviously stunted.

20. A 45-year-old man who takes a lot of anabolic steroids is scheduled for an excision of a pheochromocytoma. He has been on medication for 2 weeks, and his blood pressure seems under control.

21. A 30-year-old man who was selling Bibles on the street corner to benefit crippled children was shot in the throat. He cannot talk but can move air. Surgeons plan to explore the neck.

22. A 15-year-old Boy Scout dove into the shallow end of the pool on a dare. He has a suspected C5 fracture. He cannot move any of his extremities. Surgeons plan to stabilize his neck with a posterior approach.

23. A 68-year-old man, 2 years after myocardial infarction (MI), is scheduled for a radical retropubic prostatectomy. He says he is "the nervous type" and takes two or three Valium pills each night to sleep.

24. An 80-year-old woman with atrial fibrillation, an AICD, and a bedridden existence fell out of bed and broke her hip. Her heart rate is 140 beats/min. She can give no history.

25. Evil Knievel's cousin attempted a jump over 15 buses. He cleared 14 and is now in for repair of a pelvic fracture. He drinks, smokes, listens to country music, and has a big gun collection. The procedure will be prone.

26. A 71-year-old man who is 6 weeks out from a cerebrovascular accident (CVA) that left him flaccid on the left side is scheduled for a tracheotomy and percutaneous endoscopic gastrostomy. He has a feeding tube in his nose and is intubated.

27. A 49-year-old executive with high blood pressure has developed searing back pain. Computed tomography (CT) shows a possible type A aortic dissection. Pulses are lost in the left arm.

28. A 45-year-old woman with multiple sclerosis, who is wheelchair-bound and has intermittent bouts of psychotic behavior, is scheduled for a cholecystectomy. She is staring at everyone in the holding area and refusing to speak.

29. A 5-year-old girl is scheduled for strabismus surgery. Her first cousin had a "problem with the anesthetic gases" that led to an ICU stay.

30. A 110-kg woman is scheduled for a thyroidectomy. Her neck is huge, and the surgeon says he may have to explore the chest. She has a morbid fear of dying under anesthesia and wants to be "asleep before they give me the anesthetic." She is hoarse.

31. A fire fighter has 40% burns on his face, chest, and back and needs multiple débridements. The surgeon asks if he should go ahead and do a tracheotomy to make airway management easier during all these procedures.

32. A 2-year-old child with a brain tumor needs multiple radiation therapy treatments in the prone position. She was intubated for a month after a premature delivery and has tracheal stenosis. The physicians prefer she not be intubated for these procedures.

33. A 65-year-old man with Parkinson's disease has a halo on. He is scheduled to have an awake stereotactic stimulator placed to improve his parkinsonian symptoms.

34. A 59-year-old man is scheduled for a right parietal craniotomy for a tumor. He has been vomiting and complains of blurred vision. He takes nitroglycerin for angina.

35. A 40-year-old, 151-kg man is scheduled for a uvulopalatopharyngoplasty on an outpatient basis. He falls asleep every day at work and snores loudly.

36. A 25-year-old woman with a Harrington rod for scoliosis is scheduled for an elective cesarean section because she has active herpetic lesions.

37. A 31-year-old owner of an herbal store presents for bunionectomy. She has depression and chronic fatigue syndrome. She visits the pain clinic weekly, her acupuncturist twice each week, and her Tarot card reader daily. She wants to watch the procedure and wants hypnosis for her anesthetic.

38. In your ICU, a nurse complains she cannot get the Swan-Ganz catheter to wedge. The 59-year-old patient has had mitral valve repair. You notice the inspiratory pressures are going up, and the blood pressure drops to 70/50 mm Hg with each inspiration.

39. A 70-year-old woman broke her left humerus in a fall. She has a big bruise along the left side of her face. She had a mitral valve repair 2 years ago and is on Coumadin.

40. A 51-year-old farmer was in a tractor rollover. He has a flail chest, a depressed skull fracture, and a mandibular fracture on the left and right sides. He is in respiratory distress in the emergency room.

41. A hernia repair on a 16-year-old baseball player is going well. He has an athletic heart rate in the 60s. With all else the same, his heart rate creeps up into the 130s.

42. You are asked to consult in a medical malpractice case in which a physician did not bother to check a urine level of human chorionic gonadotropin before a carpal tunnel release. Turns out that the woman was 10 weeks' pregnant, and the child was born with an atrial septal defect. Attorneys claim the general anesthetic is to blame. They ask for your opinion.

43. A 60-year-old man is scheduled for resection of a pituitary tumor. He has obvious signs of acromegaly. Five years ago, he had a tumor resection at the base of the tongue.

44. A patient with prostate cancer metastatic to the spine is failing pain relief on narcotics. How can you help with pain relief?

45. A 4-year-old girl is in the emergency room with stridor, drooling, retractions, and a high fever. What is the diagnosis, and how can you help?

46. A developmentally delayed, 27-year-old woman needs hand surgery after putting her hand in a blender. She will need a general anesthetic, but the surgeon asks if you can help with a block after induction.

47. After a motor vehicle accident (MVA), a 45-year-old man needs his right leg amputated. He is in the ICU with acute respiratory distress syndrome, requiring 20 cm H_2O of positive end-expiratory pressure (PEEP) and 100% oxygen. The surgeon asks if it is safe to take him to the OR or if they should do the operation at bedside in the unit.

48. A 200-kg man gets claustrophobic in the magnetic resonance imaging (MRI) scanner and needs to be "asleep to hold still." Can you do this with sedation? How?

49. A patient has a type 1 dissection of the aorta. The surgeon says the aorta does not look that bad and decides to cannulate the aorta. What do you notice when you go on bypass if the aortic cannula is in the false lumen?

50. How does the scavenge system work, and what happens if it clogs up? How can the scavenge system cause negative-pressure pulmonary edema?

51. In what cases is it safe to skip the postanesthesia care unit (PACU) and send the patient directly home?

52. The catheter laboratory report told you the patient had an ejection fraction (EF) of 30%, but when you have the patient under general anesthesia, transesophageal echocardiography (TEE) clearly shows a good EF of about 50%. What about the catheter laboratory's experience could explain this discrepancy?

53. An abdominal aortic aneurysm (AAA) is scheduled for repair, and the surgeon is mad that "everyone keeps needing dialysis later." What can you do to protect the kidneys that makes a difference?

54. During cross-clamping, the blood pressure in a patient with an abdominal aortic aneurysm (AAA) rises to 220/110 mg Hg, the ST segments are elevated, and the patient develops ectopy. How do you treat this?

55. You placed a spinal for a short inguinal node biopsy. Turns out that it is an entrapped hernia, and the patient is becoming uncomfortable. This 38-year-old man had cervical laminectomy 2 months earlier for disk disease.

56. A vaginal delivery after cesarean section is going smoothly. In the middle of a forceps delivery, the patient complains of severe abdominal pain despite the epidural, her pressure drops, and she loses consciousness. The baby is halfway out, and blood pours out of the vagina.

57. A rock climber wants shoulder arthroscopy done under local anesthesia so he can "see inside." He is stocky, with a short, thick neck.

58. A 70-year-old man was rear-ended in a traffic jam, and a retinal detachment must be fixed. He had an MI 3 weeks ago, but he refused angioplasty. He has chest pain while waiting in the holding area.

59. In a medical malpractice case, an anesthesiologist taking care of a patient with a C4 fracture is being sued because he did not give any steroids during an operation to stabilize the neck. The anesthesiologist maintains, "No one told me to give it." Discuss his point and the plaintiff's point.

60. You do a routine hernia repair on a 5-year-old child and plan a deep extubation to "avoid coughing so we don't pop the new stitches." The surgeon likes the idea, but your certified registered nurse anesthetist (CRNA) thinks it is stupid. Reconcile these views.

61. An intracranial aneurysm bursts, and the surgeon screams for "the lowest possible blood pressure you can possibly give me, or this patient is dead!" What do you do?

62. A 42-year-old man with a seizure disorder and taking Dilantin is scheduled for a parathyroidectomy. His last seizure was 4 months ago.

63. A 4-kg newborn boy has difficulty breathing and no breath sounds whatsoever on the left side. His chest appears "odd" on the left side.

64. A 6-year-old child with prune-belly syndrome is scheduled for excision of a megacolon of epic proportions.

65. A 50-year-old drinker is scheduled for orthotopic liver transplantation. He is intubated in a coma resulting from liver failure.

66. A 24-year-old woman suffered postpartum cardiomyopathy and is on the list for a heart transplant. She just ate dinner and is on an infusion of milrinone. A heart just became available.

67. A 120-kg man has cancer of the left lower lobe. His airway appears difficult, and the surgeon says, "I always want a double-lumen catheter. Do not do any of that other weird stuff."

68. A woman with her jaws wired shut after shooting herself in the mouth is to have electroconvulsive therapy (ECT) for suicidal depression. How can you provide anesthesia for this procedure?

69. A patient refuses a spinal for a transurethral prostatectomy (TURP). In the middle of the case, the patient suddenly becomes bradycardic, and the abdomen starts to distend.

70. A 44-year-old intravenous drug abuser develops jaundice 2 weeks after a cholecystectomy. The surgeon blames you for interstitial fluid hepatitis: "It is just like halothane hepatitis."

71. A 5-foot, 600-pound woman is scheduled for a gastric stapling for treatment of morbid obesity. She had an umbrella placed in her inferior vena cava for recurrent pulmonary emboli.

72. A new ears, nose, and throat specialist says, "I just cannot zap those condylomas with the endotracheal tube in place." Can you provide a clear field for him by intermittent ventilation? Does this pose a fire risk? How do you avoid that?

73. A patient with a diagnosis of hypertrophic obstructive cardiomyopathy is scheduled to have a colectomy for cancer. In the middle of the case, you tell your certified registered nurse anesthetist (CRNA) to "give more halothane to get the blood pressure up." The CRNA looks at you like you are insane.

74. You just started a thoracotomy, and you forgot to turn off the patient's automatic implantable cardioverter-defibrillator (AICD). Every time the Bovie cautery fires, the patient gets shocked. Now what do you do?

75. A neonate with a tracheoesophageal fistula is scheduled for repair. How do you manage the tricky ventilation in this case? How do you address the concern about retrolental fibroplasia?

76. You placed an epidural yesterday in a woman, and today, she cannot stand up because her legs buckle every time she tries to stand.

77. A man presents to your preoperative clinic to be evaluated for treatment of alveolar proteinosis. You will be doing the case. How do you manage this?

BONUS SECTION

In this section, you still produce the exam questions, but for a few, we broke down and provided questions.

1. A 22-year-old man with severe developmental delay resulting from neonatal meningitis is scheduled for dental rehabilitation under general anesthesia. He is given ketamine (200 mg) and glycopyrrolate (0.2 mg IM) preoperatively, and anesthesia is induced with propofol (150 mg) and cisatracurium (10 mg). A 7.5-French cuffed nasotracheal tube is placed, and anesthesia is maintained with N_2O/O_2 and sevoflurane. Intraoperative hypertension is treated with boluses of esmolol and nicardipine. During emergence, his SpO_2 decreases to the mid 80s, and he becomes very difficult to ventilate.

2. An 18-month-old boy who is otherwise healthy presents to the emergency room with acute onset of cough and cyanosis. The chest radiograph shows collapse and consolidation of the right lung, and a foreign body is suspected. The child is scheduled for rigid bronchoscopy. His mother gave him cereal 3 hours earlier.

3. A 14-month-old girl with lymphoma is scheduled for a Hickman catheter to initiate chemotherapy. She has no intravenous line on arrival to the OR, and anesthesia is induced with sevoflurane in oxygen. On induction, she breathes spontaneously with ease, but controlled ventilation with the mask seems very difficult.

4. A 37-year-old woman presents at term with severe epigastric pain. Her platelet level fell from 300,000 to 50,000 over 24 hours. She had had temporomandibular joint surgery and could barely open her mouth. What do you do?

5. A 60-year-old woman with an American Society of Anesthesiologists' physical status classification of 3 (ASA 3) was scheduled for excision of an abdominal malignancy that extended into the liver. It was a monster resection. She also had carcinoid syndrome. Intraoperatively, the patient had hypoxemia, hypotension, and high pulmonary artery pressures—the real death spiral. None of the normal stuff worked. What to do, what to do? Pop in a transesophagral echocardiography (TEE) probe—what else? Lo and behold, with the amazing loading swings of this high-volume-need case, the patient unmasked a previously undiagnosed patent foramen ovale, creating a right-to-left shunt. Now what?

6. A 29-year-old, 90-kg man was involved in a motor vehicle accident (MVA) 6 hours earlier. He was scheduled for bilateral open reduction and internal fixation (ORIF) for his tibias. He was unconscious for 3 hours and now opens eyes in response to commands. He is intubated and on a vent; PEEP is 10 cm H_2O and FiO_2 is 0.6. He aspirated. His blood pressure is 100/70 mm Hg, pulse is 140 beats/min, hematocrit is 28, pH is 7.34, $PaCO_2$ is 35, and PaO_2 is 80.

   How can you tell wedge waveform? Draw a picture of it.
   The pulmonary artery pressure (PAP) is 60/20 and the pulmonary artery occlusion pressure (PAOP) is 40. What does it mean?
   The PAP is 60/20, and the PAOP is 3. What does it mean?
   How does a Swan-Ganz catheter help you in determining volume status?

7. A 100-kg, 56-year-old man has steadily increasing chest pain. He has no history of a myocardial infarction (MI), but he needs to get his vessels fixed. He is scheduled for coronary artery bypass grafting (CABG). He has

a symptomatic hiatal hernia. His medications include metoprolol, cimetidine, and acetylsalicylic acid. He has a low-intensity systolic murmur at his left sternal border. His blood pressure is 155/80 mm Hg, pulse is 50 beats/min, respiration rate is 22 breaths/min, and temperature is 37° C.

What about the murmur? Will it affect your anesthetic management?

How will mild aortic stenosis affect your management?

What about the hiatal hernia?

What about other changes in your technique?

Could you do an awake intubation?

If the patient develops tachycardia to 135 beats/min, what do you do?

After you come off pump, you are giving 4 µg/min of epinephrine, and when you start protamine, the pressure drops. What do you do? If that does not work, do you go back on pump?

Is the transesophageal echocardiography (TEE) better than the pulmonary artery catheter for managing hemodynamics? Would you use both?

What anesthetic technique would you use?

Is one inhaled agent better than another?

8. A 19-year-old parturient with preeclampsia has a blood pressure of 160/110 mm Hg.

Do you want anything before you proceed?

Which drip would you use?

Would the epidural help the hypertension?

9. An outpatient is going to have a knee operation. He requests an epidural.

Do you do it?

What agent will you use?

If you get a wet tap, what do you do?

Will you do an immediate blood patch?

Is a blood patch given for a symptomatic headache more effective than a prophylactic blood patch given before symptoms?

10. A 28-year-old, 75-kg man got second- and third-degree burns while working in the fields. This is his third trip to the OR for débridement and skin grafting. He abuses cocaine and alcohol. His blood pressure is 135/88 mm Hg, heart rate is 110 beats/min, respiratory rate is 30 breaths/min, temperature is 38.5° C, and hemoglobin level is 7.5.

Are you concerned about the hemoglobin level?

Would you transfuse?

Why is he tachycardic?

Do you want an arterial line?

If you absolutely could not get an arterial line placed, would you still do the case?

What are the risks of an arterial line?

If the intraoperative pressure goes to 70/40 mm Hg and you have already given 1500 of crystalloid, what would you do? How would you look for ischemia?

If the blood pressure is still 70/40 mm Hg, and there is no improvement, would you give ketamine for induction and maintenance?

11. A 6-year-old boy has a fishhook in his eye. He has an open eye and full stomach. His heart rate and pressure are normal; everything is normal.

How would you proceed?

If you cannot see anything and the patient aspirates, what do you do?

The ophthalmologist says, "What now?"

12. In the ICU, a patient has a PaO_2 of 60 on an FIO_2 of 0.6. You are called for a cuff leak. You push the tube in, and the PaO_2 drops. The patient's oxygen saturation is still down.

13. A 40-year-old woman is scheduled for total abdominal hysterectomy because of bleeding. She has a history of deep venous thrombosis on Coumadin. She has a small mouth opening and receding chin. Her hemoglobin level is 8.

   Preoperative questions:

   Are you going to transfuse blood before surgery?

   If patient does not have blood type and crossmatch performed before surgery, will you delay the case or go to the OR and send for the results from there?

   When do you stop Coumadin, and how do you reverse it?

   What is the onset of action of vitamin K and fresh frozen plasma (FFP)?

   How will you manage the airway?

   What do you tell the patient about awake fiberoptic intubation?

   Intraoperative questions:

   Which monitors will you use?

   Will you use a central venous pressure (CVP) line? Why or why not?

   How will you induce?

   While using the fiberoptic scope, you cannot see the anatomy because of bleeding. You try again and still cannot see. What is your plan?

   You secured the airway. You placed a CVP line, and the pressure dropped. During surgery, the line isolation monitor goes off. What does that mean?

14. A 7-year-old boy had a foreign body aspiration. He has a family history of malignant hyperthermia. What is your anesthetic plan? You tried sedation and oral/nasal intubation, but nothing worked. He has no intravenous line. What will you do?

15. During a laparoscopic hysterectomy, the patient starts breathing spontaneously. What is the differential diagnosis?

16. How do you manage the blood pressure for a patient having kidney transplantation who has a history of an aortic abdominal aneurysm (AAA)?

17. A patient with coronary artery disease had a hernia repair and is now shivering in the PACU. What are your concerns?

18. A patient is scheduled for a thoracotomy and lobectomy.

   Would you use an epidural for pain management?

   What is most common arrhythmia after pneumonectomy?

   How do you manage that rhythm?

   What are the causes of peak pressure only? What are the causes of peak plus plateau pressure?

   During ventilation intraoperatively, what are the causes of auto PEEP? Does this happen in the patient with chronic obstructive pulmonary disease?

19. A 54-year-old, obese woman with hypertension, asthma, and hypothyroidism has colon cancer. She presents with vomiting and abdominal pain.

Endoscopic laparotomy is planned. She has an enlarged thyroid (MP III), and her mouth opens 1 fingerbreadth. Laboratory results included a potassium level of 3.0 and hematocrit of 27.

Intraoperative questions:

How would you induce?

How would you anesthetize the airway for a fiberoptic intubation?

Why do they call it *transtracheal*? Isn't it in the larynx?

The patient is not cooperating with the FO. What now?

You explain and explain, but she will have nothing to do with it. You have to put her to sleep. How are you going to do it?

You put her to sleep, can see arytenoids, but cannot pass the tube. What do you do?

You have a laryngeal mask airway (LMA), a gum elastic Bougie, and a Bullard. Which do you use?

How do you know the gum elastic is in the right place?

Intraoperatively, she wheezes. What will you do? How will you know if she aspirated?

The blood pressure drops. What do you do?

Postoperatively, she is extubated, and she becomes agitated. How will you handle this?

Her arterial blood gas determination shows a pH of 7.5, with a $Paco_2$ of 30 and Pao_2 of 60. What do you think of that?

20. A 20-year-old woman is 34 weeks' pregnant. She has a history of hypertrophic cardiomyopathy.

What are the options for labor analgesia?

Are you worried about doing an epidural?

If she goes for a cesarean section, how do you handle it?

You do the epidural and get a wet tap. Now what?

Would you use a local anesthetic?

Why use fentanyl and not morphine?

21. A 2-year-old child with myelomeningocele presents for inguinal hernia repair.

How do you induce anesthesia?

You do not have an assistant. You breathe him down and place the tube and then do the intravenous line. You place a tourniquet, the patient becomes flushed, and the peak inflating pressure goes up. What drug will you give?

You do not get the intravenous line. How are you going to give the epinephrine for his latex allergy?

Is there a problem with giving too much epinephrine?

22. A 6-year-old child has a posterior fossa tumor and a history of headache, vomiting, and irritability for 2 days. He is scheduled to have a prone craniotomy. His medications are Dilantin and Decadron.

Does he have increased intracranial pressure (ICP)? Why?

Can you see increased ICP on the CT scan?

Why does increased ICP cause a headache?

The child is vomiting. What electrolyte disturbances do you expect?

Do you want a Dilantin level? What do you do if it is low?

What are the side effects of Dilantin?

What premedication do you give the child? Why not premedicate?

Would you do an inhalational induction? Why not?

If you place an intravenous line, will the kid cry, and will crying raise the ICP or central venous pressure (CVP)? Why?

How will you manage the increased ICP?

The patient is placed prone and 15 degrees head up. Are you worried about venous air embolism?

What monitors are used for venous air embolism?

Can you test the Doppler ultrasound to see if it is working?

Surgeons are working, and they have a sinus wide open. What would you do if you noticed air but no hemodynamic changes? Would you stop the case? At what blood level would you transfuse the patient?

The hematocrit is 21, and the patient is stable. Would you transfuse?

The patient bleeds a lot, and you give 5 units of blood. Should you give platelets?

Is he at risk of thrombocytopenia? Should you give fresh frozen plasma (FFP)?

Will you extubate at the end of surgery?

You extubate, and several hours later, the patient has respiratory distress and stridor. What will you do?

What is racemic epinephrine?

23. A 35-year-old woman with myasthenia gravis presents for thymectomy. Would you tell her to stop or keep taking her medications? Would you give steroids? How would you treat postoperative pain?

24. A 20-year-old man with laryngeal papilloma is in respiratory distress. How would you premedicate? How would you induce? The surgeon does not want a tube in the way. How will you manage the airway?

25. A patient with a breech pregnancy is dilated 3 cm. The obstetrician wants to cut. Would you wait until the stomach is empty? What if she had a bad airway?

26. A 76-year-old, 85-kg man is scheduled for aortobifemoral repair. He takes metformin for type 2 diabetes and metoprolol for hypertension. He smokes 2.5 packs/day. Examination revealed S_3 and S_4 sounds. The stress test result was negative (reached a heart rate of 118). He has wheezing and rales, that clear with a cough. The chest radiograph shows enlarged heart. Pulmonary artery and arterial lines are already in. His coagulation status is normal, and his heart rate is 52 beats/min.

Should he take his morning dose of metformin?

Your colleague advises tight glucose control. What do you say?

What are the benefits of combined regional and general anesthesia?

Which muscle relaxant should you use?

What are your aortic clamp concerns?

How will you improve renal perfusion during the clamp?

For postoperative pain control, is an epidural a good idea?

During placement of the epidural, you get a wet tap. Should you use a prophylactic blood patch?

How do you treat the headache?

As the surgeon pushes on his abdomen, the blood pressure goes down and palmonary artery pressure (PAP) up. What do you do for this situation?

The surgeon removes his hand and later puts it back in, and the pressure does not go down. What gives?

The oxygen saturation level drops. What do you do?

How do you differentiate rales from wheezes?

How do you differentiate a tension pneumothorax from a pneumothorax?

Do you use an epidural with narcotics and local anesthetics?

In the ICU, the patient has been extubated, and he is wheezing. What will you do? Will you intubate?

Hypoxemia develops later, and the left lung is consolidated. What now?

Should the patient begin chest physiotherapy?

27. A patient needs electroconvulsive therapy (ECT) and has a history of neuroleptic malignant syndrome.

What is it?

What are the anesthetic considerations?

Would you use suction?

How would you see the effect of the ECT?

How would you diagnose diabetic ketoacidosis?

The arterial blood gas determination shows a pH of 7.3, with a $PaCO_2$ of 22 and PaO_2 of 50. How would you diagnose diabetic ketoacidosis with that?

What do you need to do about the anion gap?

What is the treatment for this patient?

28. A 20-month-old, 14-kg boy had a sled accident. In the emergency room, he is scheduled for an endoscopic laparotomy for hepatic laceration. He has a 22-gauge intravenous line in the right saphenous vein, through which he has received 120 mL of lactated Ringer's solution. His blood pressure is 70/40 mm Hg, pulse is 180 beats/min, and temperature is 35.2° C. His skin is pale and mottled.

Will you remedy his low temperature?

What laboratory test results are needed before going to the OR?

How will you assess his volume status? Will you use Hespan?

Four units of packed red cells are given. Would you give calcium? bicarbonate?

Will you intubate the patient in the emergency room with an awake fiberoptic approach?

Direct laryngoscopy and fiberoptic intubation fail. Now what?

What protects better against aspiration: laryngeal mask airway (LMA) or a mask?

After intubation, the patient's blood pressure drops to 50/30 mm Hg. After 4 units of blood, the patient oozes. Can the thromboelastogram tell you whether to give fresh frozen plasma (FFP) or cryoprecipitate?

Should you use suction?

A colleague says to use irradiated red blood cells. What do you say?

29. A rheumatoid arthritis patient with an unstable neck is scheduled for elective surgery. No neurology or neurosurgery consult is available.

How do you intubate the patient?

Can you use regional anesthesia?

30. A patient is scheduled for a craniotomy for a benign tumor, a right parietal lesion.

Can you use N_2O? Would you use it?

Would you use desflurane or propofol/remifentanil?

17

Final Word

Parting is such sweet sorrow.

WILLIAM SHAKESPEARE

It has been fun writing this book, and I hope you got a kick out of it. Before you go, I want to pass along some points from the first edition of *Board Stiff*:

- Everyone knows someone with the intelligence of a newt who passed the exam.
- You already know that you already know this stuff; you passed the written exam!
- Keep your cool at all times! Do not become obsessed with something you do not know. Even the examiners do not know everything.
- Speak clearly, concisely, and slowly. It makes you sound more professional.
- Dress like a professional, even if you are a Bohemian Rasputin. The examiners do not care; they want you to look pretty!
- If you pretend that the stem question is a case you are about to do with no warning in the operating room and plan accordingly, you will pass the exam!
- Answer the questions *exactly* as if you were doing the case in the operating room, not the way you think the examiners want you to answer. They already know a gazillion different ways to do this.
- It is okay to say, "I don't know," as long as you do not answer all the questions that way.
- Stop speaking *immediately*, even in the middle of a sentence, when the knock comes at the door! Remember that anything you say can and will be used against you if it is wrong.

MORE THAN ANYTHING ELSE, PRACTICE MAKES PERFECT!

Say it three times fast: Practice makes perfect, practice makes perfect, practice makes perfect! Practice a billion times in front of a mirror, with your favorite fellow resident, a fellow anesthesiologist, your significant other, your mom, your dog, or strangers at a bar. The more you practice speaking clearly and concisely and sticking to your plan, the better you will become, and you will pass the oral exams!

Now, dress nicely, brush your teeth, show up sober, and pass your exam.

Index

Index